GENERAL CONCEPTS
of
HISTOLOGY AND ENDOCRINOLOGY

GENERAL CONCEPTS *of* HISTOLOGY AND ENDOCRINOLOGY

Swapan Kumar Rej MSc, PhD

Ex-Associate Professor and Head, Department of Zoology and
Guest Lecturer, Netaji Subhas Open University, Behala College, Kolkata,
Formerly Lecturer in Zoology, HSET Centre, Jadavpur University,
Guest Lecturer, Serampur College, Postgraduate Section,
Vidyasagar College, and Mahadevananda College, Barrackpore

New Central Book Agency (P) Ltd

LONDON

HYDERABAD ERNAKULAM BHUBANESWAR

NEW DELHI KOLKATA PUNE GUWAHATI

NCBA

REGD OFFICE
8/1 Chintamoni Das Lane, Kolkata 700 009, India
email: ncbapvtltd@eth.net

OVERSEAS
NCBA (UK) Ltd, 149 Park Avenue North, Northampton, NN3 2HY, UK
email: ncbauk@yahoo.com

EXPORT
NCBA Exports Pvt. Ltd, 212 Shahpur Jat, New Delhi 110 049
email: ncbaexports@ncbapvtltd.com

BRANCHES

2/27 Ansari Road, 1st Floor
Daryaganj, **New Delhi** 110 002
email: ncbadel@ncbapvtltd.com

Shop Nos. 3 & 4, Vinayak Towers
681/B Budhwar Peth, Appa Balwant Chowk
Pune 411 002
email: ncbapune@ncbapvtltd.com

Shop No. 15, Bharati Towers, Ground Floor
Forest Park
Bhubaneswar 751 001
email: ncbabub@ncbapvtltd.com

House No. 3-1-315, 1st Floor
Nimboliadda, Kachiguda, **Hyderabad** 500 027
email: ncbahydb@ncbapvtltd.com

GSS Shopping Complex, 1st Floor
Opposite College Post Office, Convent Road
Ernakulam 682 035
0484-4021054 / 53

Radhamayee Complex (Second Floor)
Opp. SBI, Panbazar, Jaswanta Road
Guwahati 781 001
email: ncbaguwahati@ncbapvtltd.com

GENERAL CONCEPTS OF HISTOLOGY AND ENDOCRINOLOGY • Swapan Kumar Rej

First Published: August 2015
Reprinted: February 2018

PUBLISHER AND TYPESETTER
New Central Book Agency (P) Ltd
8/1 Chintamoni Das Lane, Kolkata 700 009

PRINTER
New Central Book Agency (P) Ltd
Web-Offset Division, Dhulagarh, Sankrail, Howrah

TECHNICAL EDITOR
Dipan Roy

PROJECT TEAM
Somenath Ganguly and Pradip Biswas

ISBN: 978 81 7381 976 6

Price ₹ 385.00

This book is dedicated to my
reverend and beloved teacher,

Professor Amar Chatterjee, PhD, DSc, FO & G (Kansas)

This book is also dedicated to my granddaughters,

Ananya Rej and Aatreyee Rej

CONTENTS

PREFACE

The present book entitled **"General Concepts of Histology and Endocrinology"** is a revision (text) for students preparing for examinations in BSc Hons in Zoology and Medical Science of various Indian universities. However, the students of MSc will also be benefited from this book. This text is divided into two categories—Histology and Endocrinology. The study of Histology is useful to understand the correlation between the structure and functions of an organ and the central theme of Endocrinology is the role of chemical messengers, or hormones, whether they are of endocrine or neural origin, in the control of physiological processes. Although endocrine physiology has been separated from neurophysiology in the past, it is now amply documented that hormones may originate from either endocrine or neural tissue. Thus has emerged the field of neuro-endocrinology.

The style of this text is unique and will not please everyone: it is deliberately cryptic and concise and attempts to compress large areas of physiology into readily assimilable facts and concepts with a minimum of description. This is illustrated by the many flow-diagrams and summaries.

It is hoped that the present book shall fulfil the requirement of the undergraduate students (both in Zoology and Medical Sciences) of many Indian universities. Valuable suggestions and comments for further improvement of this book shall be gratefully acknowledged.

15 August 2015
Kolkata

Swapan Kumar Rej

ACKNOWLEDGEMENTS

I owe my deep sense of gratitude to Sri Amitabha Sen, Director, for giving me the opportunity to publish the book and I express my sincere thank to Sri R M Nath, for his constant encouragement and moral support. It has been my pleasure to work with Sri Prabhat Jas for his immerse cooperation. Acknowledgement is due to Sri Somenath Ganguly for typing the manuscript, Sri Dipan Roy for cooperation in proof reading and Sri Niranjan Giri for drawing the diagrams and flow charts. No thanks are sufficient for them.

The author wishes to express his deep sense of indebtedness to Dr (Mrs) Rita Chatterjee and Ms Krishna Bhuiya for encouraging him to carry out the project of writing this book.

Last but not least I am grateful to Dr (Mrs) Rakhi Roy for writing the topics, Epithelial tissue, Muscular tissue and Adenohypophysis.

I would also like to extend my appreciation to all my students who are the source of my inspiration always.

Swapan Kumar Rej

Introduction

Histology (Gr. histos = tissue; logia = knowledge) is the study of minute structure of living organisms. It is a branch of anatomy that deals with the structure of animal and plant tissues as observable with the microscope. **Stevens** and **Lowe** (1992) have defined histology as the study of the structure of biological material and the ways in which individual components are structurally and functionally related. Histology includes the consideration of cells and tissues as well as the organs. As the development proceeds, groups of cells become differentiated from one another and are built up into different patterns to form the *tissues* of the body. **A tissue is defined as a group of organised cells with a common origin, function** and **similar** or **different structures.** Tissues are the building blocks that form the organs. The human body and the body of other vertebrates are composed of different kinds of tissues. These elementary tissues are mainly classified into four major types on the basis of their structural and functional similarities and differences. These groups are mentioned below :

(1) **Epithelial tissue :** Groups of cells which cover the outer surface of the body as well as the inner free surface of the organs of a body.

(2) **Connective tissue :** The tissues of the vertebrates containing cellular and fibrous materials in its matrix in large amount and which are important for connecting different parts together and which are mesodermal in origin, are called connective tissue.

(3) **Muscular tissue :** This type of tissue has the ability to contract and relax, as a result each and every organ is associated with the movement.

(4) **Nervous tissue :** This kind of tissue which is involved in the co-ordination of the bodily functions through conduction of nerve impulses.

The study of histology is useful to understand the correlation between the structure and functions of an organ. It imparts the knowledge of normal cells and tissues and assists to distinguish them from abnormal ones with deranged functions.

The glands which have no excretory duct and whose secretions (i.e., hormones) convey directly into the blood stream, are known as endocrine glands or ductless glands. The word **'endocrine'** means **'internal secretion'** (Gr. endon = within, Krinein = to separate or to secrete) of biologically active substances; this contrasts with **'exocrine'** secretion which is secretion outside the body, e.g., through the sweat glands or ducts leading into the gastrointestinal tract. So **Endocrinology is the study of the ductless glands or tissues** and **their hormonal products.**

The endocrine system and the nervous system are the major means by which the body communicates information between different cells and tissues (Fig 1). The endocrine system uses hormones to convey its information. Thus, a **hormone** is typically defined as **an organic compound produced in the body by an endocrine gland and transported into the blood stream or tissue fluid, has some specific regulatory effect on the activity of certain organ, usually remote from the site of its origin.** These actions are mediated by the binding of the hormone to **receptor molecules,** which are the loci to which the hormones are bound in mediating their responses. The receptors must distinguish the hormone from all of the millions of other molecules to which they are exposed and transmit the binding information into the post-receptor events.

The endocrine system is diverse and complex, with varied and sophisticated mechanisms that actuate and regulate the synthesis and release of hormones, their transport in the circulation, and their metabolism and supply to the surface or the interior of the tissues upon which they work.

Hormones commonly work without ever entering the circulation. Complex interrelations exist among the nervous, immune and other systems. Molecules that are usually not considered hormones may function as hormones, and tissues ordinarily not considered to be endocrine glands may produce and release hormones. These hormones may act on the same cell in which they are formed (*autocrine*) without leaving the cell or after their release and subsequent binding to receptors in or on the cell. They may act on other target cells in their vicinity, including neurotransmitter cells without entering the circulation (*paracrine*). They may go to the target cell through the circulation (hormonal).

It has been found that hormones not only reach target tissues through the circulation but can also work logically in the vicinity in which they are released. When they work locally on cells other than those that produce them, the action is known as **paracrine**—explained by the action of sex-steroids in the ovary, angiotensin II in the kidney, and platelet derived growth factor secreted by platelets, i.e., **paracrine mechanism** where the released hormone diffuses to its adjacent target cells through the immediate extracellular space and where following the release of hormone, it may also feed back on the cell of origin by a so-called **autocrine mechanism.** The hormone can also act on the cell in which it is produced, a phenomenon referred to as **autocrine;** the hormone may be secreted by the cell and then act on it, or it may act inside the cell without ever being secreted. For example, insulin secreted by pancreatic β-cells can inhibit insulin released by the same cells and somatostatin can inhibit its secretion from pancreatic γ-cells.

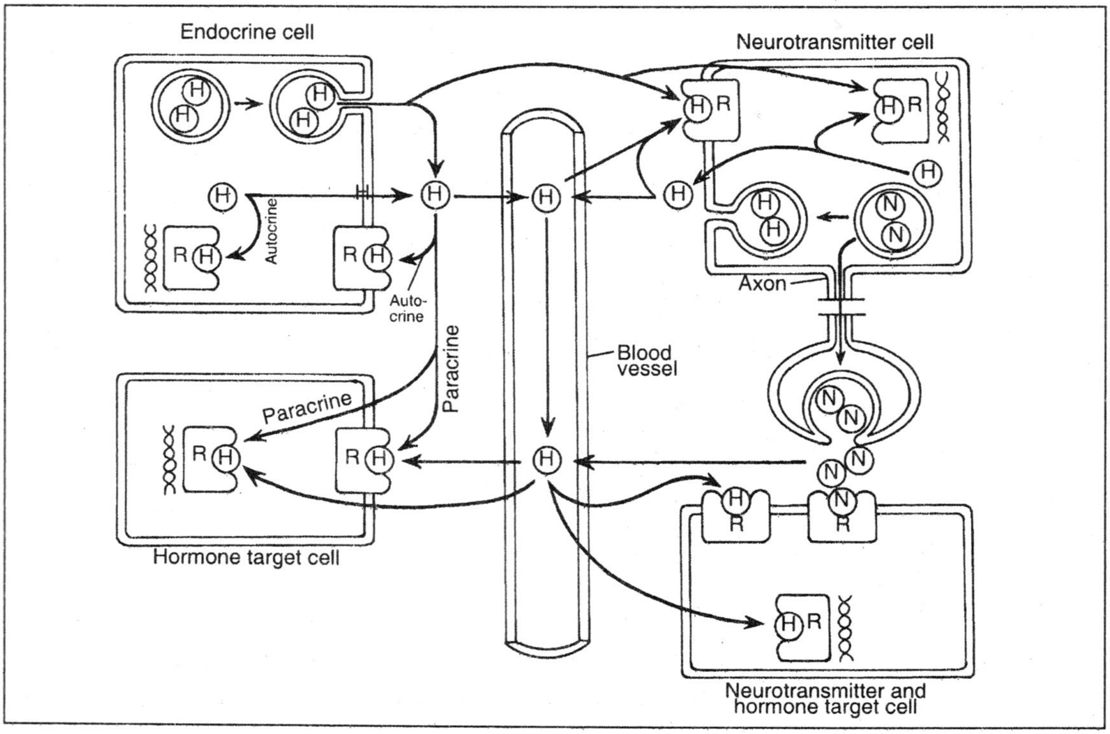

Fig 1: Actions of hormones and neurotransmitters and their interrelationships. Both endocrine and neurotransmitter cells release hormones that they synthesize either from secretory vesicles or by diffusion. These same neurotransmitters can be released to act as hormones through the synaptic junctions or directly by the cell. (H. hormone; R. receptor; N. neurotransmitter).

CHAPTER 1

Classical Histology

1(A) EPITHELIAL TISSUE

The basic structural and functional unit of body is cell. Cells remain organized in such a way that they can perform particular function. Such organized aggregation of cells of same or different origin, that commonly function in a group is called **tissue** [L. texere, to weave].

The tissue concept provides a basis for understanding the cell types present within our body. There are four main types of tissues [depending upon the general appearance, structural organization and physiological properties] :

(1) Epithelial tissue
(2) Connective tissue
(3) Muscle tissue
(4) Nerve tissue.

1.1 Meaning of Epithelia

Epithelium is one of the most important tissue of four basic tissue types, which lines the cavities and surfaces of structures throughout the body and also form many glands. In Greek, **'epi'** means 'on' or 'upon' and **'theli'** means 'tissue'.

1.2 Embryological Development of Epithelium

In general, there are epithelial tissues deriving from all of the embryological germ layers :

- from ectoderm [e.g., the epidermis]
- from mesoderm [e.g., the inner linings of body cavities]
- from endoderm [e.g., lining of the gastrointestinal tract]

1.3 Characteristics of Epithelial Tissue

(A) Presence of Basal lamina and Basement membrane

(i) All epithelial cells remain in contact with adjacent connective tissue by a sheet like extracellular material, called **basal lamina.** Sometimes, it is called **lamina densa.** This layer with five filamentous network can only be visible under electron microscope.

(ii) In between basal lamina and the cell, a clear zone present, called **lamina lucida,** which includes **fibronectin receptors** [cell adhesion molecules—members of **integrin** transmembrane protein].

(iii) The main components of basal lamina includes four group of molecules :

- Collagen type IV—monomers contain three polypeptide chains, forming a **felt-like sheet** for anchorage.
- Laminin—large glycoprotein molecules, forming **lace-like sheet,** placed with transmembrane integrin protein.

- Proteoglycans—formed of heparan sulphate and chondroitin sulphate–maintains the passage of ions across the basal lamina.
- Entactin and fibronectin.

  Entactin—a sulfated glycoprotein, having binding site for collagen type IV and binds with laminin forming a stable entactin—lamin complex.

  Fibronectin—a glycoprotein, includes binding sites for all basal lamina component and also binds to connective tissue.

(iv) In some cases reticular fibres are closely associated with basal lamina made up of type III collagen and help to anchor with type IV collagen. This forms the **reticular lamina** below the basal lamina.

(v) **Basement membrane :**

- All epithelial cells rest on a **basement membrane;** which varies in thickness in different places. It is the combination of a **basal lamina** and a **reticular lamina.**
- It is a PAS positive layer [visible under light microscope] which acts as a scaffolding on which epithelium can grow and regenerate after injuries.
- It acts as a selectively permeable membrane that determines in which substances will be able to enter the epithelium.

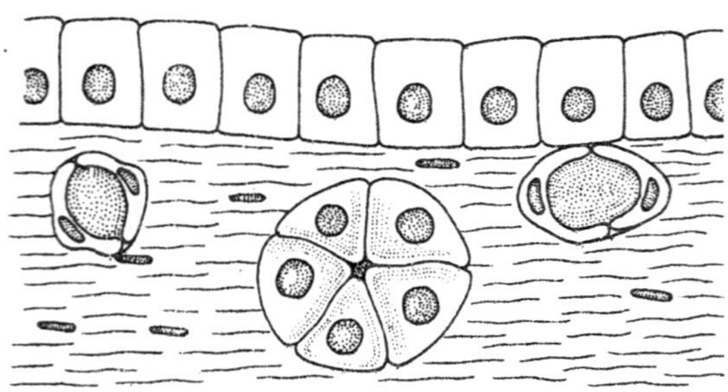

Fig 1(a).1: An extracellular basal lamina.

- Epithelial tissue is innervated but it is avascular which is being nourished by substances diffusing from the blood vessels in the underlying tissue.

(B) Intercellular junctions :

(vi) Epithelial cells are extremely cohesive, and relatively strong mechanical forces which are necessary to separate them.

(vii) The lateral membrane of epithelial cells exhibits several specializations, that in terms form various type of **intercellular junctions,** in a definite order from apex to base of the cell.

(viii) **Cell junctions** permit epithelia to form a continuous cohesive layer by which cells communicate and cooperate to achieve particular function. **Junctions** are :

- **Tight junctions/Occluding junctions/ Zonula occludens :**

These are the most apical junctions which are located just beneath the luminal surface of epithelial tissue.

The principal function of the tight junction is to form a more or less tight seal that prevents the flow of materials between epithelial cells.

- **Adhering junctions :**

These junctions are tightly bound to the constituent cells of the epithelium which act as anchorage site for cytoskeleton.

Morphologically adhering junctions are of two types—(i) zonula adherens and (ii) macula adherens or desmosomes.

(i) **Zonula adherens :**

- It locates just next to tight junctions in many epithelia forming a continuous band around the cell.
- It mainly helps to adhere one cell to its neighbouring cells.

(ii) **Macula adherens (Desmosome)** :

- It is distributed in small circular patches or spots along the lateral membranes of most epithelial cells.
- It helps to provide firm adhesion of one cell to the next.

Junctional complex : The combination of zonula occludens, zonula adherens and macula adherens together is known as **Junctional complex.**

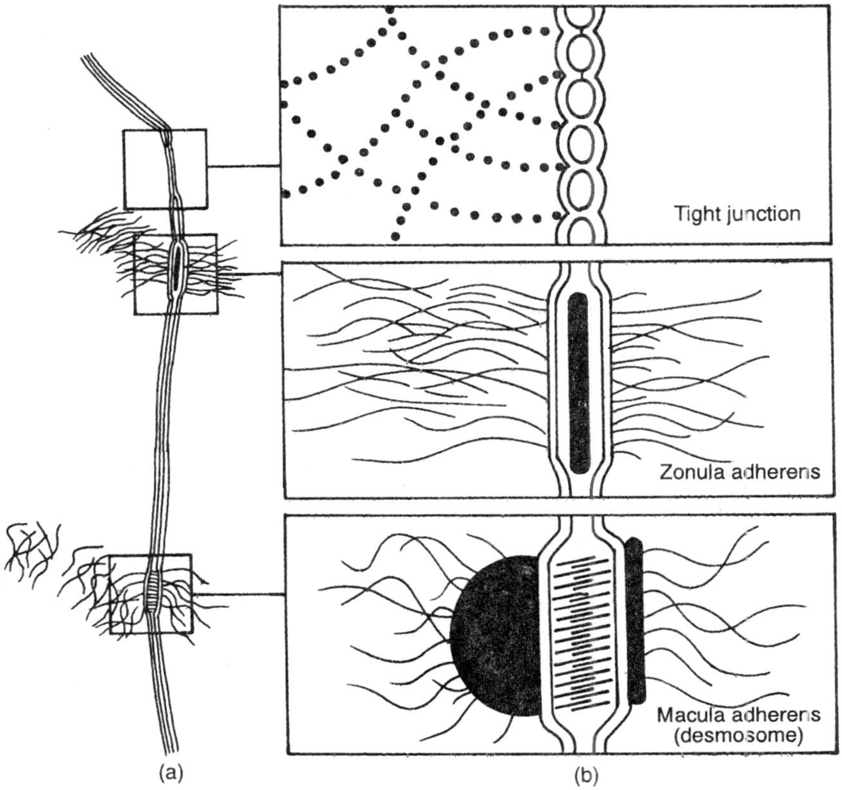

Fig 1(a).2: Intercellular junctions : (a) Schematic diagram, (b) Junctional complex, EM × 125000.

• **Communicating junction/Gap junction/Nexus junction :**

Presence of this junction occurs almost anywhere along the lateral membranes of epithelial cells where intercellular contact areas containing numbers of tiny pores to permit passage of small molecules between adjacent cells.

It permits flow of materials like ions, cyclic AMP, hormones, GMP, etc.

• **Hemidesmosomes :**

[Gr. hemi, half; desmos, band; soma, body]

It occurs in the contact zone between epithelial cells and basal lamina.

Junctional area between cells (on the basis of function)

- Adhering junction
  - Zonula adherens
  - Hemidesmosome
  - Desmosome
- Impermeable junction or tight junction
- Communicating junction or gap junction

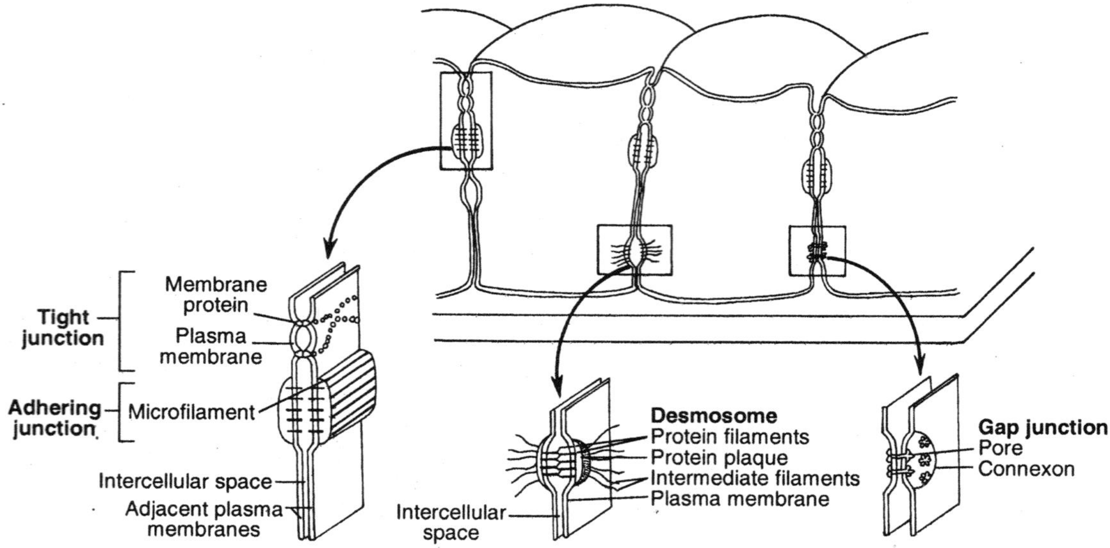

Fig 1(a).3: Junctional complexes of epithelial cells.

(C) Nucleus :

Each and every epithelial cell possesses a distinct nucleus. Shape may vary from spherical to elongated in different types of epithelial tissue.

(D) Extracellular Matrix (ECM) :

In case of epithelial tissue extracellular matrix is absent as because it is compactly arranged cells.

1.4 Classification of Epithelial Tissue

Epithelia are classified according to their **structure** and **function,** into two main groups :

A. **Covering Epithelia** and

B. **Glandular Epithelia.**

Flow chart representation of both the epithelia are presented within Table 1.1.

A. Covering Epithelia

Covering epithelia are tissue whose cells are organized in single layer or multiple layers that cover the external surface or line the cavities of the body. It forms a sheet like cellular part that separates **underlying** or **adjacent connective tissue** from the **external environment, internal cavities** or fluid connective tissue.

Covering epithelia can be classified morphologically according to number of cell layers and the morphology of the cells in the surface layer.

(1) Simple epithelia :

Epithelial tissue which is only **one cell thick** is known as simple epithelium.

Simple epithelium can be subdivided according to the shape and function of its cell.

Table 1.1

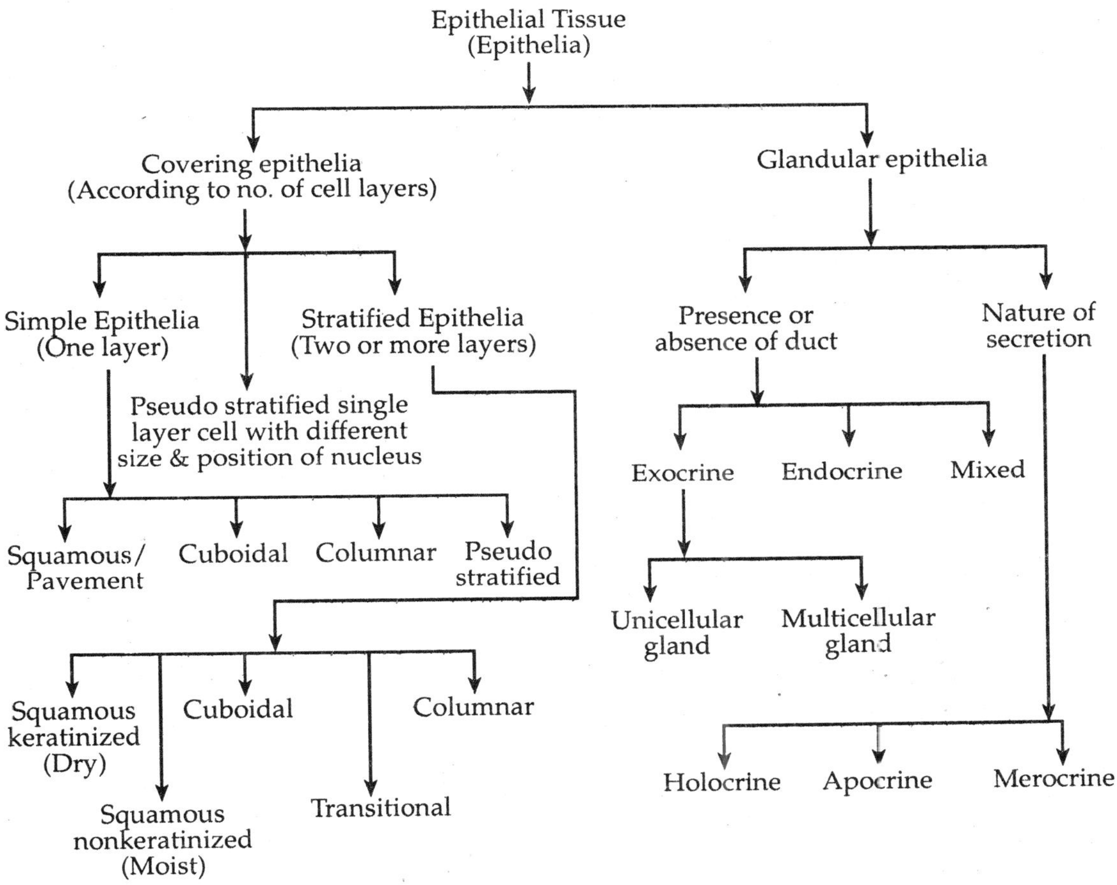

- **Simple epithelia :**

Type	Characters	Distribution	Function
Squamous/ pavement epithelium	1. Appears as thin, plate -like cells. 2. Closely fits with the tissue, provides a smooth low friction surface. 3. Special shape of nucleus is sign of identification. 4. Cells are with elliptical nuclei due to horizontally flattened appearance [Fig 1(a)4].	• Alveolar epithelium in lung • Lining of blood vessels (endothelium). • Lining of pericardium, pleura, peritoneum (mesothelium) • Lining of Bowman's capsule. • Make up the outer layer of skin. • Inner lining of mouth.	1. Facilitates the movement of the viscera (mesothelium). 2. Active transport by pinocytosis (mesothelium and endothelium). 3. Exchange and lubrication. 4. Act as barrier, specially barrier in central nervous system.

Type	Characters	Distribution	Function
Simple cuboidal epithelium	1. Cells are roughly cuboidal in shape, appearing square in cross section. 2. Spherical nucleus lies at the centre of each cell. 3. They are specialized gland forming cells. 4. Most commonly found in secretive or absorptive tissues [Fig 1(a)5].	• Small ducts of exocrine glands (secretive). • Within mixed gland (pancreas-absorptive) • Lining of the renal tubules of kidney. • Germinal epithelium of ovary (covering). • Cells of thyroid gland. • Cells of salivary gland.	1. Acts as covering. 2. Helps in absorption and secretion. 3. Provides protective barriers to the important visceral organs. 4. Takes part in excretion.
Simple columnar epithelium	1. Cells are elongated and column shaped in appearance. 2. Elongated nuclei are located near the base of the cells. 3. It lines the major part of the G.I. tract. 4. In cross sections, they are situated at the right angle to the basement membrane. 5. The luminal plasma membrane of some epithelia are with numerous minute, finger-like projections, called microvilli [Fig 1(a)6].	• Lining of stomach and intestine. • Specialized sensory receptors in nose, ear and taste buds of the tongue. • Goblet cells of duodenum, gastric glands. • Cells of gall-bladder.	1. Helps in secretion. 2. Helps to increase the absorptive surface area. 3. Acts as lubricant by secreting huge amount of mucous. 4. Helps in sensory reception in sense organ (nose—olfaction).

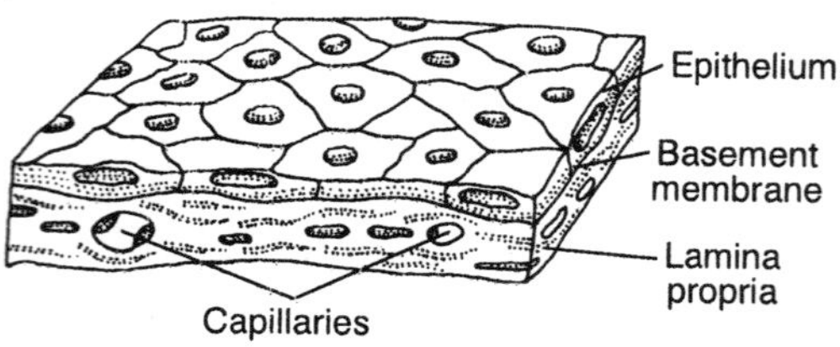

Fig 1(a).4: Simple squamous epithelia.

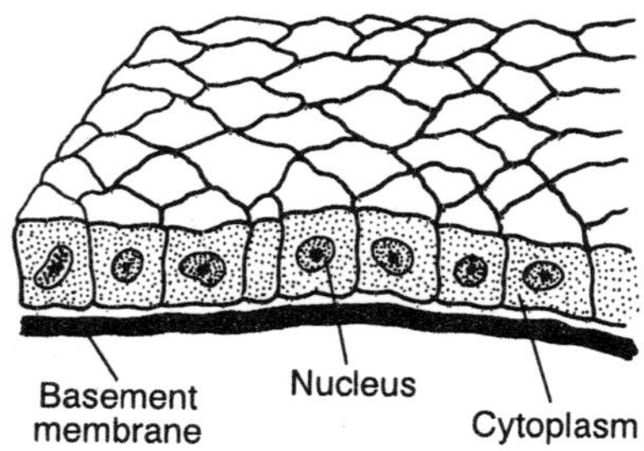

Fig 1(a).5: Simple cuboidal epithelia.

- **Pseud-ostratified epithelia**

Type	Characters	Distribution	Function
Pseudo-stratified epithelum	1. Some simple columnar epithelial cells whose nuclei appear at different heights, giving the misleading impression that the epithelium is stratified [when cells are viewed in cross section]. 2. Cells are with different sizes, not all cells reach surface but all adhere to basal lamina. 3. Some pseudo stratified epithelia posses fine 'hair' like apical extensions called 'cilia' [Fig 1(a)7].	• Lining of trachea, bronchi, nasal cavity. • Ductus deferens and efferent ductules of epididymis. • Fallopian tubes and uterus of females.	1. Protection, secretion, cilia mediated transport of particles trapped in mucus out of the air-passages. 2. Cilia propelthe ovum to the uterus. 3. Cilia are capable of energy dependent, pulsatile beating in a certain direction through interaction of cytoskeletal microtubules and connecting structural proteins and enzymes. 4. Cells are capable of cell division, provide replacements for cell lost or damaged.

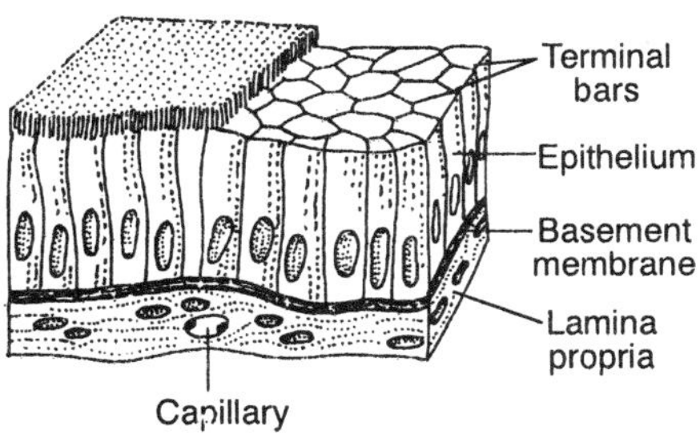

Fig 1(a).6: Simple columnar epithelium.

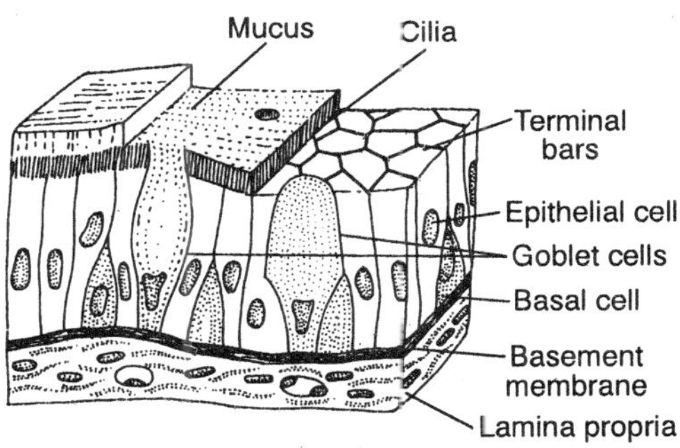

Fig 1(a).7: Pseudostratified epithelium.

(2) Stratified epithelia :

Stratified epithelia are epithelia consisting of two or more layers of cells. These cells are protective in function.

The classification of stratified epithelia is based on the shape and structure of the surface cells since cells of the basal layer are usually cuboidal in shape.

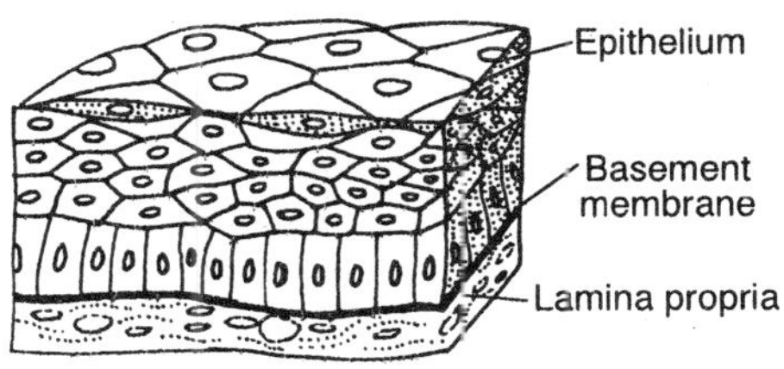

Fig 1(a).8: Stratified cuboidal epithelium.

• **Stratified epithelia**

Type	Characters	Distribution	Function
Stratified squamous (keratinized-dry)	1. The most apical layers (exterior) of cells are dead and lose their nucleus and cytoplasm. 2. Contain a tough, resistant protein called keratin.	• Epidermis • Mammalian skin.	1. Provides protection from external injury and mechanical damage. 2. Makes the epithelium water-proof, so prevents excess loss of water. 3. Cells are adopted to with-stand the constant abrasion and desiccation.
Stratified squamous (non-keratinized moist)	1. Epithelia consist of a variable number of cell layers to a flattened surface layer. 2. Basal cells divide continuously, and cells undergo first maturation. 3. It is poorly adapted to withstand desiccation [Fig 1(a)9].	• Cells of mouth oral cavity. • Oesophagus, pharynx. • Cells of larynx, anal canal. • Lines the uterine cervix and vagina.	1. Provides internal protection. 2. Prevents loss of water. 3. Helps in secretion. 4. Keep the vital parts or organs of body moist by glandular secretion.
Stratified cuboidal epithelium	1. It is a thin, stratified epithelium, usually consists of only two or three layers of cuboidal cells [Fig 1(a)8].	• Cells of sweat gland ducts. • Large ducts of exocrine glands and pancreas. • Cells of anorectal junction. • Ducts of mammary gland.	1. Helps in profuse secretion (specially in glands) 2. Provides more protection than simple cuboidal epithelium.
Stratified columnar epithelium	1. Usually consists of two or three layers of low columnar cells [Fig 1(a)10].	• Cells of male urethra and vas deferens. • Parts of the pharynx. • Cells of conjunctiva.	1. Provides protection. 2. Helps in secretion.
Transitional epithelium	1. It is like pseudo stratified epithelium. 2. It is stretchable in nature. 3. It may distend. 4. Sometimes it may be called urothelium. 5. It is a modified type of stratified epithelium [Fig 1(a)11].	• Found in urinary bladder, ureter, and renal calyces.	1. Provides protection. 2. It has distensible property. 3. It acts as barrier. 4. As surface cells do not slough off, all cells are able to modify their shape when placed under different conditions.

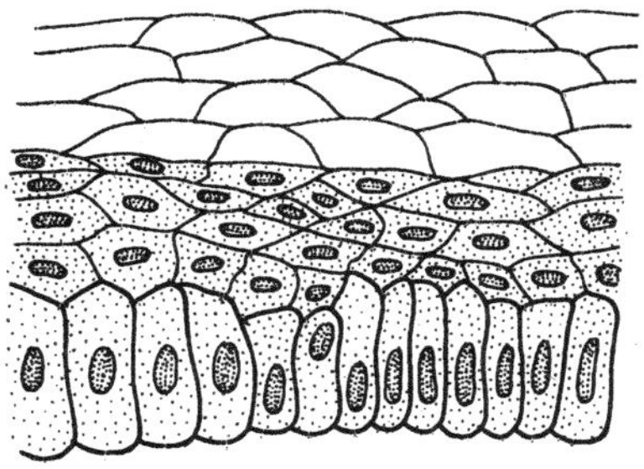

Fig 1(a).9: Diagrammatic figure of stratified squamous non-cornified epithelial tissue.

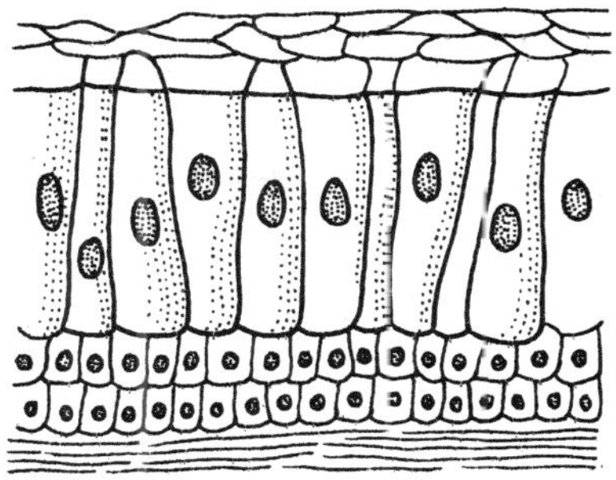

Fig 1(a).10: Diagrammatic figure of stratified columnar epithelial tissue.

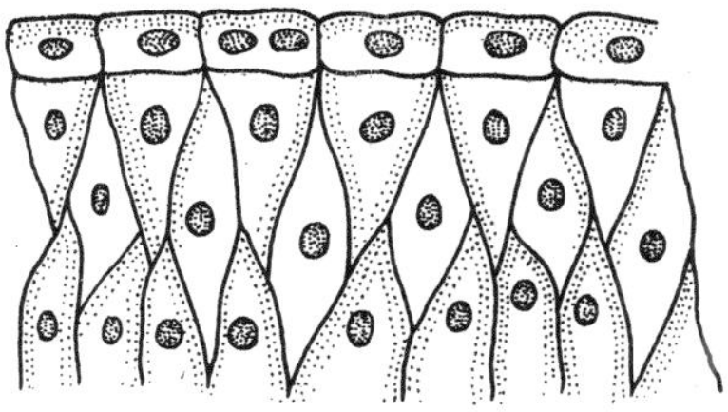

Fig 1(a).11: Transitional epithelial tissue.

B. Glandular Epithelium

Glandular epithelial tissues are those formed by specialized cells to produce a fluid secretion that differs in composition from blood or intercellular fluid. This process is usually accompanied by the intracellular synthesis of macromolecules. These compounds are generally stored in the cells in small membrane bound vesicles called **secretory granules**.

Some glandular epithelial cells synthesize, store and secrete only protein, some produce only lipids and some produce carbohydrate, proteins and lipids.

Only protein producing gland	→ Pancreas
Only lipid producing gland	→ Adrenal, Sebceous gland
Gland producing carbohydrate and protein	→ Salivary gland
Gland producing carbohydrate, protein and lipid	→ Mammary gland

• Different glands secrete their secretion in different forms :

Serous (watery) gland → Pancreatic acinar cells.

Mucous (slipper and sticky) gland → Goblet cells, Salivary gland cells.

Steroid (hormone) gland → Testes, Ovaries, Adrenal gland.

I. According to the presence or absence of ducts

Depending upon the presence or absence of ducts glandular epithelia are classified under three categories, those are as follows :

(1) **Exocrine gland :**

Glands that retain their connection with the surface epithelium from which they originate. This connection takes the form of tubular ducts lined with the epithelial cells through which the glandular secretion passes to reach the surface. Ducts either convey the secreted material in an unaltered form or modify the secretion by concentrating it [Fig 1(a)12].

- **Examples** : The secretion includes—sweat, saliva, milk, stomach acid and digestive enzymes.

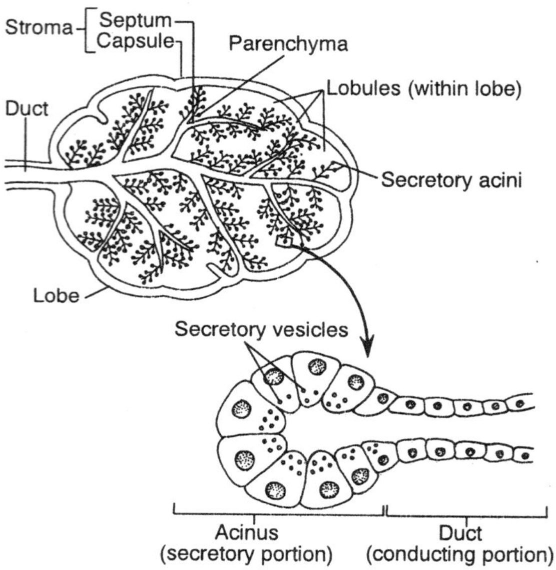

Fig 1(a).12: General structure of exocrine gland. Exocrine glands by definition have ducts that lead to an organ or body surface. Inside the gland the duct runs through connecting septa and branches repeatedly, until its smallest branches end in the secretory portions of the gland.

• Exocrine glands are classified according to their structure :

(i) **Unicellular** or **multicellular gland** describes a single celled gland or a gland made of many cells respectively. A multicellular gland consists of a group of secretory cells and a duct through which the secretions pass as they exit the gland.

(ii) **Branched** refers to branching arrangement of secretory cells in the gland.

(iii) **Simple** or **compound** refers to whether the duct of the gland does not branch or branches, respectively.

(iv) **Tubular** describes a gland whose secretory cells form a tube, while alveolar (or acinar) describes secretory cells that form a bulb-like sac.

Unicellular gland :

It is simple in structure having **single** or **unicellular secretory exocrine gland** within nonsecretory cells.

Goblet cell, a mucus-secreting cell, is a typical unicellular gland present among the columnar cells [Fig 1(a)13].

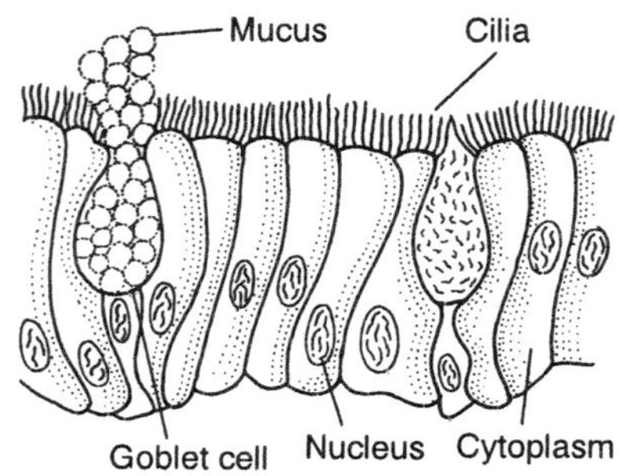

Fig 1(a).13: Unicellular goblet cells within columnar epithelium.

Goblet cells are located in the surface lining and glands of the intestine and in certain passages of the respiratory tract.

Multicellular glands :

Multicellular glands are composed of more than one cell with great complexity depending upon the **nature** and **arrangement** of **secretory cells** and **branching** of the **duct element**.

(2) Endocrine gland :

Glands that lose their connection with the surface from which they originated during development. So, endocrine glands are ductless and their secretion is directly poured into the connective tissue and transported to their site of action by blood stream to reach their target cells. The products are called **hormones.**

Example : Pituitary gland, Thyroid gland, Adrenal gland etc.

• According to the cell grouping, endocrine glands are further subdivided into two types :

Cord type—Adrenal gland.

Follicle type—Thyroid gland.

(3) Mixed gland :

In this type of gland, some cells are specialized in exocrine secretion and others are concerned with endocrine secretion.

Example : Pancreas—where acinal cells secrete digestive enzymes into the intestinal lumen by duct, while the **islet cells** secrete hormone (insulin & glucagon) into the blood.

II. According to the nature of secretion

Glandular epithelia release their secretion by different mechanisms. Specially, cells of exocrine glands exhibit different mechanisms of secretions—

1. Merocrine secretion
2. Apocrine secretion
3. Holocrine secretion

(1) Merocrine secretion (also called **eccrine secretion) :**

- Secretory products are released within the membrane-bound vesicle to the apical surface of the cell.
- Vesicles fuse with cell membrane.
- Secretion involves the process of **exocytosis** from plasma membrane.
- It is the most common form of secretion.
- Proteins are the major secretory products.

Example : Acinar cells of mixed gland of pancreas [Fig 1(a)14].

(2) Apocrine secretion :

- It involves the discharge of free, unbroken, membrane bound vesicles containing secretory product.
- The secretory product is released in the apical portion of the cell.

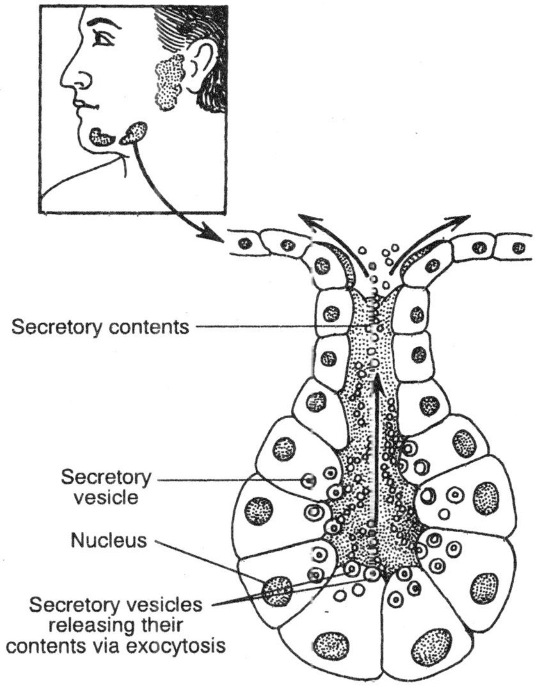

Fig 1(a).14: Merocrine gland.

- The secretary products accumulate at the free surface. It then discharges its secretion by rupturing the free surface of the cell.
- After a recovery period, the cell again recharges to repeat the same cycle.
- This is an unusual mode of secretion and applied to the lipid secretory products.

Example : Mammary gland releases large lipid droplets into the milk [Fig 1(a)15]. Sweat glands, ceruminous glands of external auditory meatus etc also act as apocrine gland.

(3) Holocrine secretion :

• Holocrine secretion involves the discharge of whole secretory cells with subsequent disintegration of the cells to release the secretory product.

• During this process of secretion, the cells undergo programmed cell death.

Example : Principally found in sebaceous gland of skin, tarsal (meibomain) glands of the eyelid [Fig 1(a)16].

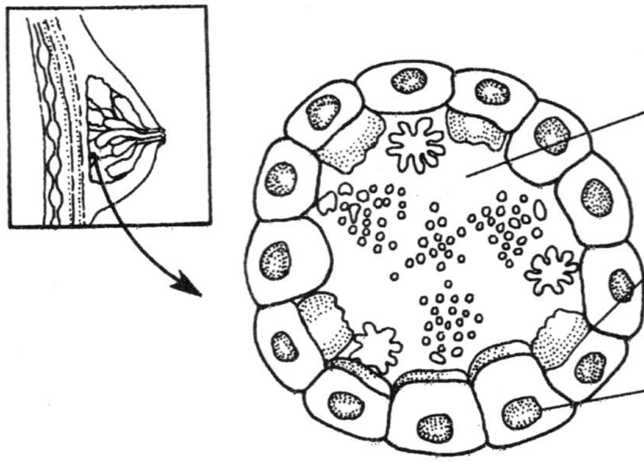

Fig 1(a).15: Apocrine gland.

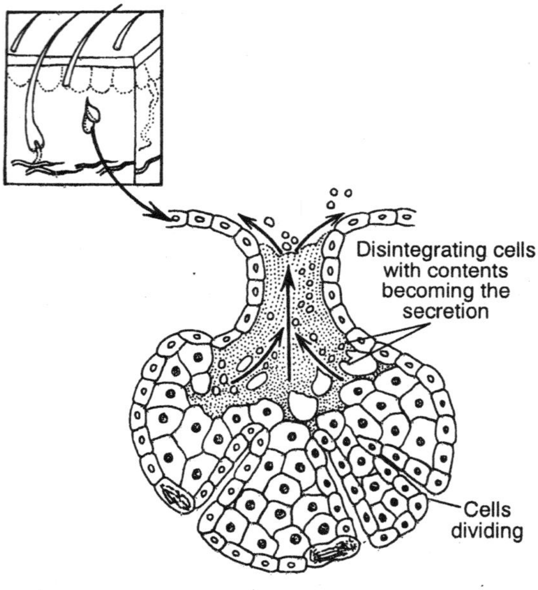

Fig 1(a).16: Holocrine gland.

Paracrine secretion :

Besides, above three mode of secretions, some epithelia secrete a substance, instead of reaching the blood-stream, it affects other cells within the same epithelium tissue. Secretory materials reach the target cells by diffusion through the extracellular space. Such secretion is called as **paracrine** secretion.

1.5 Functions of Epithelial Tissue

(1) Protection :

Epithelial cells from the skin protect underlying tissue from mechanical injury, harmful chemicals, invading bacteria and from excessive loss of water.

Transitional epithelium provides the protection to the urinary bladder.

(2) Secretion :

In gland, epithelial tissue is specialized to secrete specific chemical substances such as enzymes, hormones and lubricating fluids. Specially, the columnar epithelium of the stomach and the gastric glands also perform this process.

(3) Absorption :

Certain epithelial cells lining the small intestine absorb nutrients from the digested food and the columnar epithelium of the convoluted tubules of kidney also helps in absorption.

(4) Secretion :

Sensory stimuli penetrate specialised epithelial cells. Specialized epithelial tissue, containing sensory nerve endings are found in the skin, eyes, ears, nose and on the tongue.

(5) Excretion :

Epithelial tissues in the kidney excrete waste products from the body and reabsorb needed materials from the urinary waste products. Sweat is also excreted from the body by epithelial cells in the sweat glands.

(6) Reduces friction :

The smooth tightly interlocking epithelial cells that line the entire circulatory system reduce friction between the blood and the walls of the blood vessels.

(7) Receptor function :

Some epithelial tissue help to receive and transduce external stimuli. Taste buds of the tongue, olfactory epithelium of nasal mucosa and the retina of the eye act as receptor function.

(8) Cleaning :

Ciliated epithelium assists in removing dust particles and foreign bodies which have entered into the air passages.

(9) Diffusion :

Simple epithelium promotes the diffusion of gases, liquids and nutrients. Walls of capillaries and lungs are highly thin for the purpose of diffusion.

(10) Transport :

Epithelium with motile cilia helps in transport of materials across the epithelium to and from the connective tissue.

• **Autocrine and paracrine secretion : Paracrine mechanism** where the released hormone diffuses to its adjacent target cells through the immediate extracellular space and where following the release of hormone, it may also feed back on the cell of origin by a so-called **autocrine mechanism.**

1(B) THE CONNECTIVE TISSUES

All those tissues of the vertebrates, containing cellular and fibrous materials in matrix in large amount and which are important for constituting the framework of many organs and in binding together the various structures of the body and which are mesodermal in origin, are called **connective tissues.**

The connective tissues of the vertebrates are also called **supporting tissues** because they serve to bind other tissues and organs together, and give support to the body. The connective and supporting tissues are characterized by cells which function to elaborate and maintain a variety of extracellular materials (matrix) about themselves.

These extracellular materials are of such volume that in most cases the cells of this tissue are rather widely separated, in contrast to epithelia, where cells are closely associated. The character of the extracellular matrix is determined from region to region by the abundance and proportion of fluid, fibres, mineral aggregates and ground substance.

Characteristics :

(i) This type of tissue originates from the mesenchyme tissue of the embryo that develops from the mesodermal layer.

(ii) Usually no basement membrane is present.

(iii) The connective tissue is characterized by a paucity of cellular elements and a relatively greater abundance of intercellular substances.

(iv) In addition to cells different types of fibrous elements are found.

(v) The extracellular substance varies from a liquid consistency in blood, firm and flexible in cartilage to a solid state in bone and the bone is rigid because of the deposition of inorganic salts in the matrix.

Functions :

(i) Acts as cementing layer between two tissues.

(ii) It connects the different parts of an organ or with different organs.

(iii) This tissue makes the framework and elasticity of body.

(iv) Takes part in the formation of blood and lymph.

(v) Protects against infection.

(vi) Assists to transport nutrients.

(vii) Stores fat.

(viii) Helps movement of muscle (tendon) and bone (ligament).

1.2.1 Classification of Connective Tissue

This tissue in the mammals is classified into three major groups which are again subdi-

Connective tissue

- Connective tissue proper
  - (a) Areolar tissue
  - (b) White fibrous tissue
  - (c) Yellow elastic tissue
  - (d) Adipose tissue
  - (e) Reticular tissue
- Supporting tissue
  - (a) Bone
  - (b) Cartilage
- Vascular tissue or Fluid tissue
  - (a) Blood
  - (b) Lymph

vided according to the nature of the cellular components and intercellular substances.

A. Connective tissue proper :

This tissue consists of cells, fibres and intercellular substances or matrix. The various kinds of fibres with cells are embedded in a large amount of matrix. This matrix is secreted by the cells. The intercellular substance or matrix shows a great variety in form and nature. The connective tissue proper comprises of the following types—(a) Areolar, (b) White fibrous, (c) Yellow elastic, (d) Adipose and (e) Reticular.

(a) Areolar tissue (Loose connective tissue) : The most fundamental type of connective tissue is the Areolar tissue. The kind of connective tissue, where the plenty amount of fibres are loosely embedded in the matrix, is known as Areolar tissue. It is found all over the body, e.g., beneath the skin, where it connects the adjacent organs. It is also present between the muscles, vessels and nerves.

Areolar tissue is composed of fibres and cells. Fibres are loosely arranged bundles of white collagenous fibre and fine yellow elastic fibre. Yellow elastic fibres are few in number and these fibres cross and intercross with one another, thus form a network like structure. The spaces of the network are occupied by the jelly-like ground substance and various kinds of cells. The following types of cells are generally found in the inter-cellular ground substance—**fibroblasts**, **histiocytes** or **macrophages**, **mast cells**, **plasma cells**, **fat cells**, and **pigment cells**.

Fibroblasts : They are very common type of cells of this tissue which are responsible for fibre formation. There is evidence that they also form the ground substance. Fibroblasts are large, somewhat flattened, frequently ovoid cells, with branching processes. Their nuclei are oval and somewhat flattened, resembling the shape of the cell.

Histiocytes or **macrophages :** They are also irregularly shaped cells with processes which usually are short and blunt but occasionally are long and slender. The nucleus is more rounded and somewhat smaller and darker staining than that of the fibroblasts. They are motile and phagocytic and so they are known as macrophages.

Mast cells : These cells occur in varying numbers; being especially numerous along the course of the blood vessels. They are large ovoid cells with relatively small ovoid nuclei and numerous cytoplasmic granules which are usually basophilic. They help in the formation of haparin (anticoagulant), histamine (in allergic condition), and serotonin (a vaso-constrictor).

Plasma cells : They are infrequent and these cells are ovoid, irregularly shaped cells, smaller than histiocytes but larger than lymphocytes. The nucleus is 'spoke wheel' type and small and eccentrically placed. These cells form antibody.

Fat cells : These are small oval-shaped cells occurring singly or in clumps. Each fat cell contains a single large droplet of oil and thin rim of cytoplasm possessing a flattened nucleus at one side. The main function is to store fat in the cells.

Pigment cell : They are irregular in shape and the cytoplasm contains black or yellow pigments. These cells are found in the skin, pia mater, choroid layer of the eye, etc. They are thought to produce melanin pigments.

Distribution : This tissue is distributed throughout the body such as in the (i) subcutaneous and subserous layers, (ii) between muscles, blood vessels and nerve fibres and in the (iii) interior of other organs.

Function :

(i) Serves as a support and packing material.

(ii) The histiocytes and plasma cells in areolar tissue assist the purpose of defence of the body against the invasion of micro-organisms and others.

(iii) The fibroblasts help in fibrosis during the repair of inflammation.

• **Wharton's jelly :** Jelly-like connective tissue is the embryonic form of areolar tissue. The cell types such as macrophages, fibroblasts and lymphocytes remain scattered in a more or less homogenous jelly-like mucin ground substance. This ground substance is provided with few fibres interlacing throughout the tissue. The tissue occurs in the umbilical cord where it is called **Wharton's jelly.**

(b) White fibrous tissue : The type of connective tissue where non-contractile collagenous fibres are more than the matrix with few fibroblasts is known as white fibrous tissue. The white collagenous fibres generally course together in bundles of indefinite length and variable thickness. The bundles of fibres are wavy. Each fibre is made up of protein which is known as collagen. Fibrocytes are found between the interspaces of bundles of fibres. The fibres of the loose connective tissue follow an irregular and undulating course; this allows for movement and flexibility of the other tissues with which they are associated. The collagenous fibres themselves are flexible but so slightly elastic as to be practically nonextensible [Fig 1(b).1].

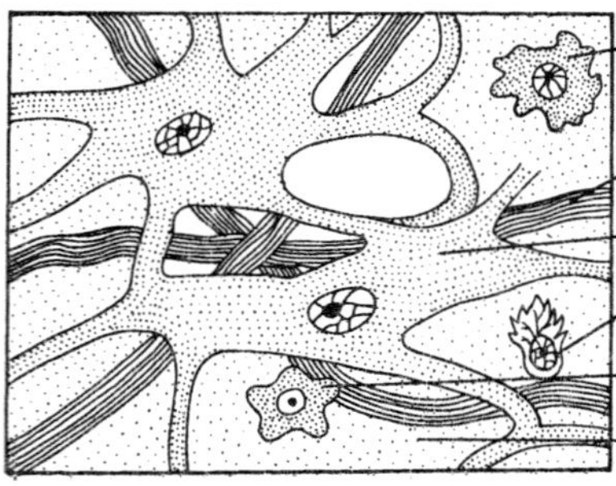

Fig 1(b).1: White collagenous connective tissue.

Distribution : This tissue occurs in tendons, ligaments, covering of the brain, i.e., dura-mater etc.

Function :

(i) Gives rigidity to the matrix and helps in wear and tear.

(ii) It provides mechanical protection against stretch and pressure.

(c) Yellow elastic tissue : The type of connective tissue which is composed of mainly by highly refractile elastic fibres with few fibroblasts is termed as yellow elastic tissue. The elastic fibres are highly refractile fibres which are as a rule thinner than the white fibres. They branch and anastomose freely, forming networks. Each fibre is composed of protein which is called elastin. Fibroblasts occur in between the elastic fibres [Fig 1(b).2].

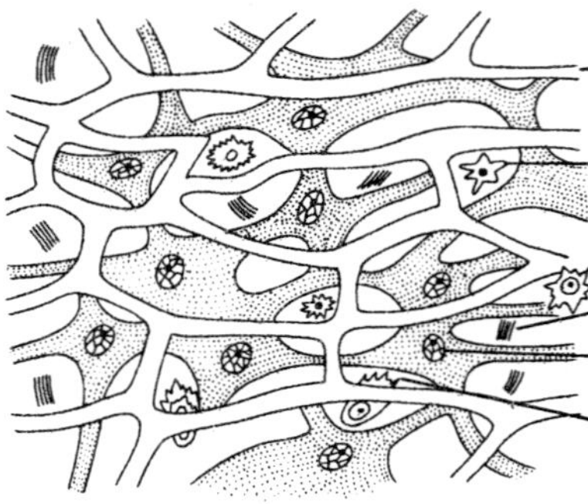

Fig 1(b).2: Yellow elastic connective tissue.

Distribution : This kind of tissue is present in the walls of bronchi, larynx, lungs, arteries, etc.

Function :

(i) It maintains the normal blood circulation and blood pressure due to its elasticity.

(ii) Acts as a strong elastic cord.

(iii) This tissue also regulates the normal expansion and contraction of lungs during respiration.

(d) Adipose tissue : The type of tissue where the large number of fat cells containing fat globules are present on a framework of loose fibres is called adipose connective

Differences between white fibrous tissue and yellow elastic tissue

Characters	White fibrous tissue	Yellow elastic tissue
Colour of the fibres	It is composed of white fibres formed by the fibroblast.	It is composed of yellowish coloured fibres.
Thickness	Fibres are thin and non-branching.	Fibres are thicker and the individual fibres are branched and the branches join to form a network.
Nature	Fibres in bundles.	The fibres run singly and also in loose bundles.
Disposition	Bundle of fibres run in a wavy way.	Bundle of fibres are not wavy but straight.
Chemistry	Made up of collagen-like protein material.	Made up of elastin-like protein material.
Function	The fibres protect against stretch and pressure.	The tissue serves as a strong elastic rope.

tissue. Fat cells are found isolated or in groups in all loose connective tissues, but in certain places they are present in such large numbers and have such an organisation as to justify the designation of adipose tissue.

Fat cells are abundant and they are enlarged owing to accumulation of neutral fat. The cells are generally round and oval in shape and those cells may be polyhedral due to the pressure of the adjacent fat cells. In the early stages the fat cells may contain isolated droplets of oily substance, which, as they grow unite into a single large fat globule and occupy the centre of the cell displacing the cytoplast to the periphery as a thin layer against the cell membrane. The cytoplasm along with the flattened nucleus are pushed to the periphery of the cell due to deposition of fat droplets. Because of the disposition of nucleus and cytoplasm at the periphery of each adipose cell, a fat cell is said to be present a characteristic "signet ring" appearance. The adipose cells are loosely attached to each other and the narrow interspaces are occupied by thin fibres which form a loose network for the support of the large fat-laden cells [Fig 1(b).3].

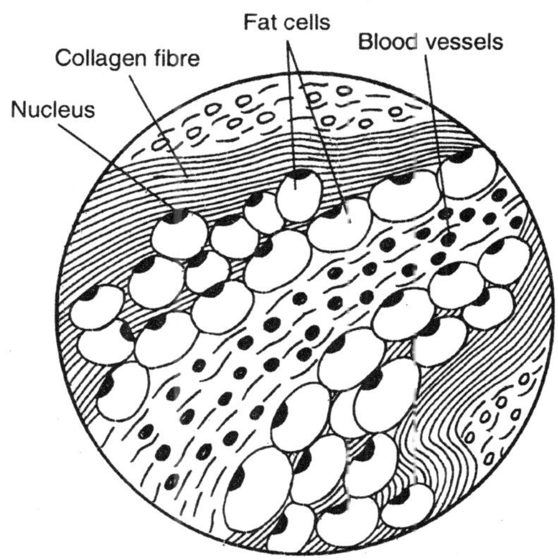

Fig 1(b).3: Adipose tissue.

Distribution : The largest deposits of fat are found in the subcutaneous connective tissue, in the kidney region, in the mesenteries and mediastinum and in the cervical, axillary and inguinal regions.

Function :

(i) Adipose tissue forms soft and elastic pads between the various organs of the body.

(ii) It gives the shape to the body and limbs.

(iii) Adipose tissue keeps the visceral organs in position and prevents them from injury.

(iv) Since fat is a poor conductor of heat, its presence just beneath the skin aids in the preservations of the body temperature.

(v) Acts as a storage of energy in the fat material.

(e) Reticular tissue : Connective tissue made of anastomosing stellate-shaped cells forming a reticulum along with fibres is called reticular tissue. This tissue consists of star-shaped reticular cells and the cytoplasmic processes of the cells are anastomosing to form the syncytium. The thin reticular fibres dispersed in the interspaces join to form a network. The intercellular space is filled with a liquid ground substance, called tissue fluid [Fig 1(b).4].

Distribution : They occur as fine networks around small blood vessels, muscle fibres, nerve fibres, lymph gland, liver, spleen, bone marrow, etc.

Function :

(i) Gives mechanical support and protection.

(ii) In addition to the mechanical support, the cells of this tissue are phagocytic in nature and play an important role in defence mechanism of the body.

(iii) The tissue may probably take part in fat and iron metabolism.

B. Supporting tissue :

The endoskeleton of the vertebrate animal is known as supporting tissue or skeletal tissue. It is regarded as a kind of connective tissue, having cells embedded in a matrix, but here the matrix is comparatively hard. **The tissue which forms the internal framework of organ and gives support is known**

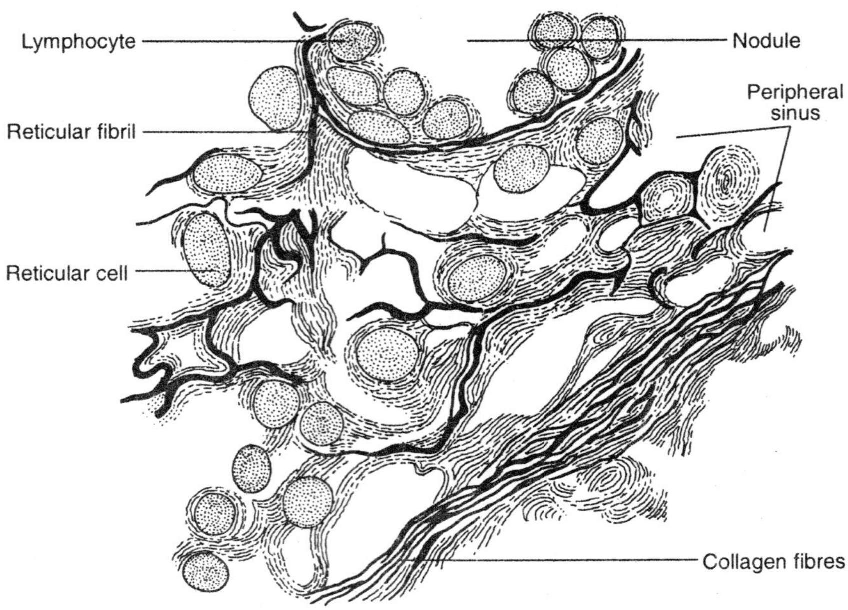

Fig 1(b).4: Reticular tissue from lymph node of monkey.

as supporting tissue. This tissue provides a resistant material for the attachment of the muscles and consequently gives rigidity. This hard tissue gives protection to delicate structures enclosed by it. The supporting tissue is classified into two groups—**cartilage** and **bone.**

I. Cartilage tissue

Cartilage is a specialised form of connective tissue compartment consisting of cells, called **chondrocytes,** and extracellular fibres embedded in an amorphous gel-like ground substance or matrix. The intercellular components predominate over the cells, which are isolated in small cavities within the matrix. Unlike other connective tissues, cartilage has no blood vessels or nerves of its own. **Cartilage is a firm and elastic non-vascular connective tissue with a solid matrix containing chondrocyte cells.** This tissue originates from mesenchyma cells. The colloidal properties of its matrix are, therefore, important to the nutrition of its chondrocyte cells and are in large measure responsible for its firmness and resilience.

Structure : Cartilage consists of large amount of intercellular substance or matrix, cartilage cells and fibres. The matrix or ground substance is called **chondrin.** This chondrin is provided with **chondromucoid** and **chondro-albuminoid** like protein substances in which a delicate network of **elastin** and **collagen** fibres can be seen. The cartilage is composed of cells, called **chondrocytes,** which lie in groups of twos, fours or eights in smaller scattered spaces, called **lacunae.** Each group of chondrocyte cells is surrounded by a common sheath, called **capsule.** The group of chondrocytes constitutes a **chondrone** which is the mechanical unit in a cartilage. The matrix is devoid of nerves and blood vessels. The cartilage is surrounded externally by a layer of dense fibro-elastic tissue covering the **perichondrium.**

Occurrence : Cartilage is restricted in the skeletal structures of cartilagenous fishes, rings of trachea, bony joints, bronchi, pinna of ear, etc.

Function :

(i) Plays an important role in the framework of the body.

(ii) Assists in firmness and elasticity of the body.

(iii) Cartilage prevents mechanical erosion in bony joints.

Types of cartilage tissue : According to the nature and visibility of fibrilar elements, cartilage is subdivided into three varieties : **hyaline, elastic** and **fibrous.** Of these, hyaline cartilage is the most widely distributed type and the others can be regarded as modifications of it.

(a) Hyaline cartilage : Hyaline cartilage appears as a bluish-white, translucent mass in the fresh condition.

This kind of tissue is mainly composed of homogenous matrix with cartilage cells. The cartilage cells or chondrocytes lie in fluid-filled spaces, called **lecunae,** within the matrix. These cells are arranged in groups of two or four in a common capsule. The chondrocytes are large with rounded angles. The cells are uni-or multinucleate with cytoplasm having few fat droplets, glycogen granules, mitochondria and occasionally some pigments. The collagenous fibres distributed throughout the matrix are not visible due to the similar refractive index with the matrix. This type of cartilage is also called articular cartilage [Fig 1(b).5].

Cartilage cells (Chondrocytes) : In the layers of cartilage immediately beneath the perichondrium the **lacunae** are elliptical, while deeper in the cartilage they are semicircular or angular. The cartilage cells, the **chondrocytes,** occupy chambers, known as lacunae. The cells appear irregularly shaped and shunt away from the walls of their lacunae. The cells fill the lacunae and the cell surface is irregular and has short processes extending into depressions in the ground substance or matrix, there is no obvious space between the cell and its surrounding ground substance. Chondrocyte cytoplasm contains, in addition to

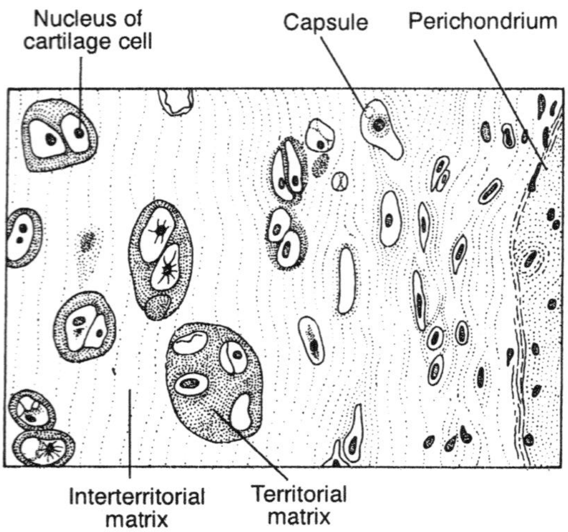

Fig 1(b).5: Hyaline cartilage from the trachea of a boy (17 years of age).

glycogen and lipid, the usual characteristics of a secretory cell. Actually, mature chondrocytes in higher vertebrates rarely if ever have processes visible with the light microscope but in electron micrographs their surface is quite irregular.

The nucleus of the cartilage cell is round or oval and contians one to several nucleoli, depending upon the species. There is a juxtanuclear cell centre with a pair of centrioles and a well-developed Golgi apparatus in regenerating cartilage. The surrounding cytoplasm contains elongated mitochondria and a well-developed granular endoplasmic reticulum with moderately distended cisternae [Fig 1(b).8(i)].

Cartilage matrix : The intercellular substance or matrix appears homogeneous in the fresh condition. The apparently homogeneous matrix contains fine collagenous fibres which are marked by a ground substance of similar refractive index. They are mostly slender fibrils of only about 100 to 250 Å in width and they usually lack the 640 Å cross banding characteristic of other collagen. The principal constituent of the matrix is chondromucoids which are composed of glycosaminoglycan complexes containing chondroitin 4-sulfate and chondroitin 6-sulfate. The ground substance also contains electron-dense granules of about 100 to 400 Å in diameter, known as **matrix granules.**

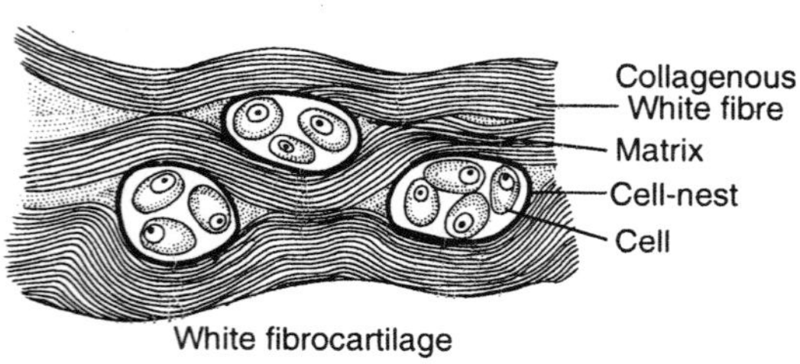

Fig 1(b).6: White fibrous cartilage.

Distribution : The hyaline cartilage is present in the articular end of the bones, at the anterior end of the ribs, etc. The cartilages of nose, larynx, trachea and bronchi, etc. also belong to this class.

Function :

(i) It is resistant to pressure and tension and as such relieves the bones and also prevents mechanical friction.

(ii) It serves to keep passage open as in trachea and bronchi and to keep the organs distended.

(b) Elastic cartilage : In mammals elastic cartilage appears more yellow and opaque than hyaline cartilage because of the large number of elastic fibres in its matrix. These branch and course to form a dense network of anastomosing and interlacing fibres. These fibres are looser and thin and the network is wide-meshed in the peripheral layers but these are thicker and more closely packed in the deeper portions.

The interstitial substance also contains collagenous fibrils, particularly in the subperichondrial region. The cells of elastic cartilage are smaller to those of hyaline cartilage; they are of the same rounded shape, are also surrounded by capsules, and are scattered singly or in isogenous groups of two or four cells. The ground substance or matrix differs from that of hyaline cartilage by being permeated by frequently branching fibres, which are positive in all staining reactions due to the presence of a protein, **elastin** in the fibrils. The elastic fibres of the cartilage continue into perichondrium [Fig 1(b).7].

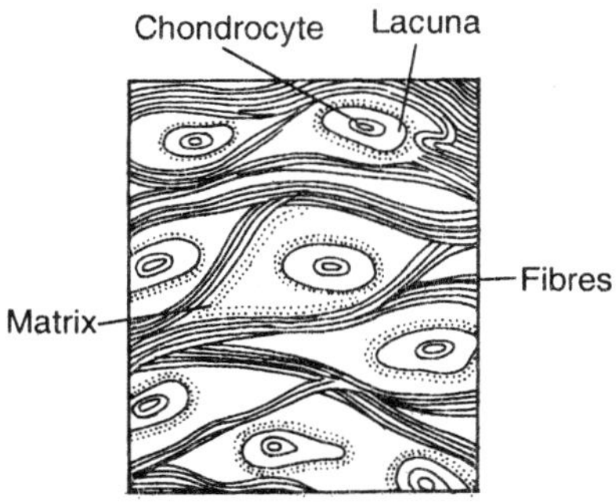

Fig 1(b).7: Elastic fibrocartilage.

Distribution : This type of tissue occurs in the external ear, the eustachian tube, the epiglottis, and some of the laryngeal cartilages.

Function :

(i) This kind of tissue gives the firmness and elasticity of the organs.

(ii) It acts as a supporting tissue where stretch and recoil is necessary.

(c) Fibrous cartilage : The type of cartilage tissue where the collagenous fibres are densely packed, i.e., fibrous cartilage is a combination of dense collagenous fibres with chondrocytes and a scanty cartilage matrix. This tissue is generally not circumscribed by a perichondrium. The relative proportion of cells, fibres and ground substance varies greatly. The cartilage cells are frequently in rows, with intervening bundles of collagenous fibres that have the characteristic 640 Å cross banding.

Fibrous cartilage is found in a few regions of the body. In small areas with poorly defined limits typical cartilage cells and a small amount of insterstitial substances occur among the abundant fibrous elements. The encapsulated cartilage cells lie singly or in pairs, or are sometimes aligned in rows between bundles of collagen fibres. The matrix is quite inconspicuous except in the immediate vicinity of the cells where its presence can be inferred from the characteristic form of the lacunae [Fig 1(b).6].

Distribution : It occurs in the intervertebral disc, mandibular joint, knee joint, symphysis, pubis, etc (Fig 1(b).8(ii)).

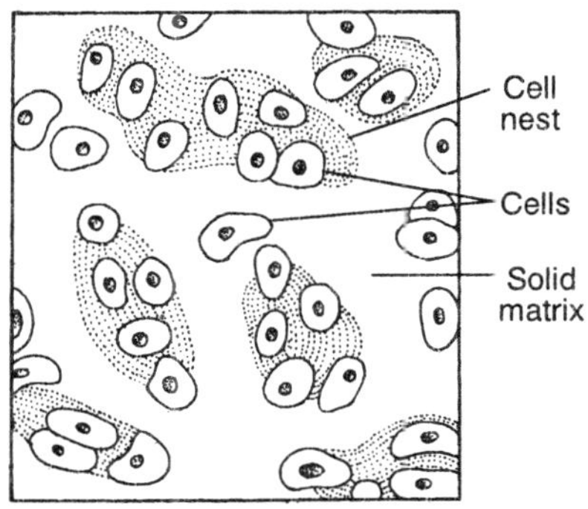

Fig 1(b).8(i): Hyaline cartilage.

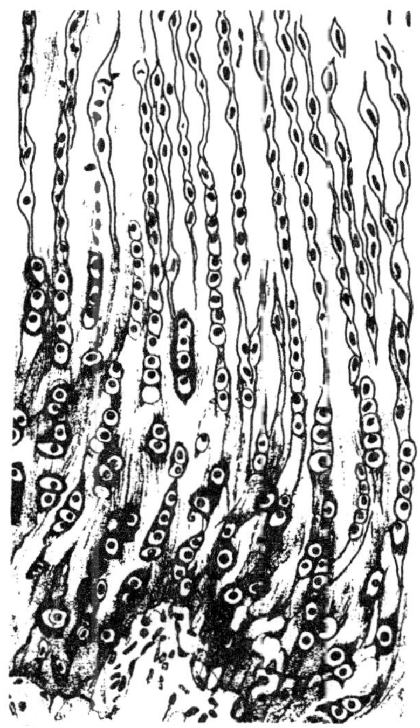

Fig 1(b).8(ii): Low-power drawing of fibrocartilage at insertion of tendon into the tibia of a rat. Note the direct transformation of rows of tendon cells (top) into cartilage cells surrounded by deeply staining matrix.

Differences between hyaline, elastic and fibrous cartilage

Characters	Hyaline cartilage	Elastic cartilage	Fibrous cartilage
1. Nature of matrix	Matrix is clear and homogeneous.	Matrix is not clear and heterogeneous.	Matrix is not clear and heterogeneous.
2. Amount of matrix	Matrix medium.	Matrix plenty.	Matrix scanty.
3. Fibres	White fibres are present.	Yellow elastic fibres are plenty and net like arrangement.	Bundles of white fibres are plenty.
4. Cartilage cell	Large no. of cartilage cells are present.	No. of cartilage cells is fewer than hyaline cartilage.	No. of cells few.
5. Capsule	Cells are encapsulated.	Cartilage cells are present in the small spaces of the network of fibres.	Cartilage cells are present in the spaces between the bundles.
6. Covering	Perichondrium is present.	Present.	Absent.

Function :

(i) It supports those structures where tensile strength and flexibility are required.

(ii) It prevents erosion from mechanical friction.

II. Bone (Osseous tissue)

Osseous tissue is a rigid form of connective tissue and is normally organized into definite structures, the bones. Bone, in common with other connective tissues, consists of cells, fibres and ground substance, but unlike the others its extracellular components are calcified, making it a hard unyielding substance suited for its supportive and protective function in the skeleton. It provides for the internal support of the body and for the attachment of the muscles and tendons essential for locomotion. It protects the vital organs of the cranial and thoracic cavities and by the attachment to the muscles acts as lever and it encloses the blood forming elements of the bone marrow. Bone is also storage place for calcium ions which can be withdrawn when needed to maintain a normal level of calcium in the body and other fluids of the body.

Gross organization of bone tissue : Bone is the hardest of all the connective tissues that constitutes most of the skeleton of higher vertebrates. Grossly, two forms of bone are distinguishable, the **spongy** or **cancellous** and the **dense** or **compact.** Cancellous bone comprises of a three dimensional lattice of branching bony spicules or **trabeculae,** delimiting a labyrinthine system of intercommunicating spaces that are occupied by **bone marrow.** Compact bone appears as solid continuous mass, in which space can be seen only by the help of microscope. The two forms of bone grade into one another without a sharp boundary.

With very few exceptions, the compact and spongy forms are both present in every bone, but the distribution and amount of each kind vary considerably. The diaphyses of the long bones consist mainly of compact tissue; only the innermost layer immediately surrounding the medillary cavity is spongy. The tabular bones of the head are provided with two plates of compact bone enclosing a marrow space bridged by irregular bars of spongy bone. The epiphyses of the long bones and most of the short bones comprise of spongy bone covered by a thin outer shell of compact bone.

Each bone, except at its articular end is covered by an outer tough membrane, known as **periosteum.** The so-called **endosteum** or inner periosteum of the marrow cavity and marrow spaces, is not a well-demarcated layer. It comprises of a variable concentration of medullary reticular connective tissue which consists of osteogenic cells that are in immediate contact with the osseous tissue.

1. Compact bone : This kind of osseous tissue is very hard having lamellated with Haversian system. This osseous tissue is covered by an outter tough membrane, the **periosteum.** The periosteum is composed of outer fibrous tissue and the inner layer of elastic tissue with **osteoblasts** and **osteoclasts.** Blood vessels, nerves and muscles are attached to the periosteum. The central hollow part of the compact bone is called **marrow cavity** or **medullary cavity** and this cavity is enclosed by a thin fibrous membrane termed as **endosteum** which is present on the inner region of the hard shaft part of the bone. The marrow cavity of long bone is filled up with **yellow bone marrow** which is composed of adipose tissue.

Compact bone is largely composed of the mineralized interstitial substance or ground substance, **bone matrix,** deposited in layers or **lamellae** 3 to 7 μm thick. Rather uniformly spaced throughout the ground substance of bone are lenticular cavities, known as **lacunae**, each is completely filled by an osseous cell or **osteocyte.** Radiating in all sides from each lacuna are exceedingly slender branching tubular passages, the **canaliculi,** that penetrate the interstitial substance of the lamellae, anastomosing with the canaliculi of neighbouring lacunae. Thus, although the lacunae are spaced some distance apart, these form a continuous system of cavities interconnected by an extensive network of minute canals. These slender passages are believed to be essential to the nutrition of the osseous cells. However, the maintenance of system of inter-communicating canaliculi provides avenues for exchange of metabolites between the bone cells and the nearest perivascular space.

The shaft, body or lamella of compact bone is disposed in three common patterns.

(i) **Haversian system :** The hard wall of the shaft is pierced by large number of minute longitudinal tunnels which are called **Haversian canals.** Each Haversian canal is provided with blood vessels, lymph vessels and nerves. The Haversian canal is surrounded by 4 to 20 concentric layers of matrix and these are called **lamellae,** and the lamellae vary in size. In cross section the Haversian systems appear as concentric rings around a circular opening. In longitudinal section, they are seen as closely spaced bands parallel to the vascular channels [Fig 1(b).9].

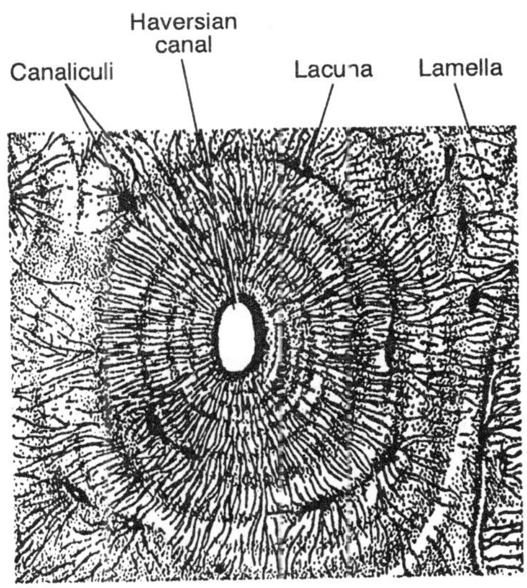

Fig 1(b).9: Magnified view of a Haversian system in compact bone.

Between the layers of lamellae there are minute fusiform-like spaces known as **lacunae** which are also arranged in circles. From all sides of each lacuna, large number of minute wavy channels are coming out and these minute wavy channels are termed as

canaliculi. The lacunae communicate with each other and also with the Haversian canal through the canaliculi. Each lacuna contains bone cell (osteocyte) and the processes of which extend into the lacunae. So the concentric lamellae of inter-cellular substance, Haversian canal, lacunae, bone cells and canaliculi form one **Haversian system** [Fig 1(b).10(i)+(ii)].

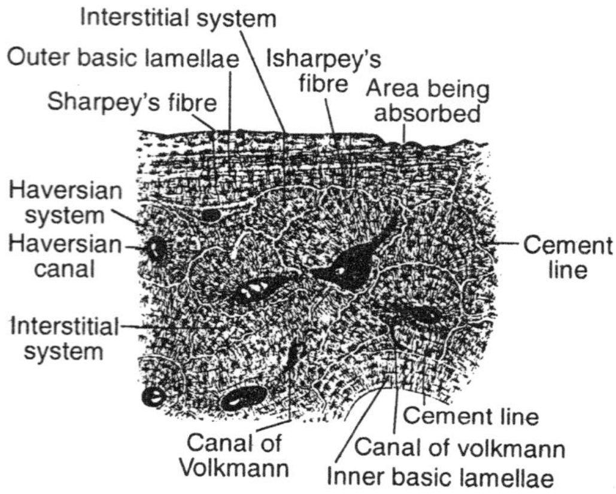

Fig 1(b).10(i): Portion of a ground cross section of a human metacarpal bone; stained with Fuchsin (After Schaffer).

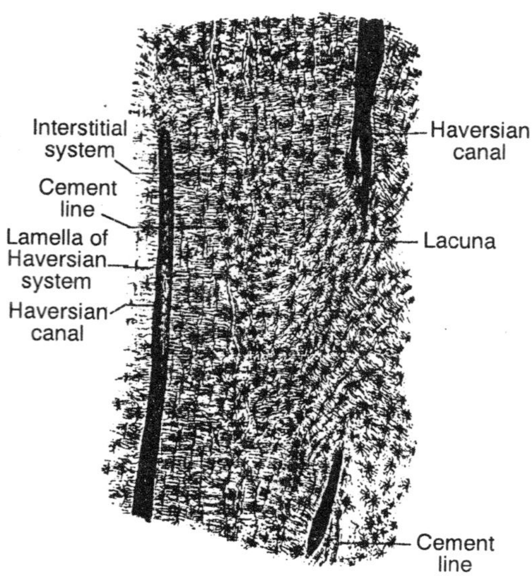

Fig 1(b).10(ii): Portion of a longitudinal, ground section of the ulna of man; stained with fuchsin. (After Schaffer).

(ii) **The interstitial lamellae :** The spaces between the Haversian systems are not lamellated in regular appearance. The bone cells and matrix are present in irregular spaces. Here the limits of Haversian systems and interstitial systems are sharply demarcated by refractile lines, called **cement lines.** In cross section, the interior of compact bone thus appears as a mosaic of round and angular pieces cemented together [Fig 1(b).11].

(iii) **Circumferential lamellae or periosteal lamellae :** These lamellae are arranged parallel to the outer and inner surfaces of the bone wall. Thus, the compact bone consists of branching and anastomosing concentric tubular lamellae, with intervals filled in by interstitial lamellae, which are coverd externally and internally by the more parallel circumferential lamellae. The perforating canals which pierce the bone from its outer and inner surface and become continuous with the central canals are not lined by concentric lamellae [Fig 1(b).12].

Two kinds of vascular channels are distinguished in compact bone on the basis of their orientation and relation to the lamellar structure of the surrounding bone. The longitudinal channels in the centres of Haversian systems are known as Haversian canals. They consist of one or two blood vessels ensheathed in loose connective tissue. The Haversian canals are connected with one another and communicate with marrow cavity and with the free surface via transverse and oblique channels, known as Volk**mann's canals**. They can be identified from the Haversian canals in sections by the fact that they are not enveloped or enclosed by concentrically arranged lamellae but traverse the bone in a direction perpendicular to the lamellae. The blood channels largely for the endosteum and to a lesser extent from the periosteum, communicate with those of Haversian system through Volkmann's canals. The vessels or channels are often larger than those in Haversian system.

Shaft or body of the long bones such as humerus, femur, etc., are compact in nature.

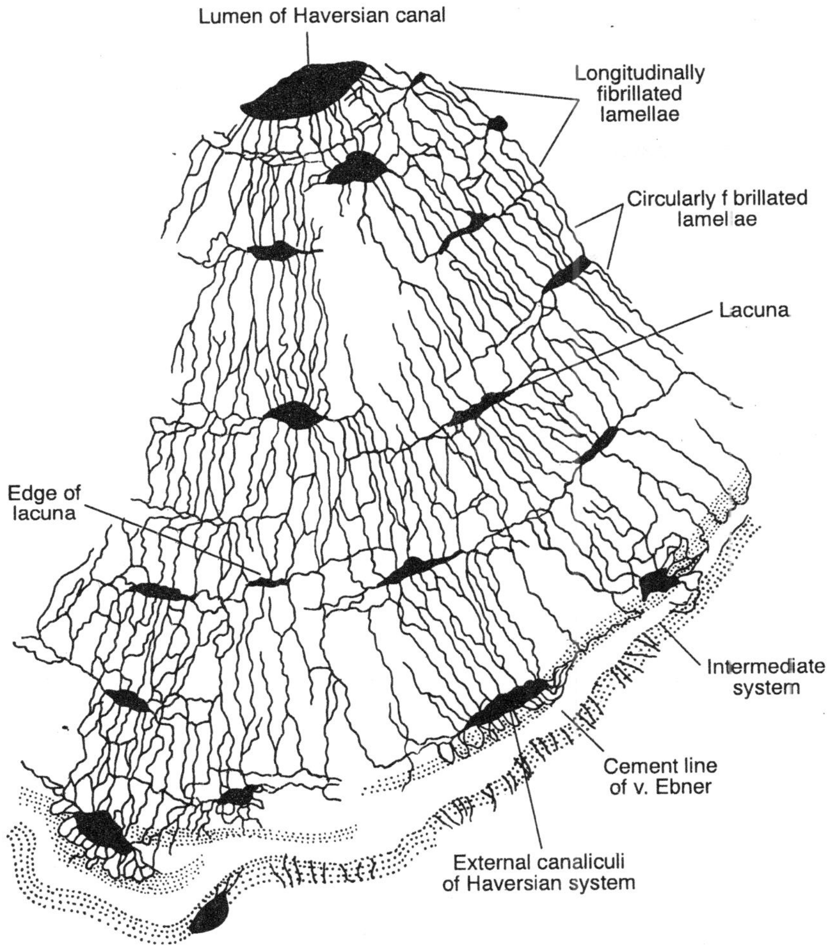

Fig 1(b).11: Sector of a cross section of a Haversian system of a macerated human h p bone. The cavities and canaliculi are filled with a dye: e, connection of canaliculi of the Haversian system with those of an intermediate system. X520. (After A. A. Maximow).

2. Spongy or cancellous bone : In this type of bone the calcification is less than the hard bone and so it is softer than compact bone. The deposition of calcium forms the lamellae which are irregularly arranged, but if trabeculae are relatively thin and are usually not penetrated by blood vessels. Therefore, there are usually no Haversian systems but merely a mosaic of angular pieces of lamellar bone. The minute spaces between the lamellae are known as lacunae from which canaliculi are developed. The osteoblasts are placed inside the lacunae. The bone cells are nourished by diffusion from the endosteal surface via the minute canaliculi that interconnect lacunae and extend to the surface. Moreover, the minute bony partitions give rise to many small spaces which are lined by endosteum and filled with red marrow. For this reason this kind of bone becomes spongy. Red marrow of spongy bones contains a certain amount of adipose tissue and mostly blood forming tissue.

Spongy bone is distributed to the inner parts of the flat bones, round ends of the long bones, the body of vertebrae, etc.

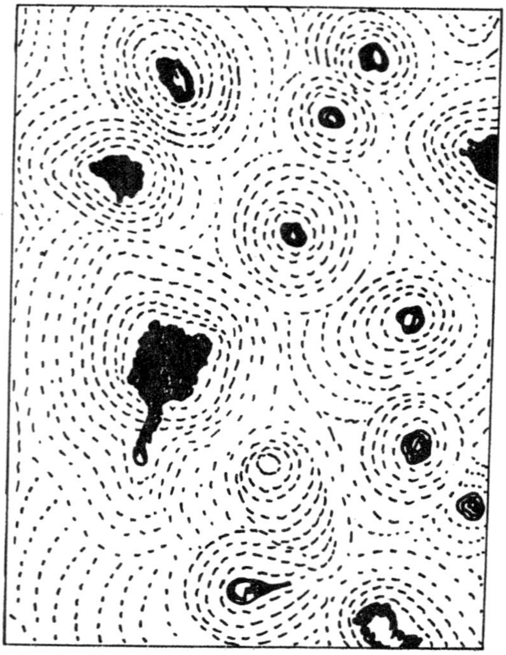

Fig 1(b).12: Ground section of bone from the midshaft of the human fibula photographed through the ordinary bright field microscope. The lacunae, the Haversian systems and interstitial lamellae are clearly shown.

Cell types in Osteogenesis : In actively growing bones four types of osteogenic cells are distinguishable : osteoprogenitor cells, osteoblasts, osteocytes and osteoclasts. Although they are usually described as distinct cell types, there is clear evidence of transformation from one to the other and it is evidently more reasonable to regard them as various functional states of the same cell type.

Osteoprogenitor cells : Like other connective tissues, bone originates from embryonic mesenchyme. In regions of the embryonic mesenchymal compartment where bone formation is beginning and in areas near the surfaces of growing bones, one finds irregularly shaped and somewhat elongated cells, which have pale staining, oval or elongated nuclei and inconspicuous acidophilic or faintly basophilic cytoplasm. They differ structurally only slightly from the mesenchymal cells from which they have arisen. The osteoprogenitor cells are active during the normal growth of bones and may be activated in adult life during integral reorganization of bone or in the healing of fractures and repair of other forms of injury. Under any of these conditions, the progenitor cells undergo division by mitosis and transform into the bone forming cells, osteoblasts, or coalesce to give rise to the bone destroying cells, osteoclasts. After multiplication of the progenitor cells, some of them change into osteoblasts, which change later into osteocytes. It seems established

Distinguish between compact bone and spongy bone

Subject	Compact bone	Spongy bone
(i) Kind of bone	(i) This kind of bone is very hard having lamellated with Haversian system.	(i) This type of bone is lamelllated without any Haversian system.
(ii) Nature of calcification	(ii) Here calcification is dense.	(ii) In spongy bone the calcification is less than the compact bone and so it is softer.
(iii) Presence of partition	(iii) Compact bone is devoid of minute partitions.	(iii) Spongy bone is provided with many minute partitions.
(iv) Occurrance	(iv) Shaft or body of the long bones such as humerus and femur, etc., are compact in nature.	(iv) Distributed to the inner parts of the flat bones, round ends of the long bones, the body of the vertebrae, etc.

Distinguish between Red bone marrow and Yellow bone marrow

Subject	Red bone marrow	Yellow bone marrow
(i) Position	Red bone marrow is found in spongy bone.	Yellow bone marrow is noticed in marrow cavity of long bones.
(ii) Composition	It contains a certain amount of adipose tissue.	It also contains more adipose tissue than that of Red bone marrow.
(iii) Function	It is provided with mostly blood forming tissue.	It has no blood forming function.

Distinguish between Osteocyte and Chondrocyte

Subject	Osteocyte	Chondrocyte
(i) Type	Bone cell	Cartilase cell
(ii) Position	Osteocyte is housed within the lacuna of bone ground substance.	Chondrocyte is located within the capsule of cartilage matrix.
(iii) Cytoplasmic process	The cytoplasmmic processes enter into canaliculi.	No cytoplasmic processes are noticed and rather they are large and rounded.
	Osteocytes are solitary.	Generally they remain in groups of 2-4 in a capsule.
(iv) Example	They remain in fully developed bone.	They are present in articular cartilage and epiphyseal cartilage.

that osteocytes can also change back to osteogenic cells in response to altered conditions in the environment.

Osteoblasts : These cells originate from mesenchyma cells of embryo. Osteoblasts are generally larger than the osteoprogenitor cells and they have a more rounded nucleus, a more prominent nucleolus and cytoplasm which is densely basophilic. The nucleus is often toward one side of the cell and the cells are clearly polarized toward the underlying bone, with a well-developed Golgi apparatus situated between the nucleus and the cell base. The mitochondria are elongated and fairly numerous. The cells have microvillous processes during early development and some of these elongate and remain as protoplasmic processes within the canaliculi as the matrix increases in amount. Small lipid droplets and membrane limited dense bodies interpreted as lysosomes are also encountered occassionally. In early part of bone development the osteoblasts help in the deposition of calcium salt in the bone matrix.

Osteocytes : The principal cells of fully formed bone are the osteocytes, which reside in the lacunae within the calcified matrix or intercellular substance. The cell body is flattened and is irregular in outline with cytoplasmic processes. It has been pointed out that they arise from osteoblasts by modulation. The nuclear and cytoplasmic characteristics at the light microscopic level are similar to those of osteoblasts except that the Golgi region is less conspicuous and the cytoplasm exhibits less affinity for basic dyes. In electron micrographs of osteocytes that have only recently been incorporated into bone, the Golgi apparatus is still rather large and the endoplasmic reticulum is quite extensive.

Mature osteoblasts give rise to adult cells as osteocytes. Osteocytes are helping in the exchange of materials from the blood.

Osteoclasts : These are multinucleated giant cells. They are frequently formed in shallow concavities in the surface of bone, called **Howship's lacunae.** The number of nuclei in osteoclasts varies greatly. The cytoplasm has a vacuolated appearance and gives a variable staining reaction. Electron micrographs show a paucity of granular endoplasmic reticulum but reveal clusters of free ribosomes. The mitochondria are relatively short and they are most numerous in the cytoplasm. There are multiple paired centrioles corresponding to the number of nuclei and also numerous Golgi complexes. Vacuoles of different sizes are abundant, as are lysosomes, which often have granules. The cytoplasm is faintly basophilic and granular.

The osteoclasts secrete proteolytic enzyme and digest collagen protein portion of bone [Fig 1(b).13].

Osteocytes—Adult bone cells.

Haversian system—Haversian canal and its lamellae.

Spongy bones—Bones without Haversian system.

Periosteum—Outer covering of bone.

Volkmann's canal—Tangential canal joining Haversian canals.

Endosteum—Membrane covering marrow cavity.

Chondrin—Matrix of cartilage containing gelatin, chondromucoproteins and other albuminous substances.

Perichondrium—Tough layer of dense fibrous connective tissue capsule and it encloses the hyaline cartilage except the articular cartilage.

Interstitial substance or bone matrix : The interstitial substance is composed of two major components, an organic matrix and an inorganic salts. The organic fraction consists

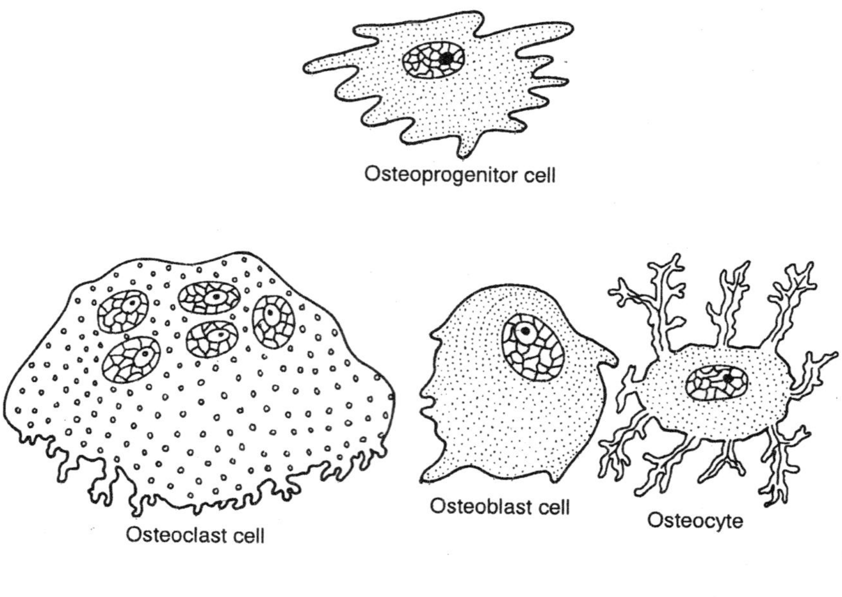

Fig 1(b).13: Different Types of bone cells—oesteoblast, osteocyte and oesteoclast.

Distinguish between Cartilage and bone

Characters	Cartilage	Bone
(i) Type	Cartilage is an elastic supporting tissue.	Bone is a kind of rigid supporting tissue.
(ii) Conversion	Cartilage is converted to bone.	Bone is not converted to cartilage.
(iii) Ground substance or Matrix	Matrix is entirely organic.	Matrix is both organic and inorganic types.
(iv) Fibres	White and yellow fibres are noticed.	Only white collagenous fibres are present.
(v) Cytoplasmic processes	Cells are without any cytoplasmic processes.	Cells are with cytoplasmic processes.
(vi) Lacuna	A group of cells are found in a lacuna.	Single cell is present in the lacuna.
(vii) Lamella	In cartilage lamella is absent.	Lamella is present in bone.
(viii) Haversian system	Absent.	Present.
(ix) Marrow	Absent.	Present.
(x) Volkmann's canal	Absent.	Present.
(xi) Blood vessels	Absent.	Present.
(xii) Covering	Perichondrium is found except white fibrocartilage.	Both periosteum and endosteum are noticed.

of collagenous fibers embedded in an amorphous ground substance. In adult mammals, about 95 per cent of the organic matrix is collagen. The matrix is acidophilic in stained section and this is due to the high content of collagen and low content of chondroitin sulfate in bone.

The inorganic component of bone is responsible for its rigidity and this inorganic matter comprises of sub-microscopic deposits of a form of calcium phosphate, very similar, but not identical to the mineral hydroxyapatite ($Ca_{10}[PO_4]_6[OH]_2$). In its final phase the calcium phosphate is found as thin plates or slender rod like crystals of 15 to 30 Å in thickness. Bone mineral contains significant amounts of the citrate ion, $C_6H_5O_7^{\equiv}$, and the carbonate ion, $CO_3^{=}$.

Thus, it is clear that the hardness of bone depends upon its inorganic constituents, while its great toughness and resilience reside in its organic substances, particularly the collagen.

Osteocalcin is a noncollagenous protein found in home and dentin. It is secreted by osteoblasts and thought to play a role in mineralization and calcium ion homeostasis. It has been stipulated that osteocalcin may also function as a negative regulator of bone formation, although its role is unknown.

In August 2007, it was reported that osteocalcin acts as a hormone in the body, causing beta cells in the pancreas to release more insulin, and at the same time directing rat cells to release the hormone adiponectin, which increases sensitivity to insulin.

C. Vascular tissue or Fluid tissue :

The connective tissue in which the interstitial fluid substance is non-fibrous and fluid in consistency is termed fluid tissue, i.e., the liquid material which flows in the body is called vascular or tissue fluid. Blood, tissue fluid and lymph are included under fluid tissue which transport various substances throughout the body of the higher animals. So they are regarded as the vascular tissue.

(a) **Blood** : Blood may be defined as opaque, slightly alkaline and highly specialized liquid connective tissue, which perform various functions.

Blood remains as a liquid condition, so it is regarded as a **fluid connective tissue** but it differs from a typical connective tissue in two important respects—its matrix is a fluid, i.e., plasma and the cellular part is represented by the corpuscles. Due to its fluid nature blood is known as liquid tissue. Various kinds of substances are transported by blood from one place to another, so blood is also known as a **vascular tissue.** Blood by its circulation connects different parts of the body and considerable amount of plasma is considered as the intercellular substance. Hence, blood is regarded as **Connective tissue.** Blood is composed of a liquid, the **plasma,** in which specialised cells, the **corpuscles** (red and white) and **platelets** are suspended.

In all other vertebrate animals, with the exception of *Branchiostoma* and *Leptocephalus*, blood becomes red in colour due to presence of **haemoglobin** which remains in red blood corpuscles (RBC). About 5 litres of blood are flowing in a healthy man. The normal pH of human blood is 7.4 which is slightly alkaline. Though in some of the higher invertebrates the blood becomes red as in earthworm (haemoglobin present in plasma) but in some cases the blood is colourless owing to the presence of a **haemocyanin** pigment in plasma as in prawn.

Composition : The blood consists of two parts, such as **plasma** and **corpuscles.** The yellowish fluid part, the plasma, which constitutes approximately 55% of the blood volume in which are suspended the **formed elements**. The formed elements are blood cells or corpuscles and platelets constitute approximately 45% of the blood volume.

Plasma : It may be defined as a fluid part of the blood without any corpuscles. The blood plasma is a light straw coloured alkaline liquid. In plasma 91-92% is water and the remaining 8-9% consists of solid materials. The solid part of plasma comprises of a mixture of inorganic and organic substances. The inorganic substances are sodium chloride, sodium bicarbonate, potassium, calcium, etc. The important organic substances are protein, glucose, fat, etc. The protein part of the plasma constitutes 7% of the chief solid constituents which are albumin, globulin, fibrinogen and prothrombin. The other non-protein nitrogenous substances are urea, uric acid, creatinine, etc. In addition

Distinguish between plasma and serum

Plasma	Serum
(i) Plasma is yellow coloured fluid part of the blood.	(i) Serum is the pale straw coloured fluid of the plasma.
(ii) In plasma different blood cells remain suspended.	(ii) Serum is devoid of cells.
(iii) It contains four types of proteins—albumin, globulin, fibrinogen and prothrombin.	(iii) It is provided with only two types of proteins only, i.e., albumin and globulin.

to this other organic substances such as bilirubin (pigment), hormones, enzymes, cholesterol, etc are present in the plasma. In some of the invertebrates such as in earthworm the plasma consists of iron containing respiratory pigment, **haemoglobin** and in prawn-like animal the respiratory pigment is copper containing pigment, the **haemocyanin.** When blood clots, the fibrinogen in the plasma forms fibrin, and the yellowish fluid part, the serum from the plasma comes out through the wound.

Functions of blood plasma :

(i) Plasma assists to transport various substances (glucose, aminoacid, lipid, urea, uric acid, CO_2, O_2, etc.).

(ii) It acts as medium for the protection of blood corpuscles.

(iii) Plasma maintains the acid-base balance of the blood.

(iv) Serum albumin and serum globulin; the proteins of plasma maintain colloidal osmotic pressure and viscosity of blood.

(v) Fibrinogen and prothrombin; other two types of proteins, help in blood clotting.

(vi) Plasma acts as a vehicle for hormones, enzymes, etc.

(vii) Plasma is acting as a protein reserve for the tissue.

Blood corpuscles : Blood cells or corpuscles are microscopic wandering cells present within the plasma. In vertebrate animals including the human being the blood corpuscles are of **three kinds** such as red blood corpuscle or erythrocyte, white blood corpuscle or leucocyte and platelet. These three kinds of blood corpuscles are collectively known as **"formed elements"** of blood. These cell types are originated from the bone marrow and they remain alive for a short period. In mammalian blood thrombocytes are absent; instead some non-nucleated cell fragments, called platelets are found. In case of invertebrates, only one type of blood corpuscle is noticed; i.e., the amoebocytes. These are phagocytic in nature [Fig 1(b).14].

1. **Erythrocyte or Red Blood Corpuscle :** They are found in large numbers and are

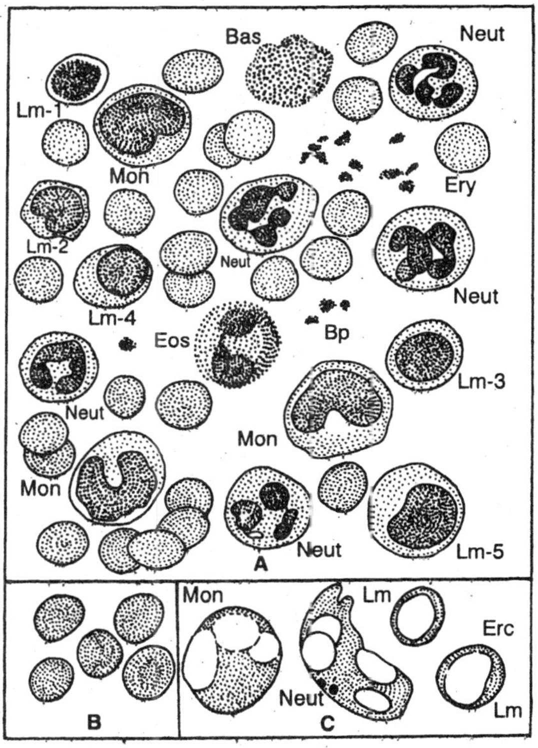

Fig 1(b).14: A. Cells from normal human blood. Wright's stain. *Bas*, basophilic leukocyte; *Bp*, aggregations of blood platelets; *Eos*, eosinophilic leukocyte. *Erc*, erythrocytes; *Lm*-1 to 5, lymphocytes; 1 to 3 are small and medium sizes and 4 and 5 are the less numerous larger forms. *Mon*, monocytes; *Neut*, neutrophilic leukocytes. B. Reticulocytes from normal human blood stained with dilute cresyl blue. C. Blood cells as seen after about 20 min of staining with neutral red and Janus green B in a supravital preparation. *Erc*, Erythrocyte; *Lm* small lymphocytes with bluish green mitochondria and a few neutral red granules; *Mon*, monocyte with mitochondria and numerous neutal red granules and vacuoles of varying size; *Neut*, neutrophilic leukocytes with staining of the neutrophilic granules and the formation of a few large vacuoles, which frequently appear after 15 to 20 min of staining.

responsible for the red colour of the blood. The RBC of vertebrates, such as birds, reptiles, camels, amphibians and fishes are oval, biconvex and nucleated. The mature human R.B.C. is a circular, biconcave, non-nucleated disc. The edges are rounded and thicker than the centre. Thus, when viewed from the side, it looks like a dumb-bell. The average diamater of RBC in man is 7.2 μm (micron) and average thickness at the rim is 2 μm. Due to biconcave nature the centre of the RBC is thinner than rim. But in all other verte-

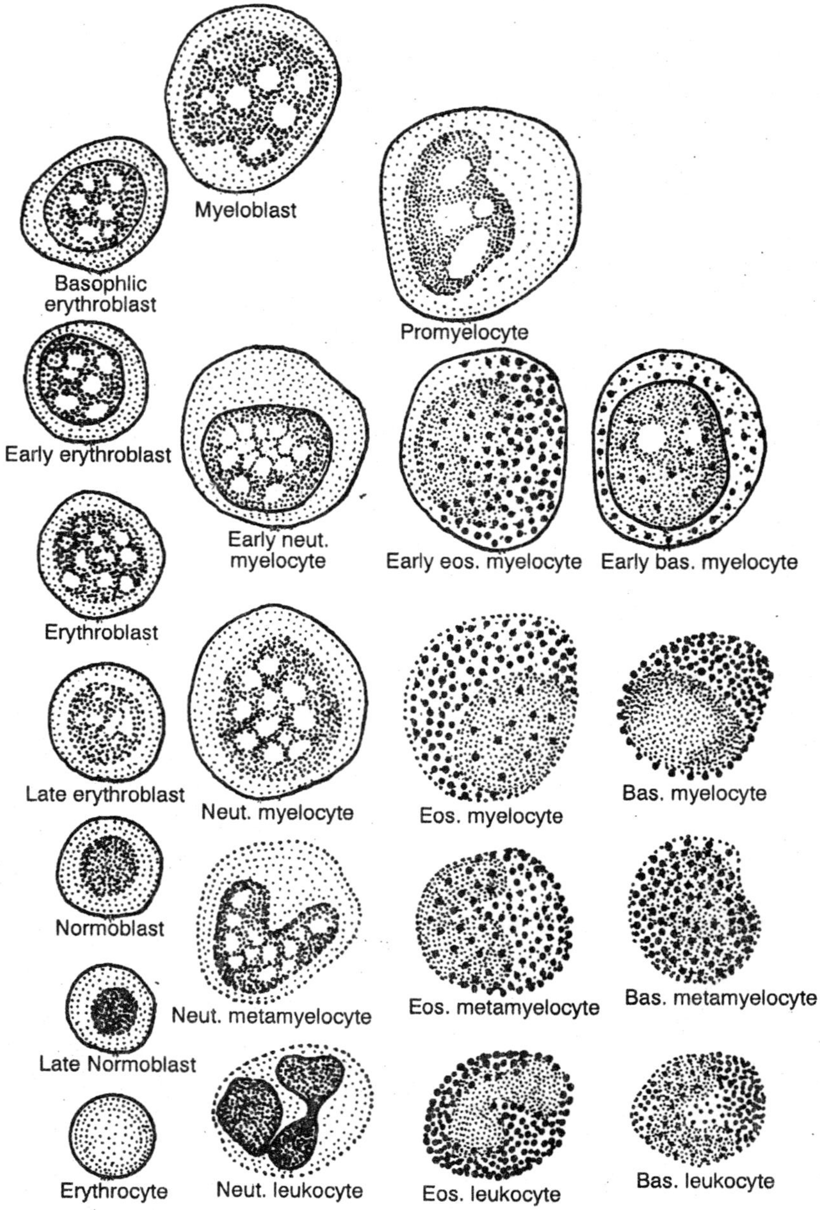

Fig 1(b).15: Various stages in blood development as seen in *dried smears* of marrow from a human rib. Wright's stain. X1560.

Differences between haemoglobin and haemocyanin

Haemoglobin	Haemocyanin
(i) Haemoglobin is a conjugated chromoprotein pigment.	(i) Haemocyanin is a blue coloured copper porphyrin pigment.
(ii) It is an iron containing pigment.	(ii) It is a copper containing pigment.
(iii) This pigment gives red colour with oxygen.	(iii) This pigment gives bluish colouration with oxygen.
(iv) This pigment is found both in plasma (earthworm) and RBC of vertebrates.	(iv) This pigment is found only in invertebrate's blood (prawn) and it is dissolved in plasma.

Differences between haemoglobin and myoglobin

Haemoglobin	Myoglobin
(i) Haemoglobin is a respiratory pigment in RBC of vertebrate's blood and in plasma of invertebrate's (earthworm) blood.	(i) Myoglobin is a respiratory pigment in muscle cell.
(ii) It carries oxygen as oxyhaemoglobin and carbon di-oxide as carbamino-haemoglobin.	(ii) Myoglobin stores oxygen in the muscle and supplies oxygen during contraction of muscle.

brates like fishes, amphibians, reptiles and birds the average diameter of erythrocytes is larger than the mammalian erythrocytes. In mammals the smallest RBCs are found in the deer tribe and the largest in the elephants. When first formed the RBCs of mammals have a nucleus, but as they mature, the nucleus is squeezed out of the cells and its position is occupied by the respiratory pigment, the haemoglobin. In the human erythrocytes mitochondria are absent. In all vertebrate animals, haemoglobin-like respiratory pigment is present in the cytoplasm of RBC. The haemoglobin contains protein which is globin in nature and haematin-like metallic pigment. This pigment contains iron. The average adult person contains 14.5 gm haemoglobin per 100 ml of blood. Each gram carries 1.34 ml oxygen. This haemoglobin has a great affinity for oxygen, and thus, helps in the carriage of oxygen and carbon dioxide. Each RBC is bounded by a thin, elastic colourless envelope of lipid and protein. The RBCs membrane comprises of inner and outer layers of protein (glycoprotein) and middle layer of lipid (lecithin, cephaline, etc). Erythrocytes, in mammals, are incomplete cells, as they lack nuclei, Golgi-network, E. R., mitochondria, RNA, centrioles and the metabolic machinery to synthesize new proteins. Thus, they can neither reproduce themselves nor maintain their normal structure for any length of time.

Number of the RBC are more numerous in comparison to other kinds of blood cells. There are about 5 million erythrocytes in a cubic millimetre of blood in a normal adult man. In female the number is slightly less, about 4.5 million per cubic millimetre of blood. The **average life span** of an erythro-

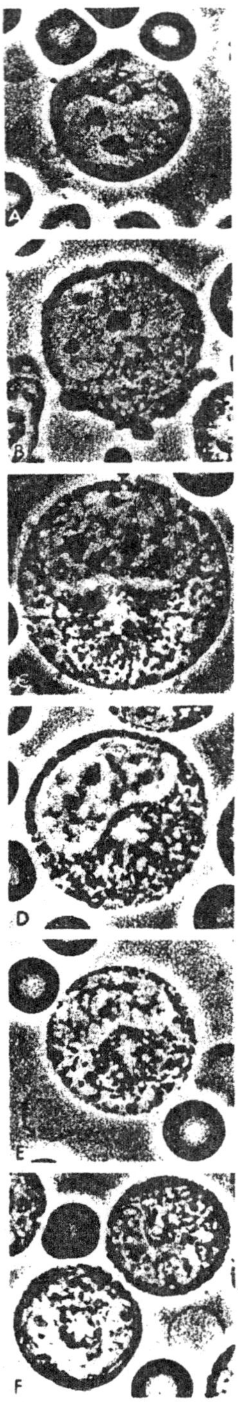

Fig 1(b).16: Phase contrast photomicrographs of promyelocytes (A, B), neutrophilic myelocytes (C, D, E) and metamyelocytes (F) from human bone marrow (Photographs from A. Ackerman, Zeitorschr f. Zeitorsch. 121, 153, 1972.

cyte is about 120 days in case of a man. They are usually destroyed in the liver, spleen, lymph-nodes, etc. by the reticulo-endothelial cells.

Functions :

(i) The main function of the RBC is to carry oxygen from lungs to form oxy-haemoglobin and supplies oxygen to the tissues; in addition, they also assist in carrying of carbon di-oxide as carbonic acid.

(ii) Erythrocyte is responsible for maintaining acid-base equilibrium of blood.

(iii) It regulates the viscosity of blood.

Formation (origin) of RBC : The process by means of which the red blood cells are formed, is called erythropoiesis. From birth till death of a vertebrate animal the erythrocytes are developed from the **haemocytoblast** of the **red marrow of bones**. After maturation, the RBC comes out from the bone marrow into the circulating blood. The erythrocytes pass through several stages of development in the red bone marrow before reaching maturity. When mature they pass from the red bone marrow into the circulating blood where they survive for 120 days. The process of RBC formation is controlled by a circulating hormone, the erythropoietin which is synthesized within the plasma probably with the help of the hormone, **erythrogenin.** This hormone is secreted by kidneys in relation to need. The formation as well as the development of a mature erythrocyte takes about a week during which the endothelial cells enlarge, divide, form haemoglobin and finally loses its nucleus. This process is known as **maturation** and it does not occur properly unless several chemical factors are noticed. The stepwise development of erythrocytes to maturity is as follows [Fig 1(b).15, 16] :

Haemocytoblast or stem cell (Endothelial cell, a big cell with a large nucleus, 18-23 μm in diameter)

↓ Proliferate by mitotic division

Proerythroblast (15-20 μm in diameter, with medium nucleus but no haemoglobin)

↓ Multiply by mitotic division

Early normoblast or erythroblast (Smaller in size, 11-17 μm in diameter, with small nucleus but no haemoglobin)

↓ Actively divides by mitotic division

Intermediate normoblast or late erythroblast (Smaller in size, 10-14 μm in diameter, very small nucleus, haemoglobin appears)

↓

Late normoblast (Size still smaller, 10-14 μm in diameter, nucleus is minute and dense, haemoglobin increases)

↓ Disappearance of the nucleus is noticed and passes into this stage

Reticulocyte (Smaller cells show a net-like structure in the cytoplasm, 7-8 μm in diameter, nucleus absent, haemoglobin increases)

↓ After maturation

Normal erythrocyte (7.2 μm in diameter, no nucleus but full of haemoglobin)

It takes about 7 days time to pass from the stage of proerythroblast (megaloblast) to that of reticulocyte, and two more days from reticulocyte to mature erythrocyte.

2. **Leucocytes or white blood corpuscles :** Amoeboid or irregular shaped blood corpuscles, having single or lobed nucleus but without any pigment, are known as white blood corpuscles. These are much less numerous than the red cells, the ratio between the two types being approximately 1 : 700. There are generally 5000 to 9000 white blood cells in a cubic millimetre of blood in the human adults, usually the WBC are circular in outward appearance but they show an amoeboid movement during ingestion of bacteria and other germs. The cytoplasm of WBC is colourless but the cell is nucleated. The WBCs are about 8 μm to 25 μm in diameter. They have their origin in the bone marrow, spleen and lymph node.

Types of WBC : On the basis of structure the leucocytes are classified into two categories—**Granulocytes** and **Agranulocytes.**

Granulocytes : The leucocytes which contain cytoplasmic granules and lobed nucleus with fine chromatin granules are called **granulocytes** or **polymorphonuclears.** The granulocytes are distinguished into three groups on the basis of characteristic features of cytoplasmic granules, such as **neutrophil, eosinophil** and **basophil.**

(i) **Neutrophil :** These constitute about 70% of the total WBC in the blood. In this type of cells the nucleus contains 2-7 lobes. But 3-lobed nucleus of neutrophil is the most common. The cytoplasm of this group consists of fine granules which are stained by neutral dye, because the cytoplasm is filled up with fine uniformly distributed granules which do not show any affinity to either acid or basic dyes and hence, the name neutrophil. Each neutrophil is about 10-12 μm in diameter. The cells are amoeboid and show phagocytosis.

They remain alive for 10 to 14 days. After that they disintegrate or are destroyed by reticulo-endothelial cells of liver and spleen.

Function : The neutrophils are responsible for providing the body with defence against invading micro-organisms.

(ii) **Eosinophil :** Eosinophils are granular leucocytes containing acidophilic granules in the cytoplasm. The diameter of the cell varies from 10-12 μm. These constitute only about 2% of the total WBC content in the blood. The nucleus of each eosinophil is 2 to 3 lobed. The cells show amoeboid movement and phagocytic power. The cells contain histamine.

The life span is about 8-10 days.

Distinguish between T-lymphocyte and B-lymphocyte

Characters	T-lymphocyte	B-lymphocyte
(i) Formation	A group of cells originate from precursor cells, migrate to thymus gland.	B-lymphocytes after coming out from the bone marrow enter into the lymph nodes.
(ii) Surface	Surface view of T-lymphocyte is smooth.	Surface view of B-lymphocyte is provided with microvilli.
(iii) Rosette formation	Rosette formation occurs.	Does not form rosette.
(iv) Mitotic division	Divides by the process of mitotis.	Mitosis does not take place.
(v) Effect on cancerous cell	Destroys cancerous cells.	Does not destroy cancerous cell.
(vi) Function	Cell mediated immunity	Blood mediated immunity.

Differences between RBC and WBC

Characters	RBC	WBC
1. Cell structure	Round, biconcave, disc shaped.	Usually the WBC are circular in outward appearance, but they show amoeboid movement during phagocytosis.
2. Size	Smaller.	Bigger.
3. Nucleus	Non-nucleated in mammalian RBC but nucleus is present in other vertebrate's blood.	Nucleus is present but nucleus is lobed in many cases.
4. Haemoglobin	Present.	Absent.
5. Number of cells	4-5 million per cubic mm.	6-8 thousand per cubic mm.
6. Type	One type.	Five types
7. Life span	120 days.	3-12 days.
8. Function	The primary function is to carry O_2 and CO_2.	The primary function is to defend the body from infection.

Differences between lymphocyte and thrombocyte

Characters	Lymphocyte	Thrombocyte
1. Kind of cell	Lymphocyte is a variety of WBC.	Thrombocyte is not a variety of WBC.
2. Nucleus	It is a nucleated cell.	It is non-nucleated blood cell.
3. Function	Lymphocyte is concerned with production of antibody and thus, acts as a body defence.	It is concerned with production of thromboplastin and thus, assists in blood coagulation.

Function : Though these are amoeboid in nature but not phagocytic in function. The eosinophil release histamine and prevent infection.

(iii) **Basophil :** The Basophil is identical to the group of connective tissue cells, known as mast cells, that is why they are also called circulating **mast cells.** Different sizes of purple blue granules are present in the cytoplasm. The nucleus is kidney-shaped or slightly lobulated. The size of these cells ranges from 8-10 μm and they constitute only 1% of the total WBC content. The basophils contain heparin and histamine. The life span is about 12-15 days.

Function : The Basophil releases a chemical substance, called heparin, which prevents the clotting of blood in the blood vessel. They are also supposed to release histamine which causes tissue damage and allergy.

Agranulocytes : The white blood cells which contain no granules and the nucleus without any lobes are called agranulocytes. Agranulocytes are of two types, viz., **lymphocytes** and **monocytes.**

(i) **Lymphocytes :** They are non-granular white blood cells. The single nucleus is never lobed and is either rounded or kidney-shaped. These leucocytes are derived from the lymphoblast of lymphoid tissue. They are 25 to 30% of the leucocyte. Lymphocytes may be small or large. **Small lymphocytes** are about 7.5 μm in diameter. The nucleus of it is large and it almost occupies the entire cell leaving only a thin peripheral cytoplasm. **Large lymphocytes** are about 12 μm in diameter and they contain round, oval or kidney-shaped nucleus and proportionally more cytoplasm.

Types of lymphocyte : There are four different kinds present in our body—**T-lymphocyte, B-lymphocyte, K-(Killer) and NK-(neutral killer) lymphocytes.**

T-lymphocyte : A group of cells after being released from red bone marrow, migrate to thymus gland and become T-cells (T-lymphocyte). These cells, after processing with thymosin hormone; take shelter in lymph node. T-lymphocytes offer specific resistance to virus, fungi, parasites, and bacteria.

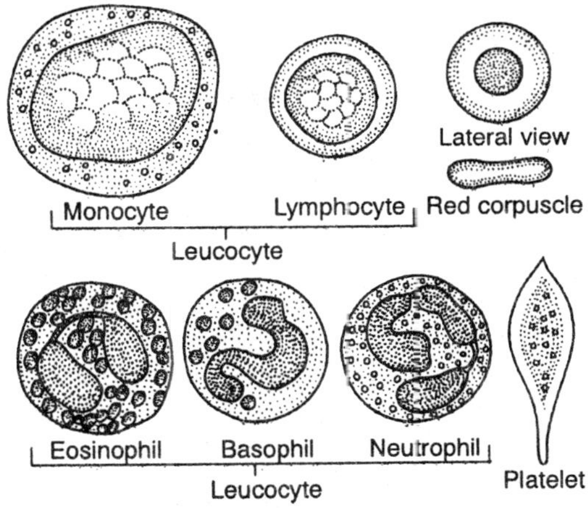

Fig 1(b).17: RBC and WBC in man.

B-lymphocytes : These are another group of lympbocytes. They do not enter the thymus gland after coming out of red bone marrow but enter into the mass of lymphoid tissues and come out into blood during infection.

B-lymphocytes are largely responsible for the development of specific immunity against foreign substances or antigen. When these cells are stimulated by an antigen they enlarge to become plasma cells and multiplly to form groups. They produce specific antibodies which act against the antigen.

Killer cells or K-lymphocytes : These lymphocytes after production from spleen or lymph nodes, migrate throughout the body and get attached to any cell carrying proper antigen. These cells inject lysosomal enzymes into the target cell. They release a factor that converts nearly non-sensitive T-lymphocytes into killer cells directed against the same antigen. They also secrete a substance that attracts macrophages and stimulates their phagocytic activity.

Neutral killer lymphocytes/NK-lymphocytes : They are produced from red bone marrow but they do not enter into lymph nodes for maturation. They destory virus infected cells and cancerous cells by secreting **interleukin.** NK cells kill antigen without prior preparation. These lymphocytes represent 5-10% of total lymphocytes.

(ii) **Monocyte :** They are the largest non-granular white blood cells with horse-shoe shaped nuclei and plenty cytoplasm. They are about 16 to 18 µm in diameter. They are 5 to 10% of the leucocytes. The cytoplasm is more abundant in relation to the nucleus and the nucleus is ovoid or kidney shaped. Moreover, characteristically the nucleus is always placed eccentrically in the leucocytes.

Function : Monocytes are actively motile and destroy the micro-organisms by the process of phagocytosis.

(iii) **Platelets or Thrombocytes :** The platelets are actually not cells but some round or oval non-nucleated fragments of large cells, called macrophages. They are very small, about 2.5 to 5 µm in diameter. There are nearly about 2,50,000 to 4,00,000 platelets per cubic mm of blood. The platelets originate from large megakaryocytes, which are found in the bone marrow. The life span is about 3 to 5 days.

Thrombocytes are small, spindle shaped and nucleated cells, found in non-mammalian blood. They are formed in the bone marrow and their life span is 2-3 days [Fig 1(b).17].

Function : Thrombocytes take part in blood coagulation.

(b) Tissue fluid : The fluid present in the intercellular space and not within vessel is called **tissue fluid.** The composition of this fluid is like the plasma except the protein content is low and a few white cells are noticed. There is a good number of lymphocytes and a small number of granulocytes but it does not contain platelets. The fluid is provided with more waste products. Its glucose and salt contents are similar to that of blood.

The tissue fluid is formed by the transcapillary exchange of components found

Distinguish between blood and lymph

Characters	Blood	Lymph
(i) Definition	Blood may be defined as a slighly alkaline and highly specialised liquid connective tissue.	Lymph may be defined as an alkaline modified tissue fluid.
(ii) Occurence	Blood flows within blood vessel.	Lymph flows within lymphatic vessel.
(iii) Types	In it erythrocyte, five types of WBC (neutrophil, eosinophil, basophil, lymphocyte and monocyte) and platelets or thrombocytes are present.	Mainly lymphocyte, somefimes monocytes, may be present.
(iv) Protein content	It contains more protein.	It contains less protein.
(v) Function	Blood takes part in nutrition, respiration, excretion, etc and in defence mechanism of the body by phagocytosis or by producing antibodies.	If supplies nutrition to the tissues and takes part in fat absorption and defence mechanism of the body.

in plasma and tissue spaces. During the process of formation plasma components move out at the arteriolar end and again tissue fluid components are absorbed in the venous end of the capillary. Exit of materials occurs through the processes like filtration, diffusion, micro-pinocytosis. Again, the entry of materials is occured by pressure dependent absorption.

Function :

(i) Tissue fluid serves as a reservoir of water and electrolytes for supply to cells.

(ii) It gives protection to various organs of the body.

(iii) Tissue fluid supplies nutrients and dispose of wastes.

(iv) It maintains the fluid balance of connective tissue.

(v) It assists to maintain the blood volume during dehydration process.

(vi) Again, tissue fluid replenishes the plasma constituents at the time of emergency.

(vii) Tissue fluid is not coagulated at all, because it does not contain fibrinogen and prothrombin.

(c) **Lymph : Lymph** may be defined as a clear or slightly opalescent alkaline fluid which is present within the lymphatic vessel. It is formed from the tissue fluid, so the lymph is regarded as a modified tissue fluid. Formation of lymph depends upon various physical factors, such as capillary pressure, permeability of the capillary wall, etc. Lymphatic tissue is present in a number of situations in the body in addition to the lymph nodes; such as the palentine tonsil, the pharyngeal tonsil, the solitary lymphatic follicle, Peyer's patches, the vermiform appendix, etc.

The lymph resembles in composition with that of the blood plasma with lower protein content. It contains 94% of water and nearly 6% of solid particles. The salts are similar to those of blood plasma. Lymph comprises of a large number of lymphocytes and monocytes and a few erythrocytes. The lymphocytes are produced in the lymph nodes and in other masses of lymphoid tissue. About 1-2 litres of lymph are present in human beings. The composition of lymph is—protein nitrogen 3.32%; non-protein nitrogen 34.80 mg/lit, urea 23.50 mg/lit, sugar 132.20% mg/lit, aminoacids 4.84 mg/lit, creatine 1.4 mg/lit, NaCl 771.00 mg/lit, phosphorus 11.80 mg/lit.

Function :

(i) Lymph acts as a conducting tissue and also functions as a defensive fluid.

(ii) Lymph of lymphatics takes part in the absorption of fat from the intestine.

(iii) It is an additional route for transport of materials of high molecular weight and fat particles.

(iv) Lymph nodes destroy bacteria and microbes.

(v) It returns back protein and hormones to the blood plasma.

Distinguish between epithelial and connective tissue

Characters	Epithelial tissue	Connective tissue
(i) Origin	Epithelial tissue generally develops from the embryonic ectoderm and endoderm layers.	It develops from the embryonic mesoderm layer.
(ii) Number of cells	Comparatively large number of cells are noticed.	In this tissue small number of cells are found.
(iii) Arrangement of cells	Here the cells are closely packed.	In this tissue cells are dispersed in the intercellular substance.
(iv) Amount of intercellular substance	Intercellular substance is scanty.	Amount of intercellular substance is plenty.
(v) Fibres	In epithelium fibres are absent.	In connective tissue fibres are generally found.
(vi) Basement membrane	This type of tissue is placed on basement membrane.	Connective tissue is devoid of basement membrane.
(vii) Blood vessels	The epithelial tissue is devoid of blood vessels	The connective tissue is provided with blood vessels.
(viii) Position	This kind of tissue is found on the outer covering of the body as well as inner covering of hollow organs.	This kind of tissue is found in the different organs.
(ix) Function	Acts as a protective tissue	Acts as a binding tissue in the different organ system.

1(C) MUSCULAR TISSUE

Physiological functions of body depends mainly on four basic tissue systems. Out of these four, muscle tissue plays pivotal role in animal movement like locomotion, eating, copulation, maintenance of posture, etc.

So, **the type of tissue which has the ability to contract and relax, as a result each and every organs are associated with the movement, is termed as muscular tissue.**

Origin of muscle tissue :

All muscles originate from mesoderm. Muscle cells lose capacity to divide, multiply and regenerate to a great extent. Study of muscle is called **myology.**

Characteristics of muscle tissue :

The muscle cells (fibres) are highly specialized elongated, slender and cylindrical or spindle shaped. They are highly contractile in nature. Muscle cells normally lose capacity to divide, multiply and regenerate to a great extent.

Muscle cells are like neurones, which get excited by chemicals or electrical impulses. Muscles have a contractile mechanism for which microfilaments and associated proteins are responsible. Some cell types generate motile forces. Those are—**myoepithelial cells, pericytes** and **myofibroblasts.**

Muscle cells differentiate by a gradual process of cell lengthening and simultaneous synthesis of myofibrillar proteins named as **actin** and **myosin.**

Classification of muscle tissue :

Muscular tissue can be classified under certain categories depending upon different parameters.

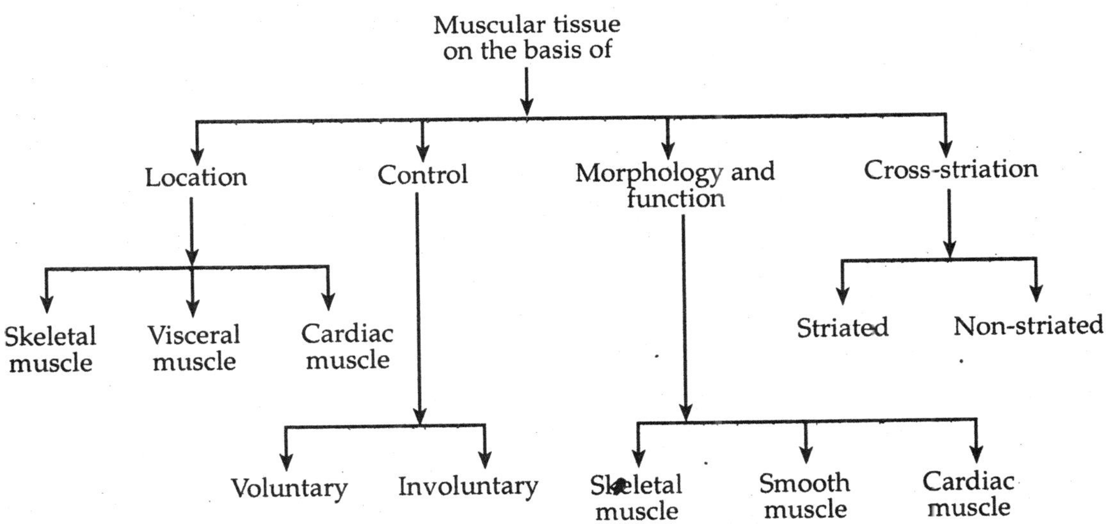

Skeletal muscle—It is a type of voluntary, striated muscle.
Smooth muscle—It is a type of involuntary, visceral, non-striated muscle.
Cardiac muscle—It is a type of involuntary, specialized, visceral, striated muscle.

I. Skeletal Muscle

These muscles are so named because they are mostly attached to bones or skeleton of the body and are involved with skeletal movements. Histologically, these muscles display a striated appearance owing to presence of cross striations; hence these are also termed **striated muscles**. Since these muscles are under voluntary control, they are also called **voluntary muscles.**

Properties of skeletal muscle :

When a muscle is activated, it either shortens or if it is attached to a rigid skeleton, it develops tension. Properties of a muscle can be investigated by attaching it to a movable lever that writes on a revolving drum **(Kymograph)**. Muscle or respective attached nerve can be stimulated by electric shocks. The nature of contraction and relaxation of muscle is exhibited by the **calf muscle** of frog **(Gastrocnemius)** on a drum by either single or repetitive shocks.

Structure of Skeletal muscle :

Attachment : A skeletal muscle is attached to a bone in at least two sites—a fixed non-movable part of the skeleton **(the origin)** and a movable part of the skeleton **(the insertion)**. It remains attached by tough, non-elastic collagen fibres called **tendons.** At one end tendon is continuous with the outer

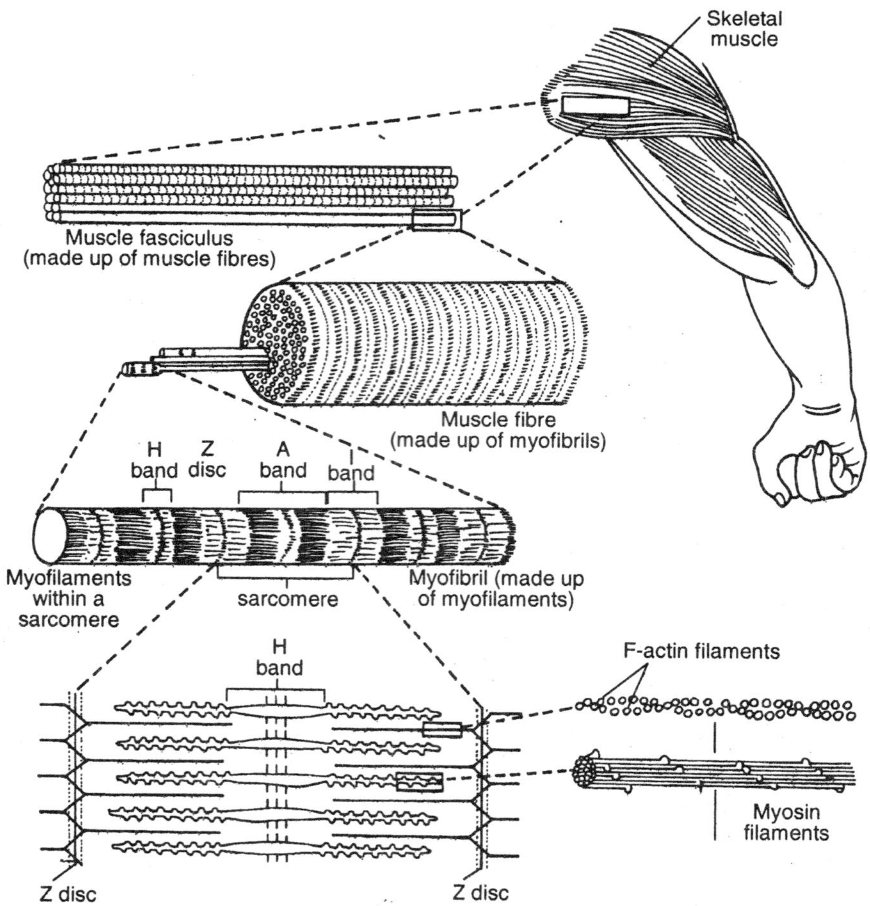

Fig 1(c).1: Organization of a skeletal or striated muscle.

covering of the muscle and the other end is attached to the outer layer of the bone, periostium.

Morphology : Skeletal muscle consists of muscle fibres, which are long, cylindrical multinucleated cells (syncytium) with diameters of 10-100 μm. Multinucleation results from the fusion of embryonic mesenchymal cells, called **myoblasts,** number of myoblasts fuse to form myotubes. Muscles are with muscle fibres, which is the structural unit of muscle. In terms, each fibre is made up of numerous parallel subunits termed myofibrils. Further, myofibrils consist of longitudinally repeated functional units, sarcomere (Gr. *sarcos,* flesh; *mer,* unit). Sarcomere represents the striations of skeletal muscle due to presence of *myosin* and *actin* protein. This also represents the unit of muscle contraction [Fig 1(c).1].

Organization : Different types of muscles are composed of bundles of fibres. Each muscle fibre (individual) is surrounded by a thin delicate connective tissue, called **endomysium.** It is composed of a basal lamina synthesized by multinucleated fibres, reticular fibres and fibroblasts.

A bundle of fibres are formed by the union of individual fibres (fascicle—L. fascicle, bundle) remain surrounded by **perimysium.** Number of such fascicles remain together and surrounded by external sheath of dense connective tissue is called **epimysium.** Finally muscles are regular bundles of muscle fibres within which thin septa of connective tissue extend inward.

Blood vessels penetrate the muscle within the connective tissue septa and form a rich capillary network in the endomysium. Lymphatic vessels and larger blood vessels are present in the outer connective tissue layer. Skeletal muscles remain attached with bones by tendons in through myotendinous junction [Fig 1(c).2].

- **Tetanus** : Tetanus is a property of skeletal muscles due to which when a muscle is repeatedly stimulated in quick succession, it attains a state of sustained contraction without intervening periods of relaxation. It occurs due to summation or overlapping of successive contractions so that the contraction caused by a stimulus begins before the completion of the previous contraction.

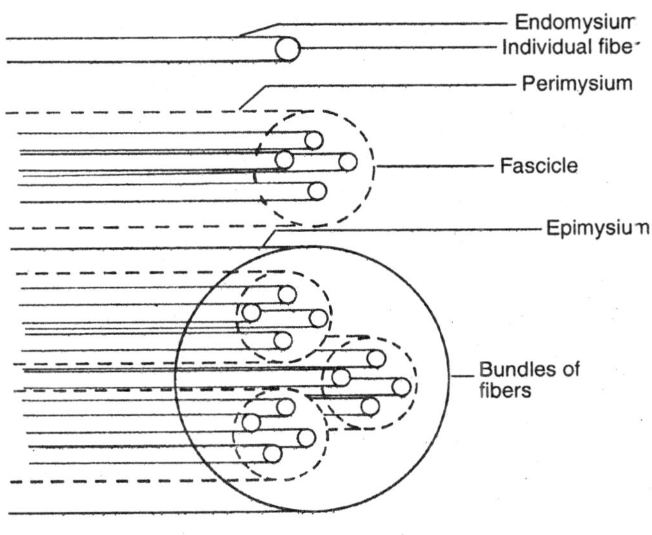

Fig 1(c).2: Organization of Skeletal muscle.

The cytoplasm of the muscle fibre is divisible into three parts—(a) sarcoplasm, (b) myofibril and (c) sarcotubular system.

(a) Sarcoplasm : It is the fluid part of cytoplasm of muscle cells similar to the cytoplasm of other cells, containing several mitochondria, small Golgi-bodies, endoplasmic reticulum, etc. The smooth endoplasmic reticulum of muscle cells is highly developed and is known as **sarcoplasmic reticulum.** Unlike the cytoplasm of other cells, the sarcoplasm of muscle cells stores glycogen and myoglobin (a haemoglobin-like pigment).

(b) Myofibril : In the sarcoplasm of muscle fibres, many special type of protein made fibrils remain arranged longitudinally and parallely. These are termed as myofibrils. The collection of myofibrils is called the **contractile system** of the muscle cell, because they are responsible for muscle contraction. Each myofibril shows the presence of alternate dark and light transverse bends along its length and it appears to be striated.

Electron microscopic structure of skeletal muscle shows striations. Striations are exhibited by the presence of two types of muscle proteins, called **myosin** (heavy protein) and **actin** (light protein).

Under electron microscope, internal structure of individual myofibrils shows straiations clearly which indicates the pattern of repetition of striations within a muscle fibre. One complete turn of striation is designated as unit structure, called one **sarcomere,** with alternate position of dark and light band, i.e., **'A' band** and **'I' band.** Two ends of one sarcomere is designated as **'Z' line** within the I Band [Ger. *Zwischenscheibe*, between disks]. In both sides of 'Z' line light band [I band] remain extended which is basically composed of only actin (light filament) protein [Fig 1(c).3].

Electron microscopic view after Haematoxylin and Eosin (H & E) preparation, further detailing of A band can be explained. At the centre of the A band a narrow dense line is present, called the **M-line.** [Ger, *mitte*, middle] The equal zone besides M-line in

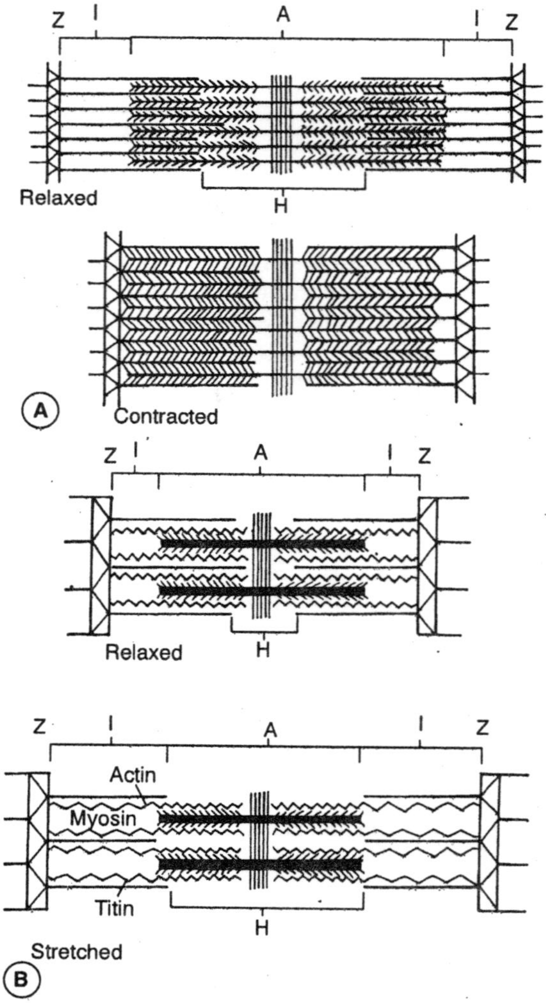

Fig 1(c).3: A. Relaxed and contracted sarcomere. In the relaxed state, interdigitation of actin and myosin filament, is not complete; the H and I bands are relatively wide. During contraction, the interdigitation of the actin and myosin filaments is increased according to degree of contraction. The length of the A band remains the same; the lengths of the H and I bands are diminished again in proportion to the degree of contraction. B. Titin, a large elastic molecule, anchors the thick myosin filaments to the Z disc.

both sides are with only myosin heavy protein, called **'H'-zone**. After H-zone, rest of the A band is occupied by the overlapping of both myosin and actin proteins. Actin protein extends further and form I band keeping 'Z' line in the middle. One 'Z' line to another 'Z' line exhibits the unit structure of one sarcomere, i.e., muscle.

(c) Sarcotubular system : The sarcoplasm of muscle cells possess a specially developed system of tubules, known as sarcotubular system. It is also designated as the conducting system of the muscle cells, because it assists in transmission of impulse all over the muscle cells. The sarcotubular system comprises of two kinds of tubules—**transverse tubules** and **longitudinal tubules.**

(i) **Transverse tubules :** The sarcolemma of muscle fibres invaginates transversely at intervals to form some tubular structures; these are termed as transverse tubules or in short **T-tubules.** In mammalian skeletal fibres, the T-tubules pass through the junction of A- and I-bands whereas in amphibian skeletal muscles, the T-tubules cross through the Z-lines.

(ii) **Longitudinal tubules :** The smooth endoplasmic reticulum of muscle cells are specially developed and modified into some tubules that remain arranged longitudinally between the adjacent T-tubules. These are called longitudinal tubules or in short **L-tubules.** The L-tubules expand to form a network at the centre of the sarcomere. Hence, they are collectively called **sarcoplasmic reticulum.** The peripheral ends of the L-tubules expand to form **terminal cisternae** that remain in contact with the T-tubules; however, there is no communication between the lumens of T- and L-tubules. The L-tubules store Ca^{++} which helps in **excitation-contraction coupling** in the muscle.

Muscular Dystrophy :

Dystrophin, is a rod-shaped cytoskeletal accessory protein with 427-KDa molecular weight. It has a short head and a long tail, end portion of the tail remains attached with **F-actin.** Absence of this particular protein leads towards the gradual muscular weakness, called Duchenne's muscular dystrophy. It is due to mutation of single gene which encodes proteins of the dystrophin-glycoprotein complex.

Treppe :

Treppe is a special phenomenon, called 'staircase' phenomenon, mostly found within the skeletal muscle. When a series of maximal stimuli is given to skeletal muscle at a frequency just below the tetanizing frequency, the tension developed during each twitch increases. After several contractions, a uniform tension per contraction is reached. This is called treppe or straircase phenomenon.

Clonus :

Clonus is incomplete tetanus, i.e., summation of successive contractions with intervening periods of incomplete relaxations. This occurs when the muscle is stimulated with repetitive stimuli of such frequency that each successive stimulus falls within the period of previous relaxation.

Rigor mortis :

This is the state of permanent rigidity of muscle after death due to complete depletion of ATP and phosphoryl creatine from muscle. During rigor mortis, myosin heads attach to actin in an abnormal, fixed and resistant way. Rigor mortis occurs 2-3 hours after death when all muscles of the body go into a state of contracting and become rigid without any stimulation (action potential). The contraction is caused by fall of ATP level in muscles owing to exhaustion of the pre-existing ATP molecules. Due to unavailability of ATP, Ca^{++} cannot be removed from sarcoplasm and thus, the cross-bridges between actin and myosin cannot be detached. As a result of this, the muscles fail to relax and remain in contracted state.

Myasthenia gravis :

Myasthenia gravis is an autoimmune disorder caused by extreme muscle weakness. In this disease, the number of functionally active acetylcholine receptors in the sarcolemma of the myoneural junction are blocked by the binding of circulating antibodies to the acetylcholine receptors in the junctional folds. Thus, the number of functional receptor sites are reduced, as a result gradual degradation of response of muscles occurs even after giving repeated nerve stimuli to it.

Skeletal muscle fibres
(Pattern of arrangement of muscle fibres in bundle)

- Parallel muscles
  - Triceps, Biceps
- Convergent muscles
  - Pectoralis muscles
- Pennate muscles
  - Rectus femoris
- Sphincter muscles
  - Sphincter

Types of skeletal muscle fibres :

Muscle fibres are of two types—**Type I** and **Type II.** Type I is red fibre and Type II is **white fibre.** Oxygen binding protein myoglobin remains in the type I fibre, so it appears as red, whereas myoglobin is absent in type II. Type I is with better endurance with slow rate of fatigue than type II fibre.

Mechanism of contraction and relaxation of skeletal muscle :

Muscles remain in two states—state of relaxation and state of contraction. Due to presence of heavy myosin and light actin protein, muscle shows contraction and relaxation phases which are primarily controlled by stimulation and nerve impulse. The gradual steps of contraction are :

1. An action potential originating in the central nervous system (CNS) reaches motor neuron, transmits an action potential to the axon.

2. The action potential propagates by activating voltage-gated sodium channels along the axon towards chemical synapse. The action potential reaches the motor neuron terminal and causes a calcium ion influx through the voltage-gated calcium channels.

3. The action potential is conducted along the whole length of the muscle fibre through T-tubule system, Z-lines and sarcoplasmic reticulum. The process by which depolarization of the muscle fibre initiates contraction is called *excitation contraction coupling*.

4. Release of calcium ions initiates the biochemical changes in muscle contraction. Action potential stimulates dystrophin protein which relays it to the calcium storage of the sarcoplasmic reticulum to release calcium ions.

5. In resting muscle troponin remains lightly bound to actin and tropomyosin covers the sites where myosin heads bind to actin. Thus, a troportin-tropomyosin complex constitutes a relaxing protein which inhibits the interaction between actin and myosin. During contraction, when the released calcium ions combind with troponin molecule, then troponin moves to the tropomyosin molecule deeper into the groove between the two actin strands, which uncovers the active sites of actin molecule to bind with the myosin head.

6. Calcium and magnesium ions act as cofactors for myosin ATP-ase present in the

Differences between three types of muscle fibres

Subject	Striated or skeletal or voluntary muscle fibres	Non-striated or smooth or visceral or involuntary muscle fibers	Cardiac muscle fibres
1. Location	Peripheral, in, proximal part of oesophagus, tongue.	Central, in hollow visceral organs.	Only in heart.
2. Shape	Long, cylindrical in appearance.	Fusiform in appearance.	Network of fibres.
3. Unit	Sarcomeres, long myofibrils placed end-to-end forming cylindrical myofibrils.	Fusiform cells with inconspicuous borders.	Oblique cross-connecting fibres make this muscle an interconnected bundle of myofibrils.
4. Nucleus	Many (syncytial) at periphery.	Single at the centre of each cell.	Many nuclei between successive end plates at central position.
5. Stripes	Dark A bands and light I bands present.	Not present	Present
6. Sarcolemma	Distinct	Absent	Absent
7. Blood supply	Rich	Poor	Rich
8. Contraction	Quick, fatigue fast	Slow, sustained contraction in heart	Rhythmic, contractions originate.
9. Intercalated discs	Absent	Absent	Absent
10. Attachment	With bones	To soft organs or viscera.	Not attached to other organs except major blood vessels which are isolated & covered by pericardium.
11. Action	Voluntary	Involuntary	Involuntary.

myosin heads. The myosin ATP-ase splits ATP into ADP and inorganic phosphate (Pi) to release the energy stored in it.

7. Now the released energy forms the actomyosin-complexes between cross bridges of thick myosin and active sites on thin actin filaments. During this interlinking, the heads are tilted, called power stroke. The energy also stimulates the rotation of heads of myosin filaments which in turn pulls the actin filaments inward. Actin filaments slide inward over the myosin filaments. This movement is supported by the **sliding filament theory,** proposed by A. F. Huxley and R. Neidergerke in 1954 and H. E. Huxley and J. Hanson in 1954.

8. According to this theory, during contraction, in each sarcomere the actin filaments surrounding the myosin filament approach toward the centre (i.e., H-band) of the myosin filament from either side. As a result of this, the adjacent Z-lines come

- Two kinds of mechanical changes are associated with muscle contraction; these are **isotonic** and **isometric muscle** contraction.

Isotonic muscle contraction	Isometric muscle contraction
1. A type of muscle contraction in which a muscle shortens in length but its tension does not rise appreciably.	1. A type of muscle contraction in which the tension of the muscle is raised but it does not shorten in length.
2. Tension is not increased considerably.	2. Tension is considerably increased.
3. During this contraction, tension is dependent on the load applied to the muscle and not on the strength of the stimulus.	3. Tension depends on the strength of the stimulus.
4. External work or movement of an organ takes place.	4. No external work or movement of an organ takes place.
5. Heat formation is less because some of the energy is utilized for mechanical work or shortening of the muscle.	5. Heat formation is greater because no energy is utilised for shortening of the muscle and the entire energy is converted to heat.
Examples : Movement of the limbs or any other part of the body, lifting of a weight, etc.	**Examples :** Suspending of a load by a hand, standing, attempt to lift or pull a heavy load, etc.

Differences between type I and type II fibres

Subject	Type I fibre	Type II fibre
1. Contraction time	Slow	Fast
2. Resistance to fatigue	High	Intermediate
3. Used for	Aerobic	Short term anaerobic
4. Size of motor neuron	Small	Large
5. Duration of work	More than an hour	Less than 5 minutes
6. Mitochondrial density	High	Medium
7. Oxidative capacity	High	Intermediate
8. Glycolytic activity	Low	High
9. Storage fuel	Triglycerides	Glycogen, creatine phosphate
10. Myosin heavy chain, human genes	MYH 7	MYH 1

closer and the sarcomere contracts and since the successive sarcomeres contract simultaneously, the whole myofibril as well as the muscle fibre contracts. The myosin filaments possess some hook-like heads that binds with some active sites of the actin filaments to form **cross-bridges.** The cross bridges are alternately broken and reformed very quickly in such a way that each head of myosin leaves one active site of actin and binds with the next site so that the actin filament is pulled towards the centre of the sarcomere.

9. Further rotation of myosin heads occurs due to hydrolysis of another ATP molecule so that actin filaments slide inward more and more and cause shortening of the myofibrils.

10. After maximum muscle contraction, sarcoplasmic reticulum begins to re-accumulate calcium from sarcoplasm by ATP-mediated active transport into the longitudinal portion of the reticulum. Dissociation of actomyosin complexes takes place due to inactivation of myosin ATP-ase enzyme and thin actin filaments swing back to their original position causing muscle-relaxation.

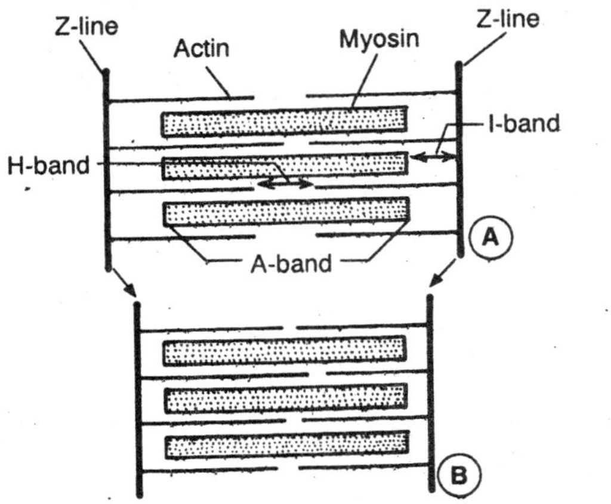

Fig 1(c).4: Contraction of a sarcomere : (A) Relaxed state, (B) Contracted state.

11. The Ca^{2+} then diffuses into the terminal cisterns, where it is stored until released by the next action-potential.

12. During relaxation, repolarization takes place, as a result, K^+ moves rapidly in the Extracellur fluid (ECF) and the sarcolemma becomes electro-positive outside and electro-negetive inside.

13. Original ionic balance is maintained by sodium-potassium pump by active transport.

Contraction : Excitation of motor nerve → Arrival of nerve impulse at the motor nerve terminal → Generation of impulse in the sarcolemma through neuro-muscular transmission and its conduction over the sarcolemma and T-tubules → Release Ca^{++} from sarcoplasmic reticulum → Combination of Ca^{++} with troponin → Displacement of tropomyosin → Exposure of active sites of actin → Formation of cross-bridges between actin and myosin → Activation of

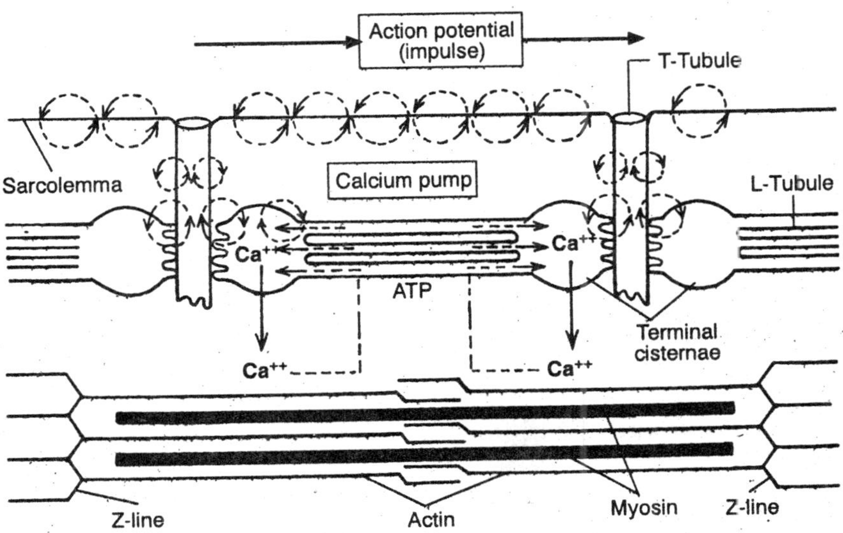

Fig 1(c).5: Role of sarcotubular system in muscle contraction.

myosin ATP-ase → Breakdown of ATP → Pulling of actin filaments towards the centre of myosin filaments → contraction of myofibril and the muscle [Fig 1(c).4, 5].

Relaxation : Cessation of excitation of motor nerve and neuro muscular transmission → Reuptake of Ca^{++} by the sarcoplasmic reticulum → Covering of active sites of actin by the joint action of tropomyosin and troponin and inactivation of myosin ATP- ase—Cessation of cross--bridge formation → Restoration of the original relaxed state.

> • **Changes in a muscle during contraction:** During contraction of muscle some changes are found in it. These are as follows : (i) The I-band is reduced. (ii) Although the A-band remains unchanged as a whole, the H-band present within the A-band is reduced and (iii) the adjacent Z-lines come closer.

II. Smooth muscle

Smooth muscles are called 'smooth' as because they lack the presence of characteristic striations of particular band pattern formed by actin and myosin filaments as unit of muscle, i.e., sarcomere.

Position of smooth muscle :

These are present in the walls of different visceral organs like alimentary canal, blood vessels, urinary bladder, ureters, genital ducts, etc. It is named as visceral non-striated muscles due to their position. Visceral muscle is also present in dermis of skin, iris and ciliary body of eye.

Structure of smooth muscle :

• **Arrangements** : They are usually arranged in layers forming sheets in the wall of visceral organs. Smooth muscles are distributed randomly within the myoplasm.

• **Shape and size :** These are small sized (0.02-0.05 mm in length), and spindle shaped having tapering ends. The size of the fibre varies in different viscera. The wall of the uterus during pregnancy shows the large sized fibres.

• **Structure :**

1. It is externally covered by plasma membrane.

2. It is uninucleate with oval shape, placed at the centre.

3. The number and size of micochondria and glycogen granules are less.

4. The myofibrils do not form dark and light bands, so-called unstriated or unstriped on smooth muscle fibres.

5. The myofibrils are formed of randomly arranged myosin and actin filaments.

6. Muscle cells possess a **contractile apparatus** of thin and thick filaments of actin and myosin II. A cytoskeleton of actin and desmin intermediate filaments are also found.

7. Thin filaments contain actin, tropomyosin and caldesmin and the thick filaments contains myosin II which is composed of two polypeptide heavy chains and four light chains.

8. A protein called desmin, is found in intermediate filaments which remain interspersed with thin filaments actin, form a part of the cytoskeleton.

9. Besides desmin filaments, vimetin filaments are also found in vascular smooth muscles.

10. Another structural specialities, called cytoplasmic densities or dense bodies, which provide two attachment sites, one with the thin filaments of the contractile apparatus along with the actin and desmin filaments; another it anchors to the sarcolemma.

11. Dense bodies contain a variety of attachment plaque proteins including α–actinin.

12. Actin and tropomyosin interact with myosin II molecules which together involved in the force generation during contraction.

13. Caldesmon is a 120-150 KDa protein which binds to F actin. The action tropomyosin and caldesmon is controlled by the calcium dependant action.

14. Besides actin and myosin, contractile apparatus of smooth muscle includes α–actinin, calmodulin and myosin light chain kinase proteins.

15. Calmodulin, a 17-KDa protein is a Ca^{+2} binding one which regulates the intracellular calcium concentration.

16. Ca^{2+} calmodulin complex binds to the caldesmon, helps in phosphorylation and release from F-actin.

17. Smooth muscle cells have a membrane system of sarcolemmal invaginations, vesicles, smooth endoplasmic reticulum (SER). Smooth muscles lack T-system.

18. Smooth muscle gets stimulation from neurons originated from autonomic nervous system (ANS). Smooth muscle is directly innervated by both sympathetic and parasympathetic nerves [Fig 1(c).6].

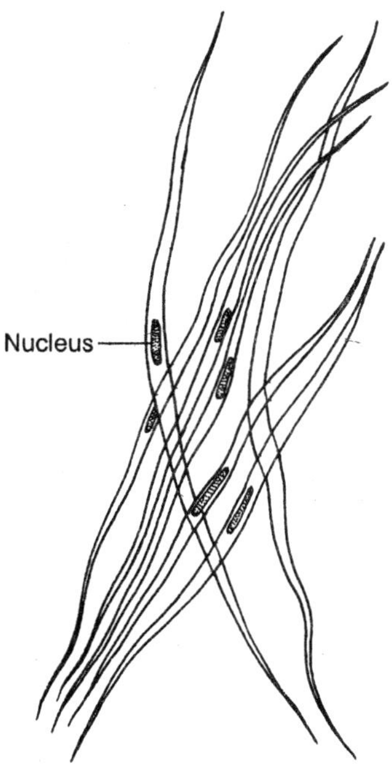

Fig 1(c).6: Structure of non-striated (smooth) muscle fibres.

N.B. : Smooth muscles which lined the wall of gastro-intestinal tract, get the source of nerve supply through enteric division of ANS to the muscular layer.

Functional aspects of smooth muscle :

Cell membrane of smooth muscle cells shows the presence of numbers of invagination. Under the plasma membrane, smooth endoplasmic reticulum (SER) remains sparsed and cytoplasmic vesicles are also present. These two release Ca^{2+} from extracellular matrix during depolarisation.

Visceral smooth muscle shows continuous, irregular and prolonged contraction without any fatigue. Their membrane potential is usually unstable and contracts like a weave in different parts of viscera.

Contraction of smooth muscle is usually regulated by postganglionic neurons of the autonomic nervous system (ANS). In absence of nerve stimuli smooth muscle exhibits a spontaneous contractile activity.

Sequence of events in contraction :

1. Contraction of smooth muscle is initiated by the involvement of Ca^{2+}. Ca^{2+} enters the cytoplasm from extra cellular fluid (ECF) via voltage-gated and ligand-gated Ca^{2+} channels.

2. Increased Ca^{2+} binds with calmodulin and forms active calmodulin-dependent myosin light-chain kinase complex.

3. Active kinase complex (enzyme) catalyzes the phosphorylation of myosin light-chain on serine at 19th position. Phosphorylation of myosin increases the activity of ATPase during contraction.

4. ATPase activity facilitates slow binding of myosin to actin and contraction of muscle takes place.

5. Smooth muscles contract slowly by Ca^{2+} influx and remain contracted for a longer period of time.

6. After that dephosphorylation of myosin takes place by myosin light-chain phos-

phatase. Myosin dephosphorylation does not immediately release myosin head from actin due to **latch-bridge** formation, i.e., myosin cross-bridges remain attached to actin for some time after the cytoplasmic Ca^{2+} concentration falls.

7. For this reason, smooth muscle contraction becomes sustained and finally when Ca^{2+}-calmodulin complex dissociates, then slowly muscle fibres relax.

of thick myosin and thin actin filaments and are covered by sarcolemma.

3. Presence of 'Z' line also shows resemblances with striated skeletal muscle.

(b) **Similarities with smooth muscle fibres :**

1. Like smooth muscle cardiac muscle is also uninucleate, small in size (85-100 μm long and 15 μm in diametere).

Distinguish between neurolemma and sarcolemma

Subjects	Neurolemma	Sarcolemma
1. **Covering**	1. This is the external covering of nerve fibre (present over thē axolemma myelin sheath).	1. This is the external covering (plasma membrane) of muscle fibre.
2. **Position**	2. It is not found in all nerve fibers (present in peripheral nerve fibres but not in central nerve fibres).	2. It is found in all muscle fibres.
3. **Presence or absence of nucleus**	3. It is provided with nucleus of Schwann cells.	3. It is devoid of nucleus.
4. **Function**	4. It helps in regeneration of damaged nerve fibres.	4. It assists in conduction of impulse in muscle fibres.

III. Cardiac muscle

Besides skeletal muscles and smooth muscles, the third type of specialized muscle tissue which is found in the periphery of heart is called **cardiac tissue.**

Position :

Cardiac muscles are found in the myocardium of heart.

Structure :

(a) **Similarities with striated skeletal muscle fibres**

1. Cardiac muscle fibres are cylindrical, with high level of vascularization.

2. Cardiac muscles are with plenty of mitochondria and glycogen granules in their sarcoplasm, also having dark and light bands i.e., striations showing similar arrangement

2. Cardiac muscles are completely involantary in response.

(c) **Special features of cardiac muscles :**

1. Cardiac muscles are branched cells and are joined end-to-end by flat, dense, zigzag junctions (cross bands) called **intercalated discs.**

2. The intercalated disc represents highly specialized attachment site between adjacent cells.

3. The nuclei of cardiac muscle cells lie at the centre of the cell.

4. Specific intercalated discs allow rapid spread of excitation from one muscle fibre to next throughout the heart. The muscle fibres are inter-connected by oblique bridges, called as syncitium.

5. Intercalated disc having transverse component which includes fascia adherens and help to hold them at their ends to form the functional cardiac muscle fibre [Fig 1(c).7].

> **• Why heart muscle cannot be fatigued inspite of continuous activity?**
>
> The heart beats continuously but the cardiac muscle is not fatigued because of the following facts : (i) the refractory period of cardiac muscle is very long allowing sufficient time for recovery so that the contractions are not summated. (ii) With every beat the cardiac muscle receives blood supply via coronary arteries which provides O_2 and food for maintaining energy supply and also washes away the waste matters.

> **• Rheobase and chronaxie of a muscle : Rheobase** is the threshold of intensity of an electrical stimulus to excite the tissue of a muscle whereas **chronaxie** is defined as the shortest duration of stimulus required to excite the muscle tissue equal to twice of rheobase. Chronaxie of a tissue is a definite measure of its excitability. A less excitable tissue has a longer chronaxie, whereas a more excitable tissue has a shorter one.
>
> Both rheobase and chronaxie are considered as the indices of excitability of the muscle. The excitability of a muscle is inversely proportional to its rheobase and chronaxie. That means, the less is the rheobase and chronaxie of a muscle, the more is its excitability.

Special junctional tissues of the heart :

Cardiac muscle consists essentially of certain specialised structures which are responsible for initiation and transmission of cardiac impulses. These specialised cardiac tissues are collectively called as the **junctional tissues** of heart. These are—(1) **Sino-atrial node (S.A. node),** (2) **Atrioventricular node (A. V. node),** (3) **Bundle of His,** (4) **Bundle bunch** and (5) **Purkinje fibres.**

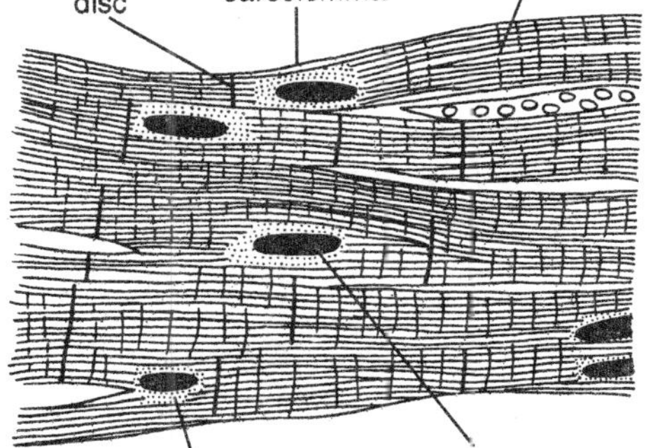

Fig 1(c).7: Cardiac muscles.

(1) **Sino-atrial node (S. A. node) :** It is situated in the right atrium at the junction of superior vena cava and the right auricular appendage. This node is made up of modified cardiac muscle fibres. The fibres are thin elongated, tapering at the ends, longitudinally striated intercrossing with one another in a plexiform manner. This nodal tissue possesses relatively few myofibrils.

(2) **Atrioventricular node (A.V. node) :** A. V. node is situated in the right atrium at the posterior part of the interatrial septum. The cells of A. V. node are cardiac muscle fibres but have a few myofibrils. It also comprises of Purkinje fibres which form a dense network.

(3) **Bundle of His :** The main trunk of this bundle is continuous with the A. V. node and passes upwards until it reaches the posterior margin of the membranous part of the interventricular septum.

(4) **Bundle bunch :** Just above the muscular part of the septum, the bundle divides into right and left branches. The bundle consists of fusiform parallel fibres with scanty striations. The fibres gradually increase in size as one proceeds onwards, and merge with the Purkinje fibres.

(5) **Purkinje fibres** : The fibres which arise from the branches of the bundle of His, spread from the interventricular septum directly to the papillary muscle and then to the lateral walls of ventricle. These fibres have got a larger diameter than the ordinary cardiac muscle fibre. It also contains relatively more sarcoplasm with large amount of glycogen [Fig 1(c).8].

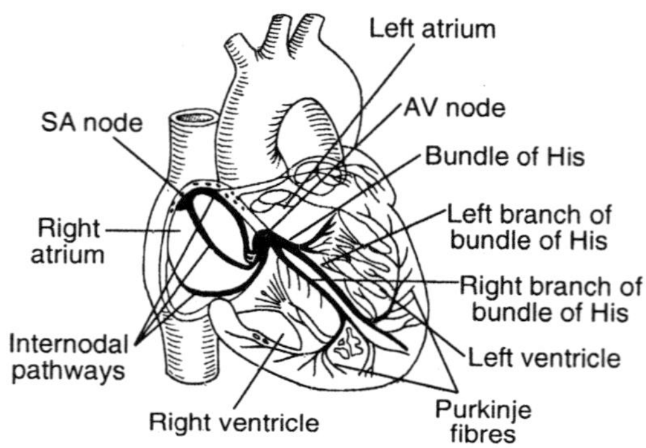

Fig 1(c).8: Junctional tissues of heart.

Mechanism of contraction and relaxation of the cardiac muscle :

The heart shows alternate contraction and relaxation throughout life. The contraction and relaxation of the heart are referred to **systole** and **diastole** respectively. A systole and its subsequent diastole are collectively called as **heart beat**; that means, the two atria and two ventricles contract and relax once in each heart beat. The number of heart beats occuring per minute is called **heart rate**.

The blood forced into the aorta by contraction of the heart produces a pressure wave which propagates through the arteries; this is known as the **pressure pulse** or simply **pulse**. Pulse is the impact felt in an artery caused by the heart beats. It can be felt easily from the radial artery in wrist or carotid artery in the neck or femoral artery in foot by placing fingers on them. **Pulse count** per minute is called pulse rate which equals to heart rate. Clinically, heart rate is often determined by counting the radial pulse per minute.

1(D) THE NERVOUS TISSUE

The nervous system comprises the entire mass of nervous tissue in the body. The essential function of this tissue is **communication,** which depends upon special signalling properties of the nerve cells and their long processes. **The kind of tissue which receives and transmits the stimuli in the animal body is known as nervous tissue.** The central nervous system (CNS) is comprised of the brain and spinal cord and consists of the **nerve cells** or **neurons** and a variety of supportive cells, called collectively the **neuroglia,** though the nerve cell or neuron is the main component of nervous tissue. Nerve impulses conveyed from all parts of the animal body over the long processes of the nerve cells, known as **axons,** come together in the CNS. The **peripheral nervous** system comprises all nervous tissue outside the brain and spinal cord and acts to keep the other tissues of the body in communication with the CNS. The activities of all parts of the animal body are thus integrated by a central "clearing house" that controls the function of the individual as a whole.

(a) **Neuron : A nerve cell with its processes that forms the structural and functional unit of the nervous tissue is called as a neuron.** The cells of the nervous system primarily involved in special functions are neurons. Each neuron has a cell body consisting of a nucleus and the surrounding cytoplasm which is known as the **perikaryon.** Typically the cytoplasm is drawn out into several short radiating processes, called **dendrites** and into a single long process, known as the **axon** or **axis cylinder.** The axis cylinder, which may attain great length, often emits branches or axon collaterals along its course and at its end may exhibit additional fine ramifications.

Structure of neuron or nerve cell : The nerve cell, or neuron, is usually large and complex in shape. Each neuron consists of three parts, the cell body or **perikaryon, dendron** and **axon**. The dendron and axon are the two kinds of **processes** which are coming out from the cell body. The processes are practically the fibre-like protoplasmic projections of the neurons.

1. **The cell body or Soma, or Centron or Cyton or Perikaryon** : The nucleated cytoplasmic portion of neuron is called cell body or soma. In each neuron there is a cell body or soma. Typically each cell body which is 100 μm in diameter may be fusiform, pyramidal, pyriform or irregular stellate in shape. In each cell body there is a single large more or less oval nucleus. This nucleus is usually centrally placed within the perikaryon. In most cases, there is a single conspicuous nucleolus as well as very fine chromatin particles. The cytoplasm of the cell body is also known as **neuroplasm.** The neuroplasm consists of the following structures : (i) Large number of dark staining ribosome granules, called **Nissl granules.** These granules are composed of ribose nucleoprotein substances. Exact function of the granules is not known. They probably may help in conduction of nerve impulse. (ii) Large number of minute microscopic filaments are present within the neuroplasm. These are called **neurofibrils.** They are present throughout the entire length of the protoplasmic processes (axons and dendrites) arising from the cell body. The cell body and its process are surrounded externally by a thin membrane, the **neuron membrane.** The cell body is with non-functional **centrosome.** In absence of functional centrosome the nerve cells do not multiply [Fig 1(d).1].

Distribution : The cell body is situated in the grey matter of the brain and spinal cord.

Function : The cell body regulates and coordinates the function of a neuron.

2. **Dendron** : The short protoplasmic processes of the cell body which receive stimulus from other neuron are called **dendrons.** Each dendron becomes branched into shorter sub-branches, called the **dendrites.** The dendrons at their origin from cell body

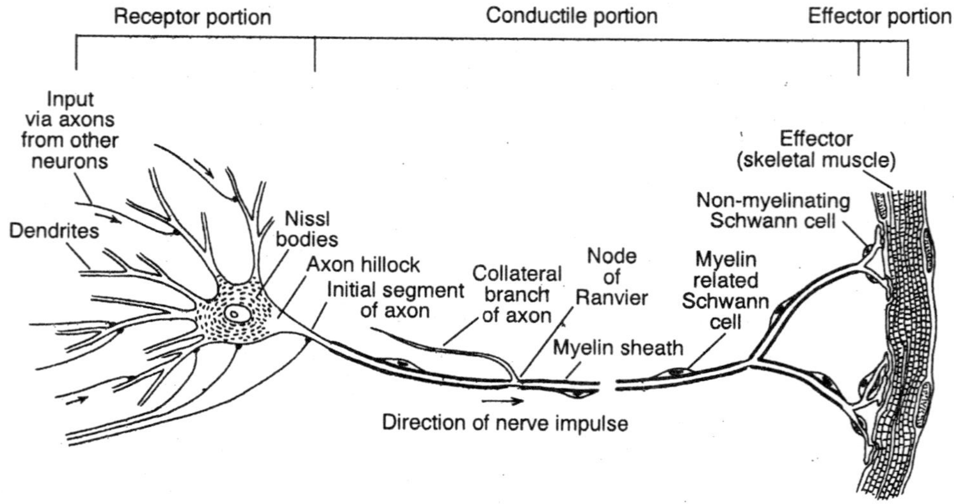

Fig 1(d).1: This diagram illustrates the receptor, conductile, and effector portions of a typical large neuron. The effector endings on skeletal muscle identify this as a somatic motor neurom; in many neurons the effector endings are applied to the receptor portions of other neurons. The presence of the myelin sheath on the conductile portion of the neuron (the axon) increases conduction velocity. The axon is shown to be interrupted, for it is much longer than can be illustrated here.

are 5-10 μm thick but gradually their thickness decreases by profuse branching. In peripheral nervous system some cell body may bear single dendron. Dendron contains Nissl granules, neurofibrils and neuron membrane.

Distribution : Brain and spinal cord.

Function : It receives nerve impulses either from the central nervous system or from another neuron through a synapse and conducts the same towards the cell body and, therefore, it is called the receptive organ.

3. **Axon :** A long and elongated generally branchless cytoplasmic process that comes out from the cell body is called **axon.** The axon arises from the cell body in a conical elevation, the **axon hillock.** Beyond the axon hillock, the axon is characterised by its smooth contour and relatively small uniform diameter. The length of axon is variable and depends on the functional relationships of the neuron. In motor neurons, the axon is much longer than the dendron but the opposite is true with most sensory neurons. The cytoplasmic portion of axon is called **axoplasm** which contains mitochondria, neurofibrils but no Nissl granules. The membrane covering the axon is known as **axolemma.** Axon can give off branches termed as **collaters** along its course, and near the end it undergoes considerable branching into numerous **axon terminals** or **end brushes,** the last part of which is enlarged, called **end bulb.** The end brush may be connected with the dendrites of another neuron forming a **synapse** or it may join with a muscle cell forming the **neuromuscular junction** or **motor end plate** [Fig 1(d).2].

Distribution : The axons are present in the white matter of central and peripheral nervous system.

Function : Axons carry impulses from the cell body of one neuron to the dendron of the next neuron, i.e., it transmits impulse away from the cell body. So it acts as an efferent process.

(b) **Neuroglia :** Neuroglia (from the Greek **neuron,** nerve, + *glia*, glue) or more simply, glia, form the non-neuronal interstitial tissue of the nervous system. Neuroglia is a collective term for the supporting cells or connec-

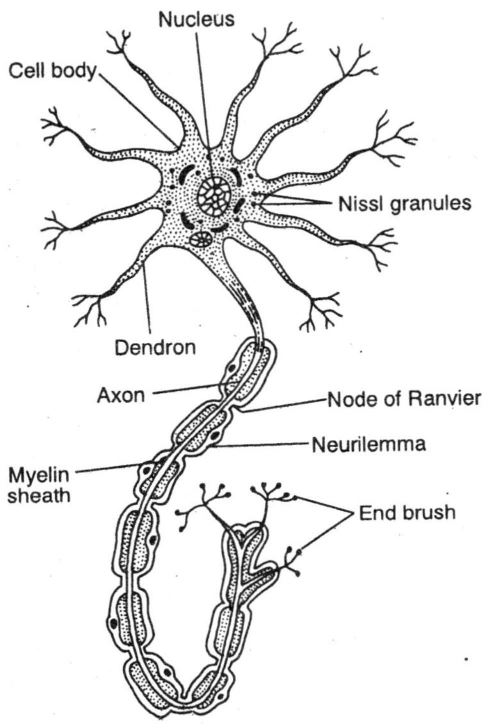

Fig 1(d).2: Different parts of a neuron.

tive tissue of the central nervous system. It is made up of four types of cells—astrocytes, oligodendrocytes, microglia and ependyma. These are the derivatives of the **neural tube glioblast population.** The **neurolemma cells** of peripheral nerves and the **satellite cells** which surround the cell bodies of spinal and cranial ganglia are the glial elements of the peripheral nervous system, the **neural crest glioblast** derivatives [Fig 1(d).3].

Distribution : Most organs of the body have an internal connective tissue framework and the peripheral nerve has such a framework of neuroglial cells and they are also present in the grey and white matters of brain and spinal cord.

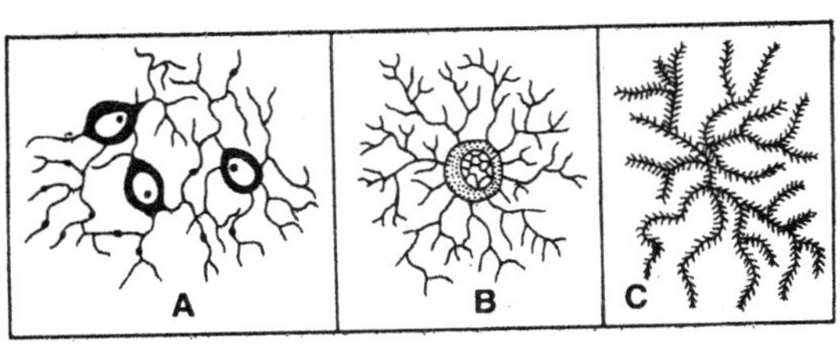

Fig 1(d).3: Neuroglia cells; (A) Oligodendroglia, (B) Astrocyte, (C) Microglia.

Function : Neuroglia cells serve to heal injury to central nervous system and play a role in the formation and maintenance of myelin sheath.

> **Neuron**—A nerve cell with all its processes that forms the structural and functional units of nervous tissue. It contains cell body, dendron and axon.
>
> **Synapse**—It is the junctional space or region between two neurons.
>
> **Neuroglia**—Connective tissue of central nervous system.
>
> **Neurilemma or Schwann sheath**—The cellular sheath around a nerve fibre and it is the unbroken tubular sheath which lies superficial to the myelin sheath.
>
> **Neurofibrils**—Fibrils embedded in the neuroplasm.
>
> **Myelin sheath**—A fatty ensheathing of some nerve fibres.

Types of neuron : Neuron may be classified into the following categories :

1. **According to the number of their processes into four groups**—

(a) **Unipolar :** When one axon and one dendrite are combined and it arises from one pole of the cell body, the neuron is called

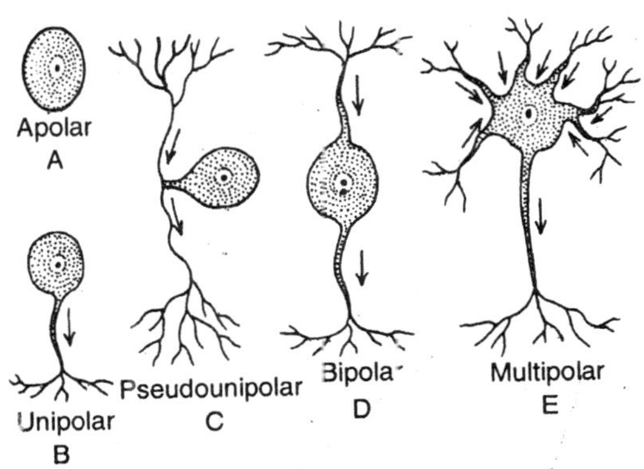

Fig 1(d).4: Different types of neuron (A) Apolar, (B) Unipolar, (C) Pseudounipolar, (D) Bipolar, (E) Multipolar.

Differences between Sarcolemma and Neurilemma

Characters	Sarcolemma	Neurilemma
(i) Position	It is a covering of a muscle fibre.	It is a covering of the axon of a neuron.
(ii) Structure	It consists of lipid and protein without cell.	It is comprised of protein and lipid with cell.
(iii) Function	It helps in conducting the muscle excitation.	It protects the nerve fibre and regenerates when the fibre is damaged. But it never transmits the impulse.

Differences between Axon and Dendrite

Character	Axon	Dendrite
1. Number	Axon is long and single which originates from the axon hillock of a cell body.	More than one short processes originate from the cell body of a neuron.
2. Branching	Generally unbranched.	More short branches are present in a dendrite.
3. Length	Longer in length.	Shorter in length.
4. Myelin sheath	Axon is myelinated.	Devoid of myelin sheath.
5. Neurilemma	In axon neurilemma is present.	Devoid of neurilemma.
6. Axoplasm	Axoplasm is seen.	Neuroplasm is noticed.
7. Schwann sheath	Sheath with schwann cell present.	Schwann sheath with cell absent.
8. Node of Ranvier	Sheath is differentiated into nodes and inter-nodes.	Absence of node of Ranvier, i.e., sheath is not differentiated into nodes and inter-nodes.
9. Nissl's granules	Absent.	Present.
10. Function	Transmits impulses received from cell body.	Receives impulses from other neuron and transmits to the cell body.

unipolar neurone, as found in lower invertebrates and vertebrates.

(b) **Bipolar neuron :** This type of neuron which has fusiform-shaped cell body and contains two poles. One pole gives origin to axon and other to dendrite, as found in retinal ganglia.

(c) **Multipolar neuron :** In this type many dendrites and one axon arise from different parts of the cell body, as found in the majority of the vertebrates.

(d) **Apolar or pseudounipolar :** Originally bipolar but because of the eccentric growth of the cell body, two processes become fused at their point of origin from the cell body to form a pseudounipolar neuron, e.g.; neuron in the cerebrospinal ganglia.

2. **According to function neurons are of three categories**, such as—sensory (afferent), motor (efferent) and inter-neuron.

(a) **Afferent or sensory neuron :** This kind of neuron carries impulses from the visceral organs to the central nervous system.

(b) **Efferent or motor neuron :** Neurons which carry impulses from the central nervous system to the peripheral organs are termed as motor or efferent neuron.

(c) **Inter-neuron :** This kind of neuron is placed between the sensory and motor neurons in the central nervous system. So they transmit impulses from one neuron to other neuron [Fig 1(d).5].

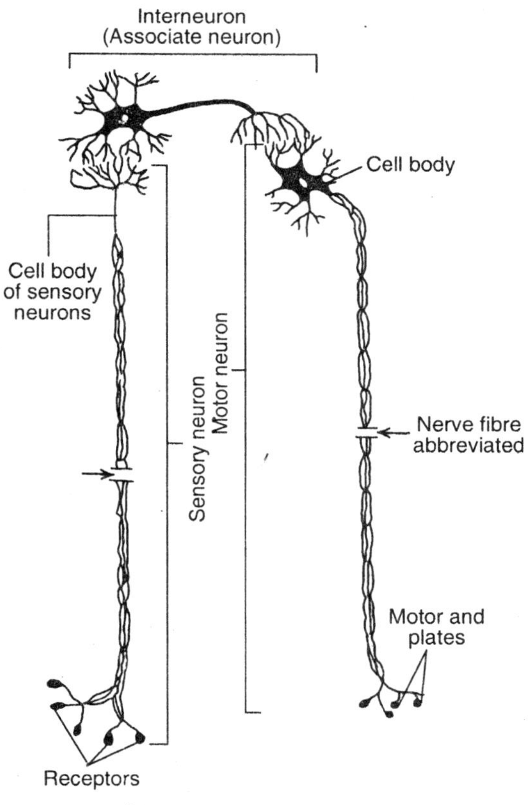

Fig 1(d).5: Diagrammatic representation of three types of neuron (basis of function).

Nerve fibres : The axon and the long dendrites of the afferent neurons in the cranial and spinal nerves are, in the anatomical sense, spoken of as nerve fibres. Practically the long processes of the neurons which invested or ensheathed by membranes are regarded as nerve fibres. On the basis of structure, the fibres are divided into two categories—(a) **Medullated** and (b) **Non-medullated.**

(a) Medullated or myelinated nerve fibres :

In this kind of nerve fibres there are two coverings outside the axolemma of axon. These coverings are myelin or medullary sheath and neurolemma. The naked axon when entering through the gray matter of the central nervous system remains uncovered. But when the axon passes through the white matter of the central nervous system, then it is covered by white phospholipid materials which are known as **myelinated** or **medullary sheath**. This medullary sheath is characteristic of medullated fibres. The myelin sheath provides both mechanical support and electrical insulation to the axon. The function of this sheath is to prevent the spread of the nerve impulse of the axon to other adjacent fibres, i.e., it acts as an insulator. These medullated fibres when come out of the central nervous system receive a nucleated covering which is called **neurolemma.** The neurolemmal covering also includes special type of cells, called the **Schwann cells.** This sheath of flattened cells, called the neurolemmal sheath, forms a thin sleeve around the myelin, which in turn surrounds the axon. The Schwann cells, like the neurons, are of ectodermal origin and represent elements similar to neuroglial cells but they are derived from neural crest and adopted to the special conditions of the peripheral nervous system.

The myelin sheath is not continuous along its whole length but is broken at regular intervals. So the outer neurolemma comes in close contact to the axon in these broken regions and constrictions are formed along the length of the fibre. These constrictions are called **nodes of Ranvier.** The neurolemma protects the nerve fibres, supplies nutrition and helps in the repairing of the damaged peripheral nerves.

(b) Non-medullated nerve fibre :

This type of nerve fibres do not contain myelin sheath. Here the axon cylinder is covered by neurolemma only. Hence, the peripheral non-medullated nerve fibres are covered by neurolemmal sheath only. Non-medullated nerve fibres are present in the autonomic nervous system.

Nerve : Bundles of nerve fibres (axons) which are covered by connective tissue along with the blood vessels are collectively known as a **nerve.** The individual axon is covered by neurolemma. The connective layer surrounding the individual axon is called **endoneurium.** Several axons are bounded together by another connective tissue sheath, **perineurium.** Again several such bundles of axons are combined together by another connective tissue layer, called **epineurium,** to form a nerve. Epineurium is the outermost covering of a nerve. Blood vessels are present both in the perineurium as well as in the epineurium.

Distinguish between medullated nerve fibres and non-medullated nerve fibres

Medullated nerve fibres	Non-medullated nerve fibres
1. Present within the white matter of brain, spinal cord, cranial nerve and spinal nerve.	1. Present within the gray matter of brain and spinal cord and autonomic nervous system.
2. Axon of this fibre is covered internally by medullary sheath and outwardly by neurolemma.	2. Axon is covered by neurolemma but medullary sheath is absent.
3. Presence of node of Ranvier.	3. Absence of node of Ranvier.

CHAPTER 2

Histology of Organs

2(A) LIVER

The liver is the largest mass of glandular tissue in the body and acts as a well-equipped biochemical laboratory where practically metabolism of all nutritional substances, viz., carbohydrates, proteins, fats, vitamins, minerals occurs as well as heat is produced. It is the largest internal organ, weighing approximately 1.5 kg and accounting for nearly 2.5% of adult body weight.

Anatomy

The liver is both a secretory and an excretory gland and is reddish brown in colour. The upper surface of liver is convex and the lower surface is concave. The liver is anatomically divided by deep grooves into a large right and a much smaller left lobe. On the inferior surface of the right lobe of liver, there lies a slate-blue pyriform sac, the **gall bladder.** It stores and modifies the bile secreted from the liver. The right and left **hepatic ducts** arising from the corresponding lobes of liver unite to form the **common hepatic duct** with which joins the **cystic duct** coming from the gall bladder to form the **common bile duct.** This in turn unites with the **pancreatic duct** and finally drains into the duodenum [Fig 2(a).1].

This anatomic division has only topographic importance because it relates lobes of the liver to other abdominal organs. Division into functional surgical segments that corresponds to the blood supply and bile drainage is more clinically important.

Development

The liver develops as an **ectodermal evagination** from the wall of the foregut to form the **hepatic diverticulum** in the embryo. The diverticulum undergoes proliferation to give rise to the **hepatocytes** which become arranged in **cellular cords,** thus producing the parenchyma of the liver. The original stalk of the hepatic diverticulum becomes the **common bile duct.** An outgrowth from this bile duct forms the **cystic diverticulum** that gives rise to the **gall bladder** and **cystic duct.**

Location

It is situated in the right side of upper abdomen and most of it is covered by the mesentary (peritoneal membrane). Practically it is located in the upper right and partially in the upper left quadrants of the abdominal cavity, protected by the ribcage. The liver is enclosed in a fibrous capsule **(Glisson's capsule)**; a serous covering surrounds the capsule except where the liver adheres directly to the diaphragm.

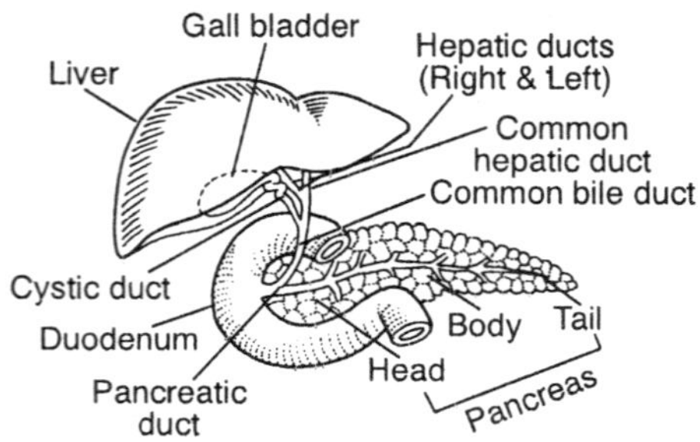

Fig. 2(a).1: Relationship between liver, pancreas and duodenum.

Histological structure

Liver is almost a solid organ consisting of several lobes. Each lobe of the liver consists of a large number of polyhedral **lobules;** thus, the hepatic lobules may be considered as the structural units of the liver. Each lobule is surrounded by a capsule made up of two layers, the outer layer being a smooth moist peritoneum and the inner a fibrous covering, known as **Glisson's capsule,** which surrounds all structures entering and leaving the liver. But this Glisson's capsule is absent around the liver lobules of men [Fig 2(a).2A].

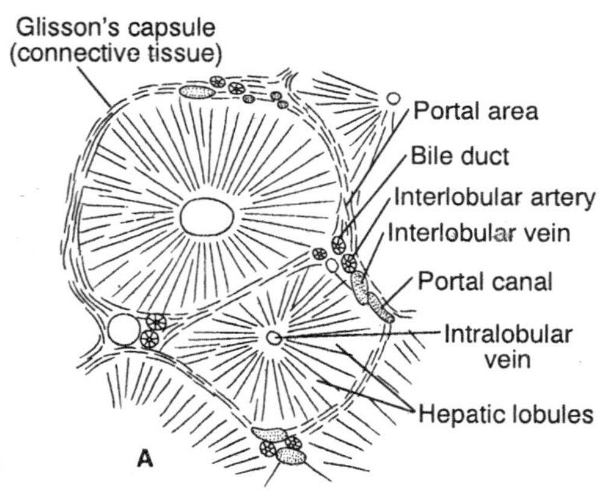

Fig. 2(a).2A: Liver of rabbit. T.S. liver to show a group of hepatic lobules and a Glisson's capsule of liver.

Classic hepatic lobule

The liver consists of a large number of hexagonal functional units, called **hepatic lobules**. Under the microscope each lobule is found to be composed of rows of **polygonal cells** radiating from the centre—like the spokes of a wheel, the periphery of the lobule being delinerated by the presence of **portal triads** or **hepatic triads,** i.e., each hepatic lobule is marked off from the neighbouring lobules by connective tissue septa through which pass groups of three tubes (each group being known as hepatic triad). The centre is occupied by the central (intralobular) vein. At the angles of the hexagons are the **portal areas** or **portal canals** which are loose stromal connective tissue characterised by the presence of portal triads or hepatic triads. Each hepatic triad contains hepatic artery, portal vein and bile duct. The portal vein and hepatic artery enter into, and bile duct and hepatic vein emerge out of the liver through a connective tissue sheath. After entering they branch repeatedly. There is a frequent hepatoportal anastomosis in between the hepatic artery and portal vein in the interlobular region. Recent studies indicate that the hepatocytes are actually as plates or sheets, one cell is thick, which forms a 'wall work' with interconnecting bridges. The cell plates are known as **hepatic laminae**. The spaces between the adjacent laminae are called **hepatic lacunae** that form a communication system of cavities. The lacunae contain blood **sinusoids** that are wider than capillaries. Sinusoids separate the sheets of hepatic cells and empty into the central veins. The lining endothelium of the sinusoids contains some specialized phagocytic cells, known as **stellate cells** or **Kupffer cells.** Electron microscope reveals that Kupffer cells may contain phagocytosed substances and they are elongated structures having irregular outline, crescent nucleus, few mitochondria and varying number of lysosomes. At the edges of the portal canal or portal areas between the connective tissue stroma and the hepatocytes, is a small space, called **Space of Mall.** This space is thought to be one of the sites where lymph originates in the liver. The narrow space separating the sinusoidal

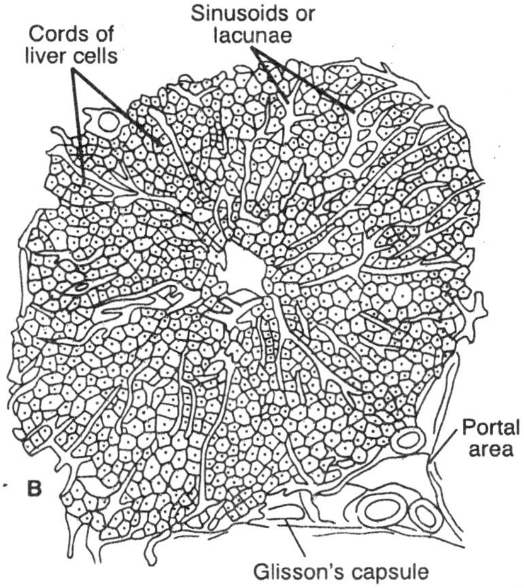

Fig. 2(a).2B: Microscopic anatomy of a lobule.

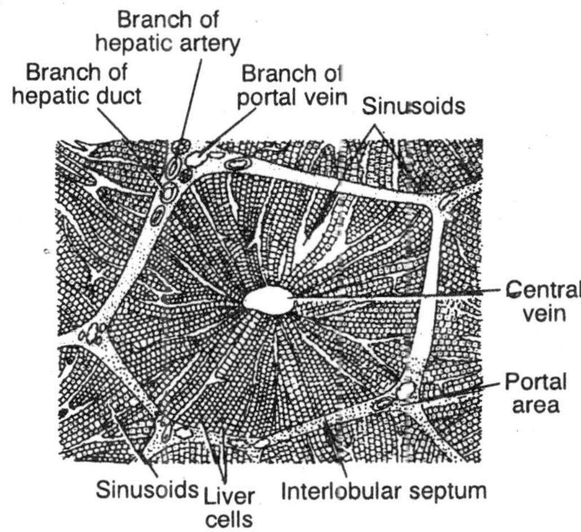

Fig. 2(a).3: T. S. of liver showing the histological structure of liver.

wall from the liver cell plates is known as **Disse's space** [Fig 2(a).2B].

The interlobular branches of the hepatic artery also end in the sinusoids directly. The central vein also passing through the long axis of the lobule, constantly receives sinusoids from all sides and ultimately leaves the lobule at its base. Hence, it joins with the central vein of the neighbouring lobules thus forming the sublobular vein which finally ends in the large hepatic vein. The liver capillaries contain numerous **mast cells** [Fig 2(a).3].

Hepatocytes

The cells of the liver are known as **hepatocytes.** Hepatocytes are large polygonal cells measuring between 20 and 30 µm in each dimension. Hepatocyte nuclei are large and spherical and occupy the centre of the cell. Many cells in the liver are binucleate; most cells in the adult liver are tetraploid. Heterochromatin is present as scattered clumps in the nucleoplasm and as a distinct bend under the nuclear envelope. Two or more well-developed nucleoli are visible in each nucleus.

The cytoplasm contains stored glycogen, fat and also basophilic material. Mitochondria, Golgi-apparatus, granular and agranular-ER and lysosomes are seen. The bile canaliculi are lined by single membrane and the membrane is protruded into canaliculus in the form of microvilli.

Under EM the border of liver cell is straight except for a few desmosomes from where microvilli project into the lumen of bile canaliculi. Hepatocytes have as many as 200 to 300 peroxisomes per cell. They are relatively large and vary in diameter from 0.2 to 1.0 µm. Peroxisomes are a major site of oxygen use. The inner invaginations of the mitochondria form cristae where most of the oxidative phosphorylation occurs. The rER in hepatocytes contain granules, ribosomes with RNA and are the seat of protein synthesis. Under light microscope, these granules are responsible for basophilia. The sER may be extensive but varies with metabolic activity. Golgi apparatus acts as a packaging site for excretion of bile and this apparatus comprises a system of particles and vesicles lying near the canaliculus.

The intervening hyaloplasm is provided with granules of lipid, glycogen and fibrils. Bile ductules are surrounded by collagen fibres..

Biliary tree

It is the system of conduits of increasing diameter that bile passes through from the hepatocytes to the gall bladder and then to the intestine. The smallest branches of this system are the canaliculi into which the hepatocytes secrete the bile.

Bile canaliculi form a complete loop around four sides of the hexagonal hepatocytes. They are approximately 0.5 μm in luminal diameter and are isolated from the rest of the intercellular compartment by tight junctions, which are part of junctional complex that also include zonulae adherentes and desmosomes. Microvilli of two adjacent hepatocytes extend into the canalicular lumen. The bile canaliculi form a ring about the hepatocyte and constitute a network that drains into small bile ducts termed as **intra-hepatic ductules or canals of Hering**. These canals are lined by cuboidal cells which are

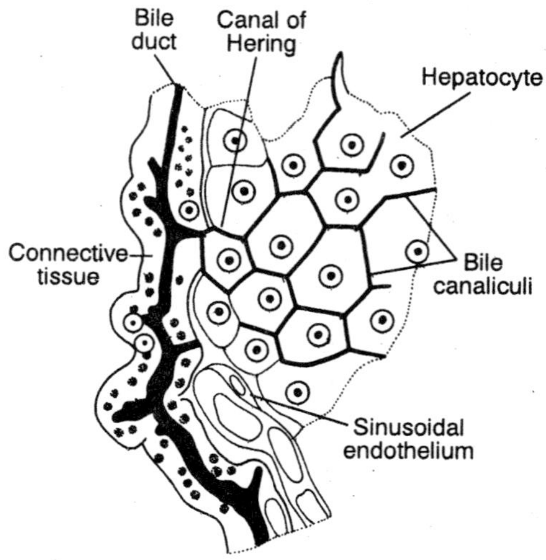

Fig. 2(a).4: Network of bile canaliculi.

- **Comparison of the classic liver lobule, portal lobule and liver acinus :**

The **classic liver lobule** has the terminal hepatic venule or central vein at the centre of the lobule and the portal canals containing portal treads at the peripheral angles of the lobule.

The **portal lobule** has a portal canal at the centre of the lobule and terminal central veins or hepatic venules at the periphenal angles of the lobule.

The **liver acinus** has distributing vessels at the equator and terminal central veins or hepatic venules at each pole [Fig 2(a).5].

- **Macrophage of the liver (Kupffer cell) :**

The macrophage of the liver is the Kupffer cell. These cells form part of monocyte-macrophage defense system and participate in the removal of spent erythrocytes and other particulate debris from the circulation.

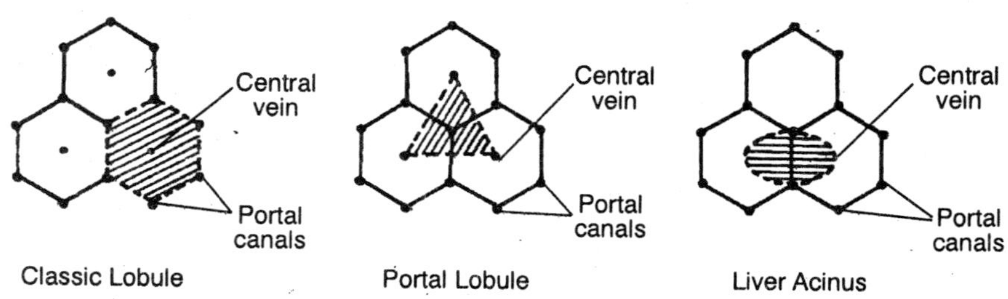

Fig. 2(a).5: Liver lobules and liver acinus.

subtended by complete basal lamina. This canal of Hering finally drains into the bile ducts of the portal canals. All bile ducts eventually fuse before leaving the liver as the common hepatic duct [Fig 2(a).4].

Functions of liver

Liver is an essential organ of the body which performs many functions :

1. In connection with blood and circulation :

(i) In foetal life RBC are manufactured by the liver.

(ii) In adult life liver stores inorganic salts of iron, copper and vitamin B_{12} and thus helps in the formation of RBC and haemoglobin.

(iii) Liver functions as a store-house for blood and regulates blood volume.

(iv) Fibrinogen, prothrombin and certain other blood coagulating factors are formed in the liver which are instrumental in blood coagulation.

(v) Mast cells form heparin and prevent intravascular clotting.

(vi) Heparin is an intravascular anticoagulant that is stored in the liver.

(vii) Manufactures all plasma proteins. Serum albumin and serum globulin are synthesized by the liver from the aminoacids derived from the protein in the diet.

(viii) The liver of the foetus is responsible for **erythropoiesis,** but this function is gradually taken over by cells of the red bone marrow.

2. Secretion : The secretion as well as excretion of liver is called bile. It is a dark green coloured alkaline fluid. Bile consists of bile salts, bile pigments, electrolytes, phospholipids, cholesterol and water. It performs various functions :

(i) Bile salts of bile emulsify the fat and activate the lipase enzyme and thus, responsible for digestion of fat.

(ii) Renders chyme alkaline for the action of pancreatic enzymes.

(iii) Bile activates the inactive lipase of pancreatic juice.

(iv) It stimulates **peristalsis** and thereby promote defecation.

(v) Bile salts convert insoluble fatty acids, cholesterol, etc. into soluble one and also increase the permeability of the absorbing epithelium of the intestinal villi. Thus, bile helps for the absorption of fat, fat soluble vitamins (i.e., Vit. A, D, E & K), iron, calcium, etc.

(vi) Certain substances like cholesterol, bile pigments, inorganic salts, some heavy metals, toxins etc are excreted through bile.

3. Antiseptic action : Bile inhibits growth of certain bacteria.

4. Choleretic action : Bile salts are potent choleretic agents i.e., they can stimulate the secretion of bile by liver thereby increasing the flow of bile.

5. Neutralizing action : The bicarbonates of bile along with those of the pancreatic juice neutralise the HCl entering into the duodenum from the stomach. This maintains a slightly alkaline pH of the intestinal contents so as to facilitate the action of pancreatic and intestinal enzymes.

6. Manufactures bile : Bile is secreted as well as excreted continuously from the hepatic cells and collected in the gall bladder. Bile contains water, bile salts, bile pigments, cholesterol, etc. **Cholesterol** is formed in the liver from active acetate. **Bile salts** are Na-taurocholate and Na-glycocholate. **Bile acids** (Cholic acid, deoxycholic acid and lithocholic acid) have been considered to be the derivatives of cholanic acid and formed in the liver. These bile acids in conjugation with glycine and taurine, form the compounds—glycocholic acid ($C_3H_{39}O_2 . CO . NH . CH_2 . COOH$) and taurocholic acid ($C_{23}H_{39}O_3 . CO . NH . CH_2 . CH_2 . SO_3 . H$) respectively. Bile salts are the Na-salts of taurocholic acid and glycocholic acid. **Bile pigments** are the biliverdin and bilirubin. These are the excretory products of haemoglobin of broken down RBC and are synthetized in the R.E system of various parts of the body. Liver, spleen, bone marrow have been considered to be the site of formation of these bile pigments.

7. **Lubricating function** : The mucin of bile acts as a lubricant for smooth passage of the intestinal contents.

8. **On carbohydrate metabolism :**

(i) Acts as a storehouse for non-consumable sugar. The sugar is stored in the form of glycogen, i.e., conversion of glucose into glycogen. It occurs in the presence of insulin hormone.

(ii) When blood sugar tends to be low, glycogenolysis occurs. It is influenced by the glucagon hormone.

(iii) Takes an important part in blood sugar regulation.

(iv) Liver is the seat of neoglucogenesis.

9. **On fat metabolism :**

(i) Liver is involved in the processing and transport of fats rather than storage.

(ii) It assists in the oxidation of fat, releasing energy in the form of ATP.

(iii) Manufactures fats from carbohydrates, proteins, etc.

(iv) It helps in the removal of cholesterol and phospholipids from the blood and their degradation.

(v) When necessary, liver can perform metabolism of steroids (including cholesterol synthesis).

(vi) It is the seat of ketone body formation.

10. **On protein metabolism :**

(i) It is the seat of deamination.

(ii) Liver is the chief seat of urea and uric acid formation.

(iii) The plasma proteins, serum albumin and serum globulin are synthesized by the liver from the amino acids derived from the protein in the diet.

(iv) Liver is the seat of nitrogen metabolism as evident from deamination process and urea synthesis (through **ornithine cycle**).

2(B) KIDNEY

The kidney is a compound tubular gland, adapted to filtering wastes from the blood, i.e., the kidneys are the main organs of urinary system. Like the lungs and liver, the kidneys retrieve essential materials and dispose the wastes. They conserve water, essential electrolytes and metabolites and remove the waster products of metabolism from the body.

Anatomy

In man, the two kidneys are located near the dorsal wall of the lower abdomen beneath the peritoneum. The right kidney is placed slightly lower than the left one, and is slightly smaller in size. The average weight of kidneys of an adult man is about 150 gm while that of an adult woman is roughly 135 gm. Each kidney measures approximately 10 cm long × 6.5 cm wide (from concave to convex border) × 3 cm thick and is covered by a fibrous capsule. The medial side of kidney is concave and contains a deep vertical fissure, called the **hilum** of the kidney through which the renal artery enters into the kidney and the renal vein and ureter emerge from it [Fig 2(b).1].

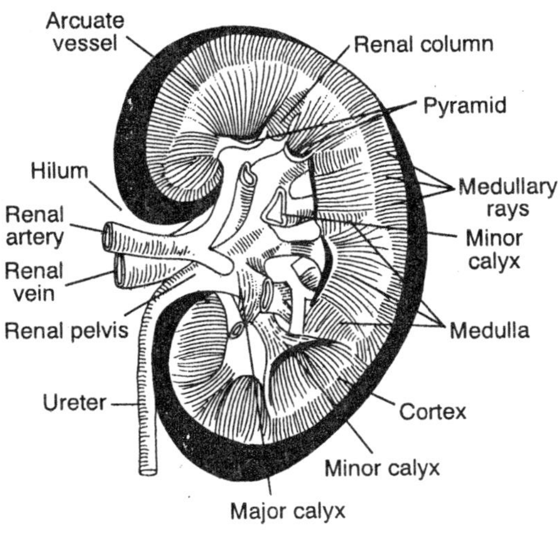

Fig. 2(b).1: Diagram of kidney structure. The diagram represents a hemisection of a kidney, revealing its structural organization.

If the kidney is sectioned along its long axis and examined, it may be seen to consist of three distinct regions.

(i) The kidney surface is covered by a connective tissue **capsule.**

(ii) The outer dark reddish brown peripheral region is the **cortex.**

(iii) The lighter region beneath the cortex is the **medulla.** Medulla is cmposed of renal tubules, connecting ducts, blood vessels and connective tissue. Within the medulla there is a hollow chamber, the pelvis of the kidney. Pelvis is formed by the expansion of the ureter. Within medulla 10-15 pyramids are found, called **renal pyramids**. The apex or papilla of each opens into the pelvis. Each pyramid is made up of a bundle of **duct of Belini,** the opening of which enters into pelvis. The pyramids are separated by strands of cortical tissue, called **column of Bertin.** The papilla of renal pyramid is fitted within a small tube called **minor calyx.** Several minor calyces joint to form a **major calyx.** At the point where the ureter leaves the kidney the renal artery may be seen entering the kidney and renal vein leaving it.

Location

The kidneys are large, reddish, bean-shaped organs housed on either side of the spinal column in the retroperitoneal space of the posterior abdominal cavity. They extend from 12th thoracic vertebra to 3rd lumbar vertebra, with the right kidney positioned slightly higher.

Histological structure

A kidney consists of the following three parts :

1. Renal capsule : The kidney surface is covered by a thin but tough connective tissue, **renal capsule.** The capsule consists of two distinct layers : an outer layer of fibroblasts and collagen fibers, and an inner layer with a cellular component of myofibroblasts.

Inside the capsule, the substance of kidney is a compact mass of **nephrons.** The renal capsule passes inward at the hilum, where it forms the connective tissue covering of the sinus and becomes continuous with the connective tissue forming the walls of the calyces and renal pelvis.

2. Cortex : The outer reddish brown part of the kidney is known as cortex. It is granular in appearance because the tubules here are much convoluted and it also contains the **renal corpuscles** or **Malpighian corpuscles.** The cortex overlies the bases of medullary pyramids and these displaced portions of cortex which invade the medullary territory are called the **renal columns of Bertin.** The cortex is not uniform in texture. It is subdivided into alternating radial tracts termed as **rays** and **labyrinths.** The rays are radially straited because they contain the straight parts of proximal tubules and the collecting ducts. Cortex also contains vertical striations that appear to arise from the medulla. These are called the **medullary rays.** A medullary ray is an aggregation of **straight tubules** and **straight collecting tubules** of nephrons. The **labyrinths** have a granular appearance because the convoluted tubules, which compose them, are cut irregularly. Among fresh tubules **glomeruli** may be seen as bright red points.

3. Medulla : Examination of a section cut through the kidney reveals a series of vertical striations that appear to emanate from the medulla. These striations are referred to as **medullary rays.** Each medullary ray is an aggregation of straight tubules and collecting ducts. They are accompanied by a capillary network, the **vasa recta** that runs in parallel with various tubules. The regions between medullary rays contain the renal corpuscles, the convoluted tubules of the nephrons and collecting tubules. These areas are called **cortical labyrinths.** Each nephron and its collecting tubule form the **uriniferous tubule.**

The tubules in the medulla collectively form a number of conical structures, the **pyramids.** The bases of the pyramids face the cortex and the apices face the renal sinus. Each pyramid is differentiated into an **outer medulla** (adjacent to the cortex) and an **inner medulla.** The outer medulla is further subdivided into an **inner stripe** and an **outer stripe.**

The caps of cortical tissue that lie over the pyramids are sufficiently extensive and they extend peripherally around the lateral portion of the pyramid forming the renal columns (of Bertin). The apical portion of each pyramid is known as **papilla** that projects into a **minor calyx.** It is a cup-shaped structure that represents an extension of the renal pelvis. The tip of the papilla, called **area cribrosa,** is perforated by the openings of the collecting ducts. The minor calyces are branches of two or three **major calyces** that in turn are major divisions of the renal pelvis [Fig 2(b).2 and 3].

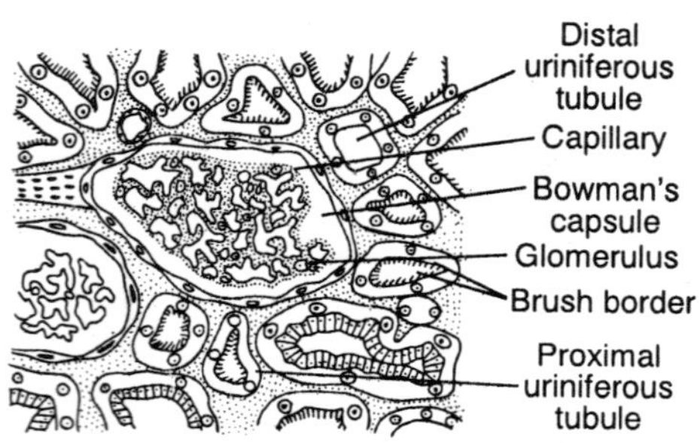

Fig. 2(b).2: T. S. of cortex of kidney of a mammal.

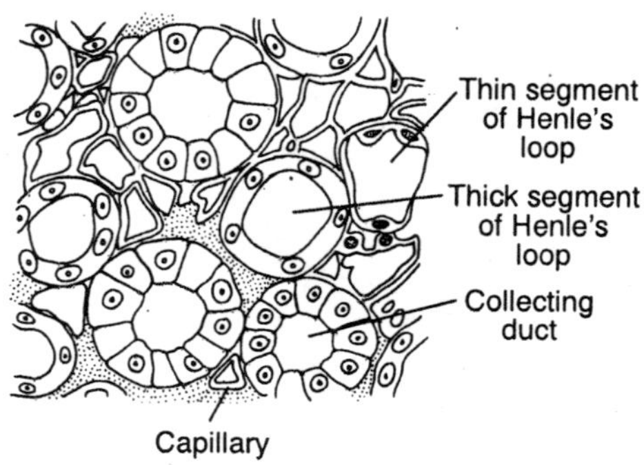

Fig. 2(b).3: T. S. of medulla of kidney of a mammal.

Uriniferous tubule (Nephron)

The nephron is the fundamental structural and functional unit of the kidney. Each human kidney contains approximately 2 million nephrons. A complete uriniferous tubule consists of two component parts : (i) the secretory tubule of nephron which is long and unbranched and (ii) the excretory portion which is a branched, tree-like system of excretory ducts.

Histologically, there are two kinds of nrephrons according to their relative position in the cortex : (i) **the superficial nephrons** occupy the outer two-thirds of the cortex and make up about 85% of the total number, (ii) and the **juxtamedullary nephrons** occupy the inner third of the cortex and constitute about 15% of the total number. The superficial nephrons are smaller in size and fully functioning under normal conditions. The juxtamedullary nephrons are large and work only in conditions of stress [Fig 2(b).4].

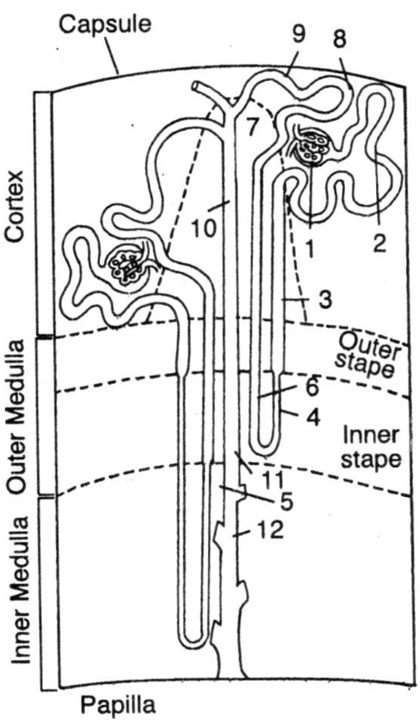

Fig. 2(b).4: Uriniferous tubule.

The wall of the uriniferms tubule consists of a single layer of epithelial cells that rests on a well-marked basement membrane.

Each nephron consists of two main parts—(1) the **renal or Malpighian corpuscle** and (2) the **renal tubule.** The structures of these two parts are completely different because they differ in their functions.

(1) Renal or Malpighian corpuscle :

This is a spheroid body consisting of a vascular tuft or **glomerulus,** enveloped by a two-layered epithelial cup, the **renal** or **Bowman's capsule.**

(a) **Bowman's capsule :** It is the blind expanded end of the renal tubule. It is a double-layered cup of squamous epithelium which envelops a capillary tuft, called **glomerulus.** Its outer layer is continuous with tubular wall and is called the **parietal layer** while the inner layer close to the glomerulus is known as **visceral layer.** These two layers are fused together at the **vascular pole** of the capsule (i.e., at the point of entry and exit of blood vessels to and from the capsule). Both the layers of the Bowman's capsule are lined by a single layer of epithelial cells placed on an underlying basal lamina (or basement membrane). The parietal epithelium of Bowman's capsule remains essentially squamous whereas the visceral layer is lined by specialised cells, called **podocytes.** These give rise to number of radiating tentacle-like cytoplasmic processes which in turn give up a large number of small branches—the **pedicels** or **endfeet.** The pedicels are actually attached to the basal lamina [Fig 2(b).5].

(b) **Glomerulus :** It is a tuft of capillaries held together by scanty connective tissue which invaginates within the Bowman's capsule. The glomerulus is derived from an **afferent arteriole** which is a small subdivision of the renal artery. The afferent arteriole on entering the Bowman's copsule breaks up into about 20-50 capillary loops. They reunite to form the **efferent arteriole** which leaves the capsule. The lumen of the efferent arteriole is smaller than that of the afferent arteriole. The endothelium of the glomerular vessels is extremely thin and

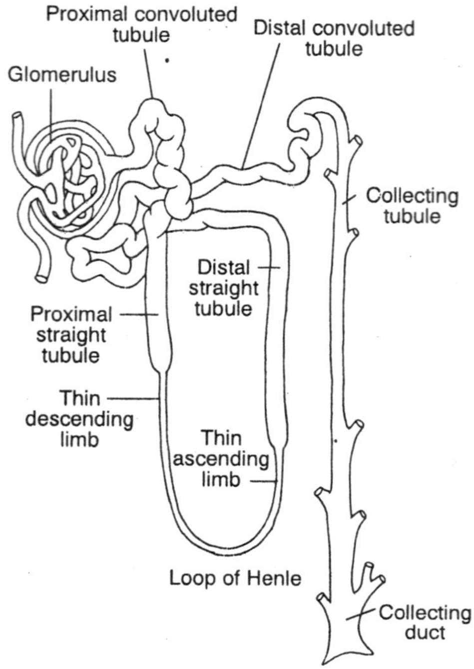

Fig. 2(b).5: Diagram showing the nephron and collecting system.

richly fenes-trated with finely pores. In majority of the glomeruli, particularly in those of the cortical nephrons, the efferent arterioles are narrower than their corresponding afferent arterioles. This arrangement helps in the maintenance of a much higher pressure in the glomerular capillaries than in capillaries elsewhere. This high capillary pressure is well adapted for the **filtration function** which the glomeruli subserve.

The cells of the endothelial lining of glomerular capillaries are flat and fenestrated lying on a basal lamina which remain fused with the basal lamina of the podocytes. Thus, the podocytes of the visceral layer of Bowman's capsule and the endothelium of the glomerular capillaries together with the common (fused) basal lamina lying in between them form the glomerular filtering membrane. Therefore, the fused basal lamina of the podocytes and endothelium are the only barrier to the passage of fluid from the capillary lumen to the cavity of Bowman's capsule and this is the actual filtering membrane of the glomerulus which functions as like a **selective filter.**

Filtering apparatus of the kidney :

(i) **Endothelium of the glomerular capillaries :** It possesses fenestrations of larger size (70 to 90 mm in diameter). These fenestrations are more numerous and more irregular in outline than fenestrations in other capillaries. Endothelial cells of glomerular capillaries possess a large number of aquaporin—1 (AQP-1) water channels that allow the fast movement of water through the epithelium.

(ii) **Glomerular basement membrane :** It is a thick basal lamina (300-350 mm) that is the joint product of the endothelium and the podocytes (the cells of the visceral layer of Bowman's capsule). The glomerular basement membrane is the principal component of the filtration barrier.

(iii) **Visceral layer of Bowman's capsule :** This layer contains specialized cells called podocytes. These cells extend processes around the glomerular capillaries. The podocytes constitute a double-layered epithelial cup of Bowman's capsule. The inner visceral layer of Bowman's capsule lies in apposition to a capillary network, the glomerulus, which forms at this site. The outer parietal cell layer forms the squamous cells of Bowman's capsule. The cup eventually closes to form the spherical structure containing the glomerulus.

(2) Renal tubule :

The long, narrow and coiled tube-like part of a nephron arising from the Bowman's capsule and ending into the minor calyx is called renal tubule. Structurally, it is differentiated into the following four parts in sequence.

(i) **Proximal convoluted tubule :** It is the first part of the renal tubule whose lumen is continuous with that of the Bowman's capsule. It lies in the cortical region and this part is highly coiled and hence it is so named. It is lined by a single layer of cuboidal or truncated pyramidal epitheloid cells, the free borders (at the lumen) of which are striated or brush-bordered. E. M study has revealed that the brush border is composed of processes or microvilli which enormously increase the surface area of the cells for absorption in the lumen of the proximal tubule. There are numerous tubular invaginations arising at the clefts between the microvilli, extending downwards into the apical cytoplasm and are called **apical canaliculi.** In the apical region, clear vacuoles of various sizes are also noted. Inside the cytoplasm there are rod-like structures of mitochondria at the basal half of the cell. The mitochondria are oriented perpendicular to the cell membrane. The cells contain a large number of enzymes and metabolically they are very active. Proximal convoluted tubule finally terminates into the 'U'-shaped loop of Henle.

(ii) **Henle's loop :** The part lying next to the proximal convoluted tubule is not convoluted and is 'U'-shaped. It proceeds towards the medulla and then again turns back as a straight tubule. It consists of a descending and an ascending limbs which are differentiated into a thick segment of descending tubule, a thin segment of descending tubule, a thin segment of ascending tubule and a thick segment of ascending tubule.

Thick segment descending tubule is a straight tubule. It has the same structural features with the proximal convoluted tubule. The thin portions of Henle's loop are lined by squamous epithelial cells having a few irregularly oriented microvilli. The cells are seated on a distinct basement membrane and each cell possesses a flattened nucleus, mitochondria, Golgi-apparatus and vacuoles. The thick segment of ascending limbs of Henle's loop consists of cuboidal cells which are tall with striated basal portion (due to the presence of vertically arranged rod-shaped mitochondria) but they are not brush-bordered, i.e., absence of microvilli. The apical cytoplasm contains a pair of centrioles; from one of the two centrioles a single flagellum may arise and project into the tubular lumen. The lining epithelium of the thin segment is of pavement type; the cells are flattened and thin except in the nuclear region which bulges into the lumen.

(iii) **Distal convoluted tubule :** The portion of the renal tubule next to the ascending limb of Henle's loop again becomes convoluted and hence, it is named distal convoluted tubule. It is present in the cortex. The distal tubule is lined by cubical epithelium with striated appearance in the basal part and without any brush border. Electron micrograph reveals that the luminal surface of the cells may have a few short microvilli. These cells also contain a number of mitochondria.

The proximal part of the distal tubule while returning to the cortex meets with the juxtaglomerular cells of the afferent arteriole in front of the renal or Malpighian corpuscle. The tubular surface in this region presents an elliptical disc of larger cells (40 to 70 microns) with closely packed nuclei termed as **macula densa.** Thus, granular juxtaglomerular cells of the afferent arteriole, macula densa of the proximal part of the distal convoluted tubule and agranular **lacis cells** constitute the **juxta-glomerular apparatus** which plays a significant role in the thermodynamics of the kidney.

Collecting tubule : This is a straight tubule extending from cortex to medulla. During its course, it receives the distal tubules of several nephrons. It is lined by simple cuboidal epithelial cells. In the medulla, the collecting tubules join successively to constitute a large wide duct, known as **duct of Belini**, which ultimately opens into the renal pyramid. The duct of Belini consists of tall columnar cells [Fig 2(b).6 and 7].

Formation of urine

(1) **Functions of Malpighian corpuscles or glomerular filtration :**

The Malpighian corpuscles by virtue of their structural peculiarity work like filters

Juxtaglomerular apparatus : It is a specialised secretory structure of kidney formed by macula densa cells of distal tubule, juxtaglomerular cells of afferent arteriole and lacis cells of the vascular angle of glomerulus.

Role : This juxtaglomerular apparatus works as a volume receptor sensitive to fall of blood volume. On being stimulated by low volume, the juxtaglomerular apparatus secretes a proteolytic enzyme-like renin which splits a plasma protein fraction (i.e., angiotensinogen) to form a peptide known as **angiotensin.** It performs the following activities—(i) secretion of aldosterone from adrenal cortex, (ii) release of ADH from posterior pituitary, (iii) thirst sensation and (iv) vasoconstriction. Thus, it assists to maintain blood volume and blood pressure. Provides feedback control of extracellular fluid volume and glomerular filtration rate by activating the renin-angiotensin system.

- **Podocytes** are modified epithelial cells lining the visceral layer of Bowman's capsule.
- **Lacis cells** are modified glandular cells present at the vascular angle formed by the afferent and efferent arterioles.
- **Macula densa cells** are specialised glandular cells present in the part of the distal convoluted tubule forming the juxtaglomerular apparatus.
- **Juxtaglomerular cells** are the specialised glandular cells of the afferent arterioles entering into the glomeruli.

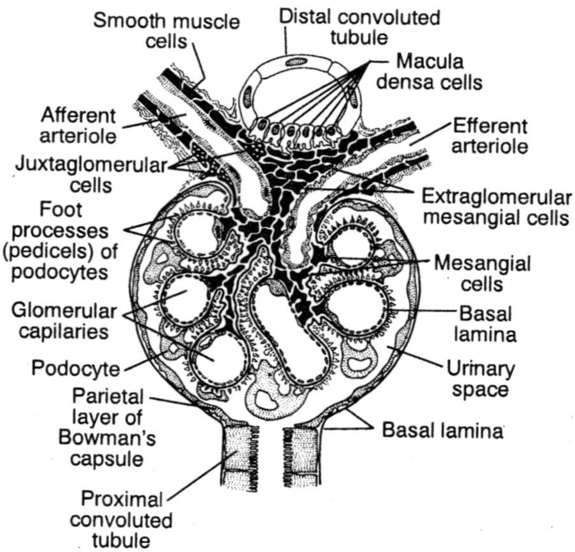

Fig. 2(b).6: This schematic diagram shows the organization of the renal corpuscle and the structures associated with it at the vascular and urinary poles. Mesangial cells are associated with the capillary endothelium of the glomerulus and the glomerular basement membrane. The macula densa cells of the distal tubule are shown intimately associated with the juxtaglomerular cells of the afferent arteriole and the extraglomerular mesangial cells.

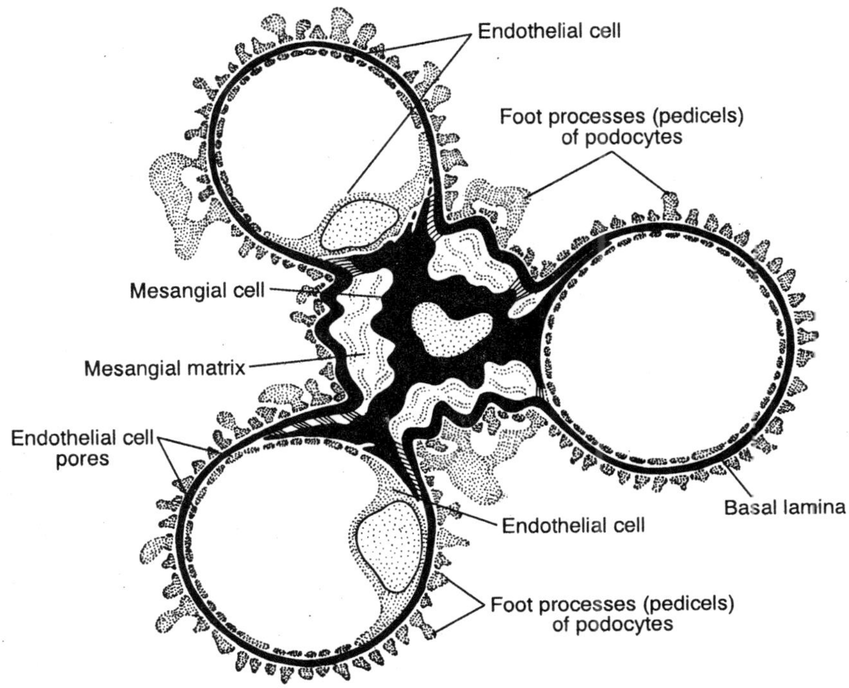

Fig. 2(b).7: Schematic diagram showing the relationship between the intraglomerular mesangial cells and the glomerular capillaries. The mesangial cell and its surrounding matrix are enclosed by the basal lamina of the glomerular capillaries. Note that the mesangial cells are in the same compartment as the endothelium and that they can be intimately associated with the basal lamina as well as with the endothelial cells, (Modified from Sakal T. Kriz W. *Anat Embryol* 1987; 176 : 373-385)

carrying out a special type of filtration which is referred to as **ultrafiltration**.

The process of urine formation involves **filtration** through the walls of the glomerular capillaries of Malpighian corpuscles and **reabsorption** in the renal tubules. The glomerulus acts as ultrafilter by which water and all substances dissolved in the plasma with the exception of colloidal macro-molecular compounds (proteins, fats, etc) are filtered into the Bowman's capsule from blood flowing along the glomerular capillaries. In the glomerulus filtration takes place through the endothelial perforations. The size of the filtering pores is such that only those components of plasma having molecular weights up to 68000 are allowed to pass from the glomerular capillaries to the capsular cavity. Again, the process of filtration is a simple mechanical or passive process in which expenditure of cellular energy is not required. The blood pressure in the glomerular capillaries is the sufficient force that effects filtration.

The glomerular ultrafiltration is governed by the glomerular blood pressure (GBP), plasma protein osmotic pressue (PPOP) and the intracapsular hydrostatic pressure (ICHP). Among these, the GBP is the driving force of filtration while the PPOP and ICHP are the forces opposing filtration. The difference between the driving force and the sum of two opposing forces represents the effective filtration pressure (EFP) which determines the rate of glomerular filtration.

The average blood pressure of glomerular blood pressure is 75 mm of Hg. This pressure is counteracted by plasma protein osmotic pressure (PPOP) which is about 30 mm of Hg and intracapsular hydrostatic pressure

(ICHP) or pressure in Bowman's capsule which is about 20 mm of Hg. Thus, the effective filtration pressure (EFP) is equal to GBP minus (PPOP + ICHP), i.e., EFP = GBP – (PPOP + ICHP); 75– (30 + 20) = 25 mm of Hg which is the active force by which filtration can occur. In men, about 170 litres of filtrate is formed per day by the two kidneys.

(2) **Functions of renal tubule :**

When the glomerular filtrate passes through the renal tubule, some of its constituents are removed and returned to blood while some materials are added (or secreted) to it as a result of which the filtrate is converted to urine. Thus, in the process of urine formation, the renal tubule performs two functions—**reabsorption** and **secretion.**

(a) **Tubular reabsorption :** By reabsorption capacity the renal tubule eliminates only 1 to 1.5 litres of **glomerular filtrate in the form of urine** from 170 litres of glomerular filtrate and the remaining part is returned back to the blood. The epithelial cells lining the renal tubule take up various materials from the tubular fluid (i.e., the glomerular filtrate) and transfer them to blood through the peritubular blood capillaries. This phenomenon of returning back of constituents from tubular filtrate to blood is known as reabsorption to distinguish it from 'absorption' that occurs in the intestine. This tubular reabsorption is very essential bacause without this phenomenon various useful substances like glucose, salts, etc that are needed for proper functioning of the body would be lost through urine.

The tubular reabsorption has two characteristic features. Firstly, all materials present in the glomerular filtrate are not reabsorbed; the renal tubules reabsorb only those substances which are essential and useful for the body. Secondly the rate of reabsorption of different materials are not same. Some substances are normally reabsorbed entirely so that they are not eliminated through urine at all; such substances are called **threshold substances.** On the other hand, some substances (e.g., salts) are reabsorbed only to such extents that are sufficient to maintain their normal blood levels. So, it is apparent that the renal tubules reabsorb the substances according to their need in the body. Hence, this phenomenon is also called **selective reabsorption.** The renal tubules reabsorb water and other dissolved substances from the lumen of the tubule back into the blood stream. The reabsorption is differential and purposefully selective. Each substance is reabsorbed to a particular degree. The more useful substances are reabsorbed to a higher degree than the less useful ones.

The tubular reabsorption may be active or passive process. The active reabsorption requires expenditure of energy (ATP) and may even take place against a concentration gradient, whereas the passive reabsorption includes a gradient of concentration or electrical potential without requiring energy. The proximal convoluted tubule is the principal site of reabsorption as it contains brush-bordered cells having a large surface area. These cells also contain a large number of mitochondria for generation of energy which is needed for active reabsorption.

Normally the **glucose** present in the capsular filtrate is completely absorbed from the proximal convoluted tubule by an active process so that no glucose is found in urine. Small quantities of **plasma proteins** may be filtered in the glomeruli. However, they are not allowed to pass out through urine and are completely reabsorbed from the proximal tubule by a **pinocytic process.** Na^+ is also reabsorbed by active process. Most of the filtered sodium is reabsorbed by the renal tubule and only a small quantity of it is excreted in urine. Reabsorption of chloride, bicarbonate and phosphate anions are generally linked with simultaneous reabsorption of cations, mainly the sodium. Again, chloride and bicarbonate ions are reabsorbed from both proximal and distal tubules whereas the phosphate ions are reabsorbed mainly from the proximal tubule.

Again, reabsorption of K^+ occurs completely from the proximal convoluted tubule by an active mechanism. But some amount of K^+ is secreted within the distal tubule which is observed in urine and this secretion of K^+ is linked with the reabsorption of Na^+.

Most of the water filtered in the glomeruli (about 168.5 litres out of 170 litres per day) is reabsorbed from the proximal, distal and collecting tubules. The reabsorption of water is a passive process which occurs due to osmotic gradient caused by the active reabsorption of sodium salts. That's why the volume of the glomerular filtrate is reduced tremendously before it is converted to urine. When water content is decreased in the body, secretion of ADH from the posterior pituitary gland increases. ADH enhances the permeability of water and thus, increases the reabsorption of water from the proximal and distal convoluted tubules and to some extent from collecting tubules.

Podocyte : Podocytes are located around the glomerular capillaries. They have long cytoplasmic extensions called primary processes which embrace the capillaries giving rise to short secondary foot processes (pedicles) which interdigitate with those of other primary processes. The secondary foot processes are directly applied to the basement membrane and bound to it by fine filaments. The gaps between adjacent secondary foot processes, known as filtration slits, are of uniform width (25 mm) and bridged by a delicate electron dense diaphragm. The ultra-structural features of the podocyte cytoplasm suggest phagocytic and secretory functions.

• **Types of nephrons :** Histologically there are three kinds of nephrons, based on the location of their renal corpuscles in the cortex.

(i) **Subcapsular or cortical nephrons** occupy the outer two-third of the cortex and make up about 85% of the total number. These nephrons have their renal corpuscles located in the outer part of the cortex. They have short loops of Henle, extending only into the outer medulla. These are typical of the nephrons where in the hairpin turn occurs in the distal straight tubule. They are smaller in size and fully functioning under normal conditions.

(ii) **Juxtamedullary nephrons** occupy the inner third of the cortex and constitute about 15% of the total number. Their renal corpuscles occur in proximity to the base of a medullary pyramid. They have long loops of Henle and long ascending thin segments that extend well into the inner region of the pyramid. These nephrons are large in size and work only in conditions of stress.

(iii) **Intermediate or mid-cortical nephrons** have their renal corpuscles in the mid-region of the cortex. Their loops of Henle are of intermediate length.

(b) **Formation of some new substances and secretion :** During maximum reabsorption of NaCl and water, glucose, amino acid, etc., certain new substances such as NH_3, inorganic phosphates, hippuric acid, etc. are also synthetised in the proximal convoluted part of the renal tubule. K^+, H^+, NH_3, hippuric acid, etc. are secreted from the distal convolted tubule. In this region Na^+ are replaced by K^+, H^+ or NH_3. H^+, hippuric acid, etc. are secreted actively but NH_3 is secreted passively (by diffusion). Due to addition of hydrogen ions, the urine becomes acidic in the distal convoluted tubule.

(c) **Secretion :** Tubular reabsorption removes substances from the filtrate into the blood and the tubular secretion adds materials to the filtrate from the blood. So these products of metabolism which are not all required by the body, they are rather injurious to health, are secreted out by the tubular epithelium in the tubular filtrate. The secreted substances include potassium, hydrogen, NH_3, creatine, uric acid, para-amino hippuric acid, etc. A certain amount of CO_2

normally diffuses from the peri-tubular blood into the cells of distal tubules and collecting ducts. Inside the epithelial cells, the CO_2 combines with water to form H_2CO_3, which then dissociates into H^+ ions and bicarbonate (HCO_3^-) ions. A low blood pH stimulates the cell to secrete the hydrogen ions into the urine. The H^+ ions, secreted into the tubular filtrate combine with HCO_3, HPO_4 and NH_3 to form H_2CO_3, HPO_4 and NH_4 respectively. Such reactions, therefore, fix up the H^+ ions in the tubular fluid and prevent their reabsorption.

Functions of kidney and glomerulus :

(i) It eliminates toxic substances and metabolic waste products, particularly nitrogenous substances.

(ii) Maintains water balance of the body and thereby plasma volume.

(iii) Helps to maintain the normal hydrogen ion concentration of body fluids and electrolytes.

(iv) Regulates blood pressure and osmotic pressure in blood and tissues.

(v) Plays an important role in vitamin D metabolism.

(vi) Helps in the regulation of erythropoiesis (formation and maturation of RBC) through the formation of erythropoietin hormone.

(vii) Manufactures certain substances like NH_3, hippuric acid and inorganic phosphates.

(viii) Helps in the regulation of blood pressure during hypoxia, in condition of emergency through the liberation of renin from the juxtaglomerular apparatus.

2(C) THE SPLEEN

The spleen is the largest lymphoid tissue of the body and specialised bean-shaped organ for filtering blood. The spleen is about the size of a clenched fist and is the largest lymphatic organ. In the adult, spleen weighs around 150 gm, though this varies with nutritional status and physical health. A large part of the reticulo-endothelial tissue of the body is also concentrated in it. There is no afferent lymphatic vessels.

Anatomy

The spleen is covered by the peritoneum; immediately beneath this is the **capsule.** Many **trabeculae** or **septa** radiate from the capsule and extend into the substance of the organ. The trabeculae consisting of dense connective tissue branch and anastomose within the gland substance [Fig 2(c).1].

Location

The spleen is a highly vascular haemopoietic organ situated in the left hypochondrium directly beneath the diaphragm, above the left kidney and descending colon.

Histology

Structurally, it consists of (i) **capsule** with its outer covering the **peritoneum,** (ii) **trabeculae** with blood vessels or without blood vessels, (iii) **hilus** (hilum), (iv) **white pulp,** (v) **red pulp,** (vi) **reticular mesh work,** (vii) blood vessels. Spleen consists of the following two main structures :

I. Capsule : The spleen is enclosed by a dense connective tissue capsule from which trabeculae extend into the parenchyma of the organ. This connective tissue capsule is again enveloped by a serous membrane, the peritoneum. The peritoneum is closely adherent

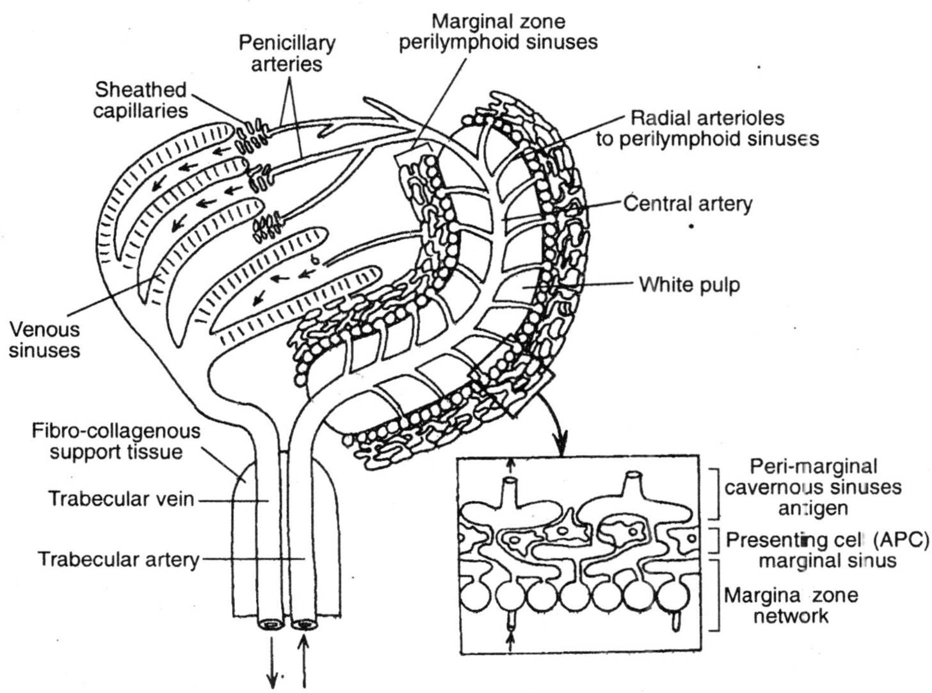

Fig. 2(c).1: Diagram showing vascular anatomy of the spleen.

to the outside. The connective tissue of the capsule and trabeculae contains **myofibroblasts.** These contractile cells also produce extracellular connective tissue fibres. The capsule is deeply indented of the medial aspect of the organ and this indentation is known as **hilus** (hilum) of the spleen. Blood capillaries, nerves and lymphatics pass through the hilus.

2. Reticular framework and splenic pulp : The spleen contains a mesh of reticular cells and reticular fibres. The parenchymal tissue which is enclosed within the capsule is the **splenic pulp.** The splenic pulp is of two distinct types—(a) White pulp and (b) Red pulp.

(a) **White pulp :** The white pulp consists of lymphatic tissue mostly white coloured lymphocytes. The white pulps are scattered all throughout the red pulp as grey patches. These grey patches at early periods were described as **Malpighian bodies.** The white pulp is the accumulation of lymphatic tissue surrounding a major arterial vessels of the spleen. This lymphatic tissue is provided with lymphocytes, plasma cells, macrophages or free cells lying in the mesh of reticular fibres.

In H & E—stained sections, white pulp appears basophilic because of the dense heterochromatin in the nuclei of the numerous lymphocytes. Branches of splenic artery course through the capsule and trabeculae of the spleen and then enter the white pulp. Within the white pulp the branch of the splenic artery is known as **central artery.** Those lymphocytes that aggregated around the central artery constitute the **periarterial lymphatic sheath (PALS).** The PALS has a roughly cylindrical configuration that conforms to the course of the central artery. In cross sections, the PALS appears circular and

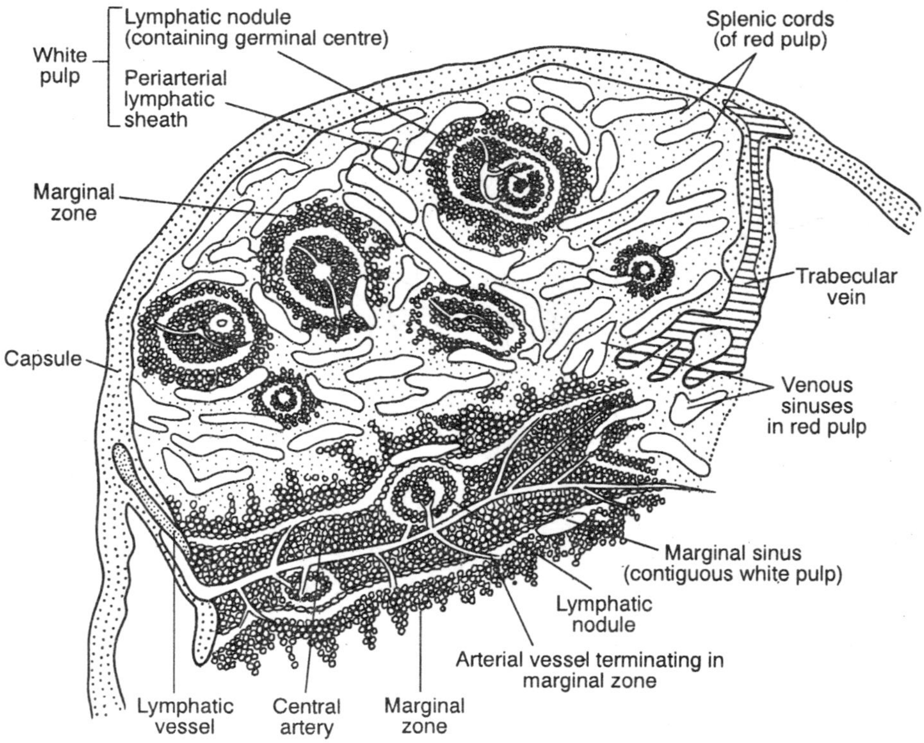

Fig. 2(c).2: Schematic diagram outlining those features of splenic structure that are evident in histologic section.

may resemble a **lymphatic nodule.** They appear as localised expansions of the PALS and tend to displace the central artery to an eccentric position. The lymphatic nodules are the territory of B-lymphocytes; other lymphocytes of the PALS are chiefly T-lymphocytes that surround the nodules. Thus, lymphoid sheath may be regarded as **thymus dependent zone** similar to the deep cortex of a lymp node. The nodules usually contain germinal centres and may become extremely large and visible with the naked eye. These enlarged nodules are called **splenic nodules** on **Malpighian corpuscles** (not to be confused with the renal corpuscles that have the same name) [Fig 2(c).2].

cords are comprised of loose mesh of reticular cells and reticular fibres that contain a large number of erythrocytes, marcrophages, lymphocytes, plasma cells, and granulocytes. Splenic macrophages phagocytose damaged erythrocytes. The iron from destroyed erythrocytes is reutilized in the formation of new RBC. **The process of haemoglobin breakdown and iron reclamation started by the splanchnic macrophages.**

The splenic and venous sinuses are special sinusoidal vessels lined by rod-shaped endothelial cells. The venous sinuses form an anastomosing network penatrating the whole of the red pulp. The sinus has a wide lumen

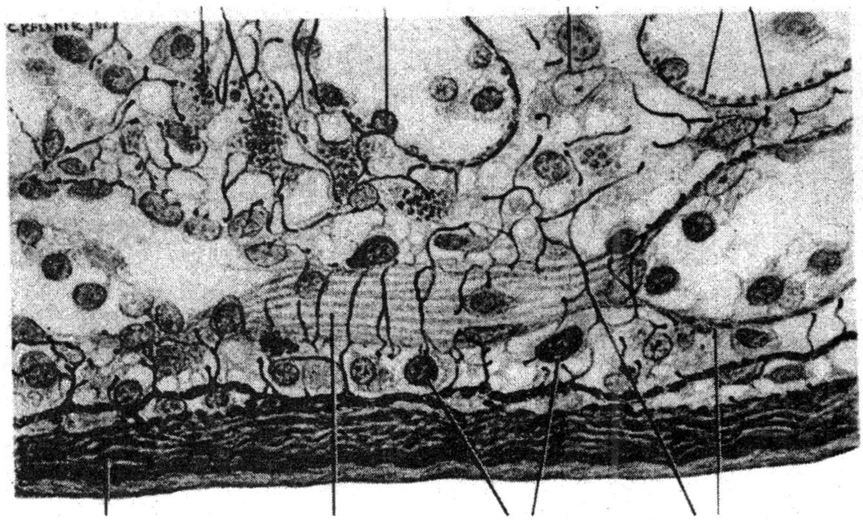

Fig. 2(c).3: This low-magnification photomicrograph of the spleen reveals the same components shown in the previous drawing. Note the capsule with several trabeculae projecting into the substance of the spleen. In the centre, there is a trabecula containing a trabecular vein through which blood leaves the organ. The red pulp constitutes the greater bulk of the splenic tissue. The white pulp contains lymphatic tissue that follows and ensheathes the central artery. Expansion of the white pulp creates the splenic nodules × 45.

(b) **Red pulps :** The red pulp is a dark red mass containing a large number of red blood cells. Essentially, red pulp consists of **splenic sinuses** which are separated by **splenic cords** (cords of **Billroth**). The splenic and its outline is fluted in appearance. The sinus wall is not endothelium; it is made up of phagocytic **fixed macrophages** supported externally by reticulin fibres. There are small slit-like openings in the sinus wall

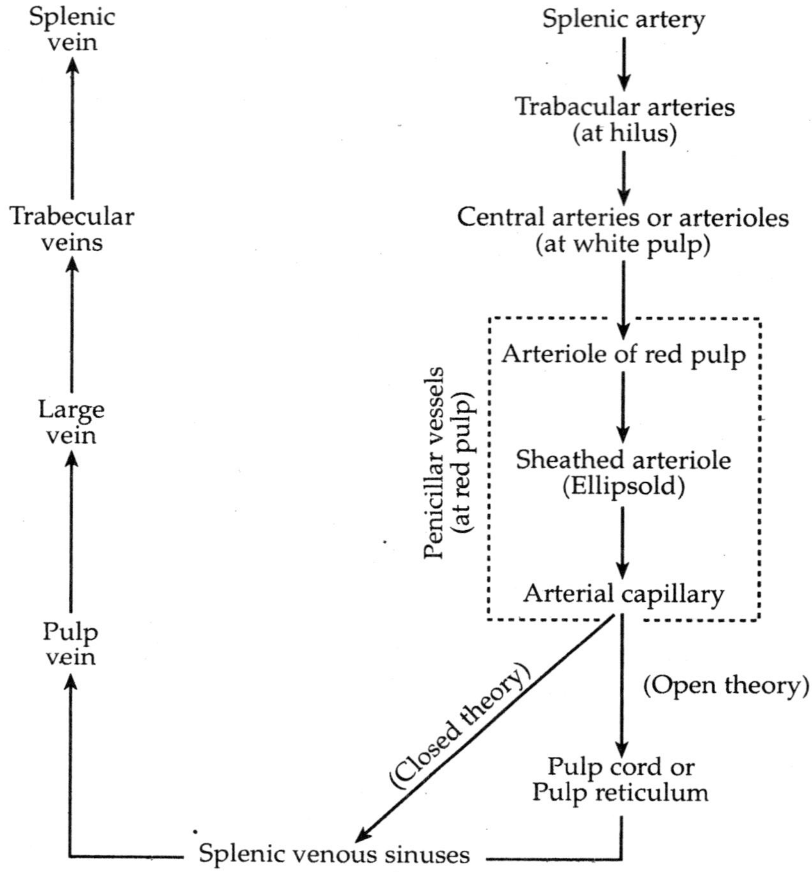

Fig. 2(c).4: Schematic representation of the anatomy of circulation in spleen.

through which blood cells pass freely. The venous sinuses drain into the veins, which ultimately join to pass into the trabeculae.

Marginal zone : It is the junctional region in between the white pulp and the red pulp, and consists of a mesh of branched reticular cells in association with extracellular reticulum, into which many arterial vessels open.

Splenic circulation : At the hilus of the spleen, arteries enter and divide into several interlobular branches which pass along the trabeculae and finally enter the splenic parenchyma. The splenic artery loses its adventitia within the parenchyma and takes the character of reticular tissue and afterward become infiltrated with lymphocyte. Now the vessels are ensheathed with lymphocyte forming the periarterial lymphatic sheath. A greater infiltration of lymphocyte constituting the splenic nodule of white pulp occurs at various points along the blood vessels.

Thus, after leaving the trabeculae as a series of **central arteries** surrounded by T-lymphocytes pass through the white pulp where the central arteries give off several branches. From here the central arteries enter the red pulp through a series of specialised vessels (such as penicillar vessels and sheathed arterioles) to drain into the splenic parenchyma. The blood then percolates through spaces between the reticular cells forming the **splenic cords** and squeezes through narrow slit spaces to enter the **splenic venous sinuses.**

There are two theories regarding the opening of the arterial capillaries into sinuses. According to **open theory** the arterial capillary drains into the pulp reticulum or pulp cord and then blood gradually filters into the splenic venous sinuses. According to **closed theory** some of the blood from the sheathed capillaries passes directly to the splenic sinuses of the red pulp. The splenic venous sinuses have got irregular anastomosing tunnels throughout the red pulp. Now the blood from these sinuses empty into the **pulp vein** which combines to constitute the large veins and finally blood comes back in the **trabecular vein.** In the hilus many trabecular veins unite to form **splenic veins** and as such leave the spleen [Fig 2(c).4].

Functions of spleen :

(1) **Formation of blood :** During early foetal life the spleen acts as a haemopoietic organ of some importance but in normal adult life it never functions in the formation of RBC.

(2) **Blood destruction :** The large amount of reticuloendothelial tissue in the spleen is of importance for the assimilation of the fragments of RBC. These fragments are phagocytosed by the free and fixed macrophages of the red pulp and lining cells of the sinuses. Thus, in the postnatal life, spleen acts as a filter, which removes the old useless corpuscles and allows only the young active corpuscles to pass into the circulation. So, in brief, the spleen acts as removal and destruction of senescent, damaged and abnormal erythrocytes and platelets.

(3) **Reservoir for blood :** Spleen acts as a reservoir of blood. It is observed that the spleen may release about 150 ml of blood (mainly RBC) to circulation.

(4) **Formation of antibodies :** Plasma cells found in the red pulp of the spleen help in the production of antibodies against antigen present in circulating blood.

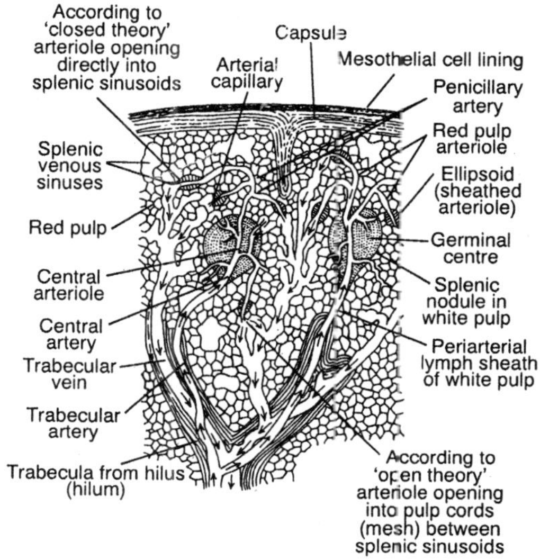

Fig. 2(c).5: Anatomy of circulation in a splenic lobule slowing both closed circulation and open circulation (diagrammatic).

(5) **Act as lymphatic organ :** Proliferation of lymphocytes and differentiation of B-cells and plasma cells, as well as secretion of antibodies occur in the white pulp of the spleen, in this regard the white pulp is equivalent pulp to other lymphatic organs.

(6) **Storage of iron :** Retrieval of iron from erythrocyte haemoglobin, i.e., the iron moiety of the haemoglobin which is freed from the stroma of the destroyed erythrocyte is stored in macrophages until it is required by the body for the resynthesis of fresh haemoglobin.

(7) **Defensive action :** (i) It exhibits antigen presentation by APCs (= antigen presenting cells) and initiation of immune response. Many pyroninophil cells (probably plasma cells) are noticed in the splenic red pulp and hence, the spleen is principal site of immune body formation.

(ii) The R.E. cells engulf bacteria, parasites like those of *Leishmania donovani* of kala-azar and foreign particles.

CHAPTER 3

Endocrine Glands and Hormones

The endocrine system is comprised of certain specialised ductless (endocrine) glands or tissues which manufacture certain chemical substances into the blood stream through which they are carried to different parts of the body and they produce regulatory effects on specific target tissues. Endocrinology (Gr. endo = within; crin = to secrete; logos = study of) is the science which is concerned with the structure and functions of the endocrine glands and the diagnosis and treatment of disorders of the endocrine system. **The glands which are devoid of ducts, and have to depend upon the blood stream and to some extent upon the lymph, to carry their secretions (hormones) to various parts of the body are called endocrine glands.** Their secretions are called **hormones**.

The endocrine glands exhibit the following characteristics :

(i) The glands must be ductless and highly vascularised.

(ii) These glands must be able to synthesise a definite chemical messenger or hormone which is transported into the blood stream leaving the organ.

(iii) The material secreted must have certain important physiological functions.

Types of endocrine glands

Vertebrate endocrine glands can be classified into following categories :

A. Classification on the basis of nature of secretion :

(i) **Classical endocrine glands :** These are typical ductless glands and they secrete the hormones into the blood stream which act on some target tissues, e.g., adenohypophysis, thyroid, adrenal cortex, etc.

(ii) **Mixed endocrine glands :** The glands, which are both structurally and functionally exocrine (with duct) and endocrine (ductless) in nature, are called mixed endocrine glands, e.g., pancreas, testis, ovary.

(iii) **Neuroendocrine glands :** There are some endocrine glands which are provided with neural tissues. The secretion of those glands is called **neuro-hormones**. The neuro hormone is produced within the specialised nerve cells and is secreted from the nerve endings into the circulation. The functioning of the neuro-endocrine glands is closely linked to that of the pituitary and adrenal glands.

B. Classification of endocrine glands on the basis of position :

(i) **Cranial endocrine glands :** These glands are housed within the cranium, e.g., pituitary gland, hypothalamus, pineal gland.

(ii) **Pharyngeal endocrine glands :** These endocrine glands are situated in pharyngeal region or neck region; e.g., thyroid gland, parathyroid gland, thymns gland.

(iii) **Abdominal endocrine glands :** These endocrine glands are found in the abdominal region; e.g., pancreas, adrenal gland, ovary, testis.

C. Classification on the basis of number of endocrine glands :

(i) **Unilateral endocrone glands :** These endocrine glands are single in number, e.g., pituitary gland, pancreas, pineal gland.

(ii) **Bilateral endocrine glands :** These endocrine glands are paired in number, e.g., thyroid gland, adrenal gland, parthyroid gland.

D. Classification on the basis of secretion :

(i) **Telecrine glands :** Hormones are secreted by specialised endocrine tissue into the extracellular space and are then transported by blood to the distant target cells. Examples—thyroid gland, pituitary gland, adrenal gland, etc.

(ii) **Paracrine gland :** Where the released hormone diffuses to its adjacent target cells through the immediate extracellular space, such as, in Islets of Langerhans, somatostatin is released from δ-cells that reacts on adjacent α-and β-cells. Secreting cells are termed as neurosecretory cells. They pour the neurohormones into the blood strean which act at a distant site. Examples of those glands are neurohypophysis, adrenal medulla, hypothalamus, pineal gland, etc.

(iii) **Specialised endocrine organs :** These organs are not endocrine organs as a whole but they are provided with some specialised endocrine tissues. They help in the production of some hormones or hormone-like chemical messengers. Examples of such organs are thymus, kidney, etc.

Ordinary glands (having an excretory duct) secrete their products into the duct through which the secretions are drained into the site of their action; these are termed as **exocrine glands,** e.g., salivary gland, sweat gland, liver, etc. On the other hand, since the endocrine glands do not possess any duct, the secretions of those glands (pituitary, thyroid, pancreas, etc) are conveyed directly into the blood stream. Thus, the hormones are transported throughout the body by the circulating blood, and they exert regulatory influence on various tissues.

Differences between Exocrine and Endocrine Glands

Exocrine Gland	Endocrine Gland
(i) Exocrine glands are those glands which have ducts to discharge their secretions into the body surface or the cavities in the body; hence, they are also called **ductular** glands.	(i) Endocrine glands are those glands which lack ducts for the transportation of their secretion but pour them directly into the blood stream. Therefore, these glands are called **ductless** glands.
(ii) The secretions are conveyed to specific parts of the body through the ducts where they exert their action.	(ii) The secretions (i.e., hormones) are carried throughout the body by the blood (circulating medium) but they exert their actions on specific tissues.
(iii) The exocrine glands are not concerned with regulation of various systems and coordination between them.	(iii) The endocrine glands are concerned with regulation and coordination of the activities of various systems.
(iv) The glands secrete digestive enzymes or excretory materials.	(iv) These glands secrete hormones that are metabolic regulators.

Mammalian endocrine system

A number of endocrine glands are found in the vertebrate animals including human beings. These include hypothalamus, pituitary, thyroid, thymus, pineal, parathyroid, adrenals, islets of Langerhans (in pancreas), testes (in male), ovary (in female) and hormonal tissues of gastro-intestinal tract (Fig 3.1).

HYPOTHALAMUS

Hypothalamus is a part of the fore brain. Its hypothalamic nuclei (masses of gray matter having neurons) are housed within the white matter of the third ventricle (cavity) of brain. The neurons of hypothalamic nuclei produce chemicals which are released into the blood. The venous blood of hypothalamus is drained by a portal vein which passes through the stalk of pituitary (hypophysis) and supplies the adenohypophysis. The hormones of hypothalamus stimulate the cells of adenohypophysis to release various hormones. Hence, these neuro-secretions or hormones are known as **'releasing factors'.**

Hormones and chief functions

The hormones secreted by the hypothalamus are called **neurohormones.** The

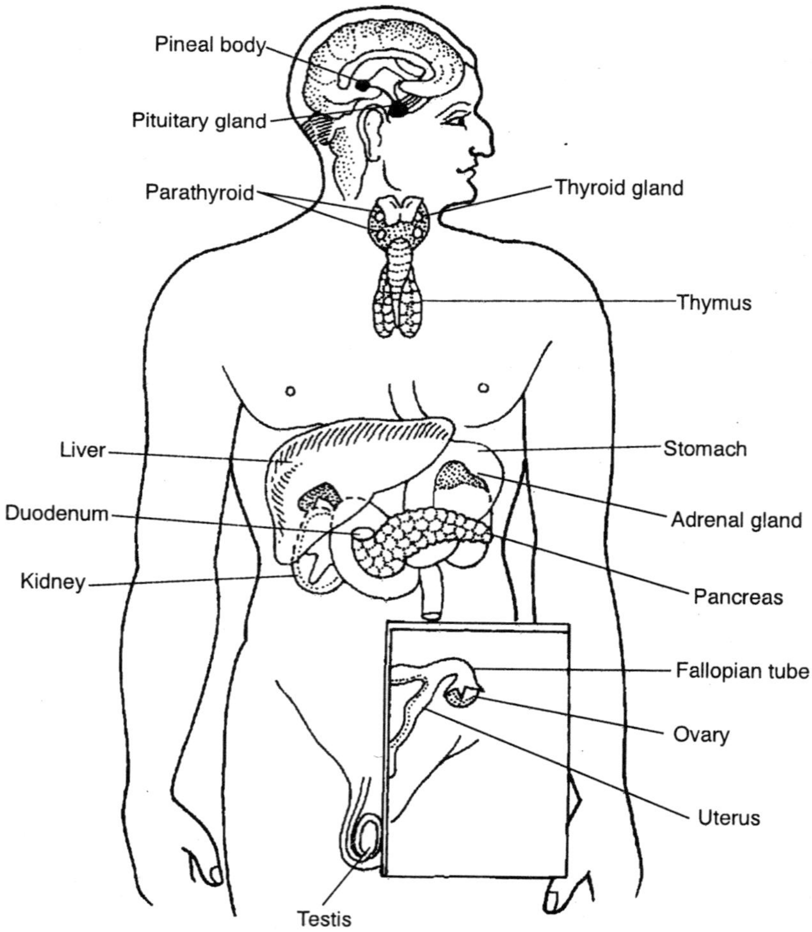

Fig. 3.1: Diagram showing approximate location of endocrine glands.

neurohormones are carried by the portal vein to the adenohypophysis to release its hormones. So hypothalamic hormones are also known as **releaser hormones** (RH). Certain hypothalamic hormones inhibit the action of some of the pituitary hormones. Such hormones are termed as **inhibitory hormones or factors** (IH or IF).

(i) **Thyrotropin releasing factor (TRF)** stimulates adenohypophysis to secrete TSH.

(ii) **Corticotropin releasing factor (CRF)** stimulates adenohypophysis to secrete ACTH.

(iii) **Prolactin releasing factor (PRF)** stimulates to release prolactin hormone.

(iv) **Somatostatin** inhibits the secretion of GH from anterior pituitary.

(v) **Growth hormone releasing factor (GHRF)** controls the release of GH.

(vi) **Follicle stimulating hormone and Luteinizing hormone releasing factor (FSH and LHRF)** induce adenohypophysis to release FSH and LH.

PITUITARY GLAND (HYPOPHYSIS)

Pituitary gland is also known as **hypophysis** (Gr. **Hypo,** under; **Physis,** growth) because it is located under the brain. It is enclosed within a small bony cavity, the sella turcica, of the sphenoid bone. A small stalk, called pituitary stalk, attaches the pituitary with the hypothalamus. The pituitary gland is a reddish, small, rounded or oval, unpaired structure about the size of a large pea. It weighs 0.5 to 0.6 gm in adult human beings.

> **Pituitary gland** secretes some trophic hormones, which perform a master role to control the functional activities of almost all endocrine glands of the body; hence, it is known as the **master gland** or the **endocrine king**.

Anatomically in most vertebrates, the pituitary gland consists of two parts : **adenohypophysis** or **anterior lobe** and **neurohypophysis** or **posterior lobe.**

I. Adenohypophysis or **anterior pituitary :** It is the glandular part of the pituitary and has three subdivisions, anteriorly the **pars distalis,** medially the **pars intermedia** and superiorly the **pars tuberalis.** Pars distalis is the only functionally active part of the adenohypophysis. Histologically it comprises of six different kinds of cells which secrete six different types of **trophic hormones.**

> • **Trophic hormones :** Those hormones which regulate the functional activities of other endocrine glands (i.e., target glands) are called **trophic hormones.**

Secretory hormones and chief functions

(i) **Somatotrophic hormone (STH) or growth hormone (GH)** regulates growth of the body tissues in general.

(ii) **Thyroid stimulating hormone (TSH) or thyrotrophin** stimulates thyroid to secrete thyroxin.

(iii) **Adrenocorticotrophic hormone (ACTH)** is essential for the growth and secretion of the adrenal cortex to release steroid hormones (corticosteroids).

(iv) **Follicle stimulating hormone (FSH)** is essential for the development of the ovarian follicle, i.e., maturation of the graafian follicle and secretion of estrogens. In male it stimulates spermatogenesis.

(v) **Luteinizing hormone (LH) or Interstitial cell stimulating hormone (ICSH)** is necessary for the development of corpus luteum and controls the secretion of progesterone. In male, it stimulates the interstitial cells of Leydig in testis to secrete the male sex hormone, testosterone into the blood stream.

(vi) **Lactogenic hormone or prolactin or Luteotrophic hormone (LTH)** is one of the gonadotrophic hormone secreted by the pituitary gland and it controls proliferation of the mammary gland tissue to initiate the secretion of milk.

Pars intermedia is an intermediate lobe of adenohypophysis which secretes a protein hormone, called **melanocyte-stimulating hormone** (MSH) or **intermedin**. This hormone controls skin pigmentation in amphibians.

II. Neurohypophysis : It is the neural division of pituitary and comprises of **pars nervosa** (the principal part), **median eminence** (upper expanded part of neural stalk) and **infundibular stem**. Anatomically, the pars nervosa and pars intermedia are together known as posterior lobe of pituitary.

The posterior pituitary releases two specific neurohormones; **oxytocin and vasopressin (antidiuretic hormone).**

> • **Neurohormones** : The chemical substances which are secreted or released from the neurosecretory cells of hypothalamus are called neurohormones. After secretion they are transported through the axons of neurons, it then passes into posterior pituitary from here into the blood to the distant places.

Secretory hormones and specific functions :

(i) **Oxytocin** causes a stimulating effect on the uterine contraction and thus helps in parturition. It also causes a contraction of the ducts of the mammary gland and helps in the expulsion of milk.

(ii) **Vasopressin or antidiuretic hormone (ADH)** stimulates reabsorption of water through the renal tubules and reduces water loss in urine. A decreased secretion of ADH causes diuresis and the condition is known as **diabetes insipidus.**

THYROID GLAND

In human, the thyroid gland is a bilobed structure, situated on either side of the trachea, and each lobe is joined with the other by an isthmus. This gland occupies the position in front of the 2nd, 3rd and 4th tracheal rings, slightly below the larynx.

The thyroid is covered by two layers of fibrous connective tissues. The weight of the thyroid gland of the adult varies between 20 to 25 gm. The thyroid gland consists of two almost symmetrical lateral lobes. The two lobes are joined together by a narrow strip of tissue, called **isthmus** or middle lobe. Each lobe is provided with many follicles of variable size. Each follicle is lined by single layer of granular cubical cells and filled with homogeneous gelatinous substance, called colloid. In between the follicles, there are blood vessels and connective tissues. In this region there are some specialised secretory cells containing lesser number of high cubical **mitochondria-rich cells.** These cells are called **parafollicular cells.**

Secretory hormones and chief functions :

(i) **Thyroxine or tetraiodothyronine (T_4)** and **triiodothyronine (T_3)** are the two hormones which are the iodinated derivatives of tyrosin. These two hormones are secreted by the chief follicular cells of thyroid. They are generally referred to as **thyroid hormones.** In human beings the main functions of thyroid hormones are to increase cell metabolism and energy production. They also regulate growth and sexual maturity.

(ii) **Thyrocalcitonin** is another hormone which is secreted by the parafollicular cells of thyroid. It helps to decrease the blood calcium level by preventing reabsorption of bone.

THYMUS

Thymus is a lymphoid organ which is situated in the thoracic region in the anterior and posterior mediastina behind the sternum.

It lies between the posterior part of the thyroid gland and the anterior end of the pericardium. Thymus is made up of two elongated and flask-shaped asymmetrical lobes, the left one is smaller than the right one. Thymus gland is large during childhood but shrinks after the onset of adolescence. So in adults, the thymus is composed largely of fat and connective tissue and probably it remains nonfunctional. This gland is made up of lymphoid tissue (lymphocytes) and is structurally similar to lymph gland.

Secretory hormones and chief functions : Thymopoietin or thymin and **thymosin** are two peptide hormones which are secreted from this gland.

(i) **Thymosin** increases the formation of lymphocytes and initiates production of antibodies.

(ii) **Thymin** influences neuromuscular transmission by inhibiting the release of acetylcholine from motor nerve endings.

PINEAL GLAND

The pineal gland is a small, pea-sized, conical pinkish body, situated on the dorsal surface of the brain in between the cerebrum and the cerebellum. This neural gland is connected with the roof of the fore-brain by a hollow stalk. It is made up mainly of parenchymatous cells, called **pinealocytes,** and some star-shaped supporting cells.

Secretory hormones and functions : The chief hormone of this neuro endocrine organ is an amine, called **melatonin.** The physiological function of melatonin in man is not clear. In rats and hamsters, it acts as an inhibitor of ovarian growth and estrus incidence. The melatonin causes a marked lightening of the skin.

PARATHYROID GLAND

In man there are four small oval brownish-red bodies embedded in the posterior surface of thyroid glands.

Each parathyroid is made up of masses or columns of epitheloid cells and numerous blood sinuses in between them. The epitheloid cells can be distinguished into two types—**chief or principal cells** and **oxyphil** or **eosinophil cells.** The chief cells are agranular, present in large number and are responsible for secretion of the hormone of this gland. The oxyphil cells are granular, very few in number and their function is unknown.

Secretory hormones and chief functions : Parathyroid secretes **parathormone (PTH).** It is a protein hormone secreted from the chief cells. PTH increases blood calcium and accelerates excretion of phosphate.

ADRENAL GLAND

The human adrenal glands are roughly triangular in shape, two in number, and each gland is situated at the top of each kidney like a cap. For this reason the gland is also known as **supra-renal gland.** The average weight of each gland in adult is about 5 gm.

The adrenal gland is covered by a fibrous capsule. The glandular tissue of adrenal is divisible into two distinct parts, outer adrenal cortex and inner adrenal medulla.

I. Adrenal cortex : It is made up of polyhedral cells containing prominent nucleus, mitochondria, golgi body and numerous lipid granules. These cells are arranged in three layers from outside inwards—**zona glomerulosa, zona fasciculata, zona reticularis.**

Secretory hormones and chief functions : A number of cortical hormones are secreted from the adrenal cortex. They are grouped into three categories :

(i) **Glucocorticoids** take part in regulation of carbohydrate, protein and fat metabolism, example—cortisol, cortisone, corticosterone, etc.

(ii) **Mineralocorticoids** increase sodium retention, potassium elimination and water retention; example—aldosterone.

(iii) **Sex steroids** influence the sex organs and secondary sex characters. Thus, sex steroids maintain the sexual activity of an individual; example—androgen, estrogen, progesterone, etc.

Aldosterone escape : It has been shown that aldosterone influences the increase of Na^+ reabsorption in kidney. But there is some limitations, beyond which an increase in aldosterone level cannot increase Na^+ reabsorption. So, even in presence of sufficient aldosterone, Na^+ passes out through urine; this is termed as **aldosterone escape.**

II. Adrenal medulla : The innermost part of the adrenal gland is called adrenal medulla. It is comprised of densely packed polyhedral cells surrounded by blood sinuses. The cells are provided with a large number of granules, **chromaffin granules.** Hence, the cells are known as **chromaffin cells.**

Secretory hormones and chief functions : The chromaffin cells of adrenal medulla secrete two hormones of **catecholamine** group, mainly **adrenalin or epinephrine** and to a smaller extent **noradrenalin** or **norepinephrine.**

Epinephrine increases blood pressure, blood sugar and heart rate; inhibits gestrointestinal tract; hastens blood coagulation; decreases glycogen in liver.

Except for a few instances, the actions of epinephrine and norepinephrine are same. Norepinephrine is more closely sympathomimetic than epinephrine.

• **Catecholamines** are amine derivatives of catechol compounds derived from the phenolic amino-acid tyrosine. They include adrenalin, noradrenalin and dopamine which act as neurohormones or neurotransmitters. Catecholamine are stored within the adrenal medulla and sympathetic postganglionic nerve endings. The adrenal medullary hormones (epinephrine and norepinephrine) assist the body to fight against, i.e., to adjust with the emergency conditions. That's why the hormones are aslo known as **emergency hormones.** They are responsible for production of physiological reactions such as palpitation, piloerection, papillary dilation, etc in conditions of emotion (i.e., fear, anger, pleasure).

Differences between Glucocorticoids and Mineralocorticoids

Subject	Glucocorticoids (Gc)	Mineralocorticoids (Mc)
1. Origin	Originate from all the three layers of adrenal cortex but mainly from zona fasciculata.	Originate from zona glomerulosa (outermost layer) of adrenal cortex only.
2. Actions	(i) Exert potent effect in carbohydrate, protein and fat metabolisms.	(i) Exert less potent effect on carbohydrate, fat and protein metabolisms.
	(ii) Less effective in raising blood volume and blood pressure.	(ii) Very effective in raising blood volume and blood pressure.
	(iii) Less potent in stimulating reabsorption of Na^+ from renal tubules of kidney.	(iii) Much potent in stimulating Na^+ from kidney tubules.
3. Regulation	The secretion of glucocorticoids is controlled by ACTH of adenohypophysis.	The secretion of mineralocorticoids is controlled by kidney through renin-angiotensin mechanism.

Differences between Corticotrophin and Corticoids

Subject	Corticotrophin	Corticoids
1. Origin	Secreted from corticotroph kind of basophil cells of adenohypophysis.	These are released from the adrenal cortex.
2. Chemical nature	It is a peptide hormone.	These are three kinds—glucocorticoids, mineralocorticoids and sex steriods.
3. Type	It has no types i.e., it is a single hormone.	These are steroid hormones.
4. Actions	(i) Acts through cell membrane receptors and cAMP. (ii) Maintains the structure and function of adrenal cortex and thereby affects the tissue metabolism indirectly.	(i) Acts through intracellular receptors and protein synthesis. (ii) Affects the tissue metabolism by modifying the enzymes in the tissues.

ISLETS OF LANGERHANS (PANCREAS)

Pancreas is a composite or compound racemose (mixed) gland. It is a pink coloured gland and lies in the abdominal cavity, in between the stomach and duodenum. It is composed of both **exocrine** and **endocrine** glandular cells. The endocrine tissues of pancreas are called **Islets of Langerhans** that remain scattered here and there in between the acinar tissue. Three main kinds of endocrine cells are found in the islets of most vertebrates which secrete hormones. These are α-cells or A-cells, β-cells or B-cells and δ-cells or D-cells. Among these, β-cells are most abundant, α-cells are relatively fewer and δ-cells are least in number.

Secretory hormones and chief functions : The pancreatic islets secrete polypeptide hormones. Separate hormones are formed from each of the three cell types found in the Islets of Langerhans. The β-cells secrete **insulin,** the α-cells secrete **glucagon** and the δ-cells secrete **somatostatin.**

(i) **Insulin** plays a vital role in the regulation of level of glucose in blood. On reaching the liver, insulin promotes glycogenesis, i.e., synthesis of glycogen from glucose.

(ii) **Glucagon's** action is just opposite to that of insulin. Glucagon increases the amount of glucose in the blood. It stimulates glycogenolysis, i.e., conversion of liver glycogen into glucose.

Thus, insulin and glucagon together control the carbohydrate metabolism of the body.

(iii) **Somatostatin** stimulates gastric motility and inhibits the secretion of insulin and glucagon. It also reduces the secretion of gastrin and secretion from the gastro-intestinal mucosa.

TESTIS

Testes are the primary reproductive organs in male situated outside the body cavity, enclosed within a sac like structure, the scrotum. Each testis is an oval glandular organ covered by a tough, compact, fibrous capsule, the **tunica albuginea**. The gland is divided into a number of conical lobules by trabeculae, which descend from the tunica albuginea. The lobules are filled with highly convoluted tubular structures, called **seminiferous tubules.** Each seminiferous tubule is lined internally by five layers of spermatogenic cells from outside inwards. These are

Distinguish between Insulin and Glucagon

Subject	Insulin	Glucagon
1. Origin	1. Insulin is secreted from β-cells of Islets of Langerhans.	1. Glucagon is secreted from the α-cells of Islets of Langerhans.
2. Chemical structure	2. It is a polypeptide made up of 51 amino acids having 2 chains joined by disulfide (s-s) linkages.	2. It is a single chain of polypeptide having 29 amino acids and is devoid of (s-s) linkage.
3. Functions	3. (i) It is an anabolic hormone. (ii) It lowers blood sugar level. (iii) It stimulates glycogenesis. (iv) It inhibits neoglucogenesis.	3. (i) It is a catabolic hormone. (ii) It increases blood sugar level. (iii) It stimulates glycogenolysis. (iv) It stimulates neoglucogenesis.

spermatogonia, primary spermatocyte, secondary spermatocyte, spermatid and spermatozoa. Groups of polyhedral cells, comprise of endocrine tissue and found in isolated clusters in the spaces between the seminiferous tubules, are known as **interstitial cells of Leydig. Sertoli cells** are elongated cells lying in between the spermatogonia.

Secretory hormone and chief functions :

(i) The interstitial cells of Leydig secrete male sex steroid hormone, called **testosterone.** Testosterone regulates the growth, maturity and functions of the primary sex organ. It stimulates the development of secondary sex characters like hairs on face (moustache and beards), axilla, pubis, chest, other parts of the body, breaking of voice (hoarseness), etc.

(ii) **Inhibin** is secreted from the sertoli cells of testis. It controls FSH secretion in male.

OVARY

The primary organs of the female reproductive system are a pair of ovaries. These are the two oval or bean-shaped ovaries situated on either side of the uterus on the lateral wall of the pelvic cavity. The normal ovary consists of six layers of **germinal epithelium, tunica albuginea, stroma, ovarian follicles, corpus luteum** and **interstitial cells.**

The germinal epithelium forms the outermost covering and gives rise to the ovarian follicles. Tunica albuginea forms a thin layer beneath the germinal epithelium. Stroma is the connective tissue network which lends support to the ovarian tissue. Ovarian follicles are known as graafian follicles. Graafian follicle produces ovum and secretes oestrogen. Corpus luteum is yellowish coloured endocrine body formed by the ruptured graafian follicle. After ovulation the ruptured graafian follicle transforms into corpus luteum. Interstitial cells are derived from the stroma cells or the unruptured ovarian follicular cells.

Secretory hormones and chief functions : Overy secretes four hormones—**oestrogen, progesterone, relaxin** and **inhibin.** Oestrogen is secreted from the ovarian follicles specially the graafian follicle. Progesterone and relaxin are secreted from corpus luteum. Inhibin is secreted from the follicular cells.

(i) **Oestrogen** promotes the development of the secondary female sexual characteristics—development of mammary gland, enlargement of genital organs and development of fat deposition around the body of female. It also participates in the regulation of menstrual cycle.

(ii) **Progesterone** is essential for the maintenance of pregnancy, i.e., embedding of ovum, formation of placenta, etc.

(iii) **Relaxin** : The main function is to facilitate the expulsion of foetus from the uterus by causing relaxation of the pelvic ligaments and cervix.

(iv) **Inhibin** helps in feedback regulation of FSH secretion from pituitary by inhibiting it.

PLACENTA

The **placenta** is purely temporary endocrine organ which is formed in early pregnancy and is expelled at birth. The name placenta has been derived from the Greek word meaning a 'flat cake'. Human placenta is a round flattened structure from which the name placenta is derived.

The embryo, specially in Eutherian mammals, becomes implanted to the uterine wall. The process of implantation involves tissue interaction and establishment of connection between the uterine wall and the extra embryonic membranes. The region of attachment between the embryonic tissue and the uterine wall is known as **placenta** and the process involved in nidation is called **placentation.** So placenta is usually defined as an apposition or fusion between uterine and embryonic tissues for physiological exchange of materials.

Structurally the placenta has two parts—a **maternal part** and a **foetal part.** The materal part comprises a few large blood sinuses. The maternal blood passes through these sinuses, arterial blood entering via uterine arteries and venous blood passing out through the uterine veins. The foetal part consists of numerous finger-like processes, the **chorionic villi,** projecting into maternal sinuses. These villi contain foetal capillaries. So the foetal blood invades into chorionic capillaries through the umbilical artery and returns to foetal body through the umbilical vein. It is to be noted that the chorionic villi remain covered by trophoblast cells. The maternal and foetal bloods come in close contact with the placenta for physiological exchange of materials, i.e., supply of O_2 and nutrients from mother's blood to foetal blood and excretion of CO_2 and other metabolic wastes from the foetal blood to the mother's blood. In addition, the trophoblast cells of placenta secrete some hormones which help in maintenance of pregnancy as well as growth and maturation of the foetus.

Hormones of placenta, and their chief functions : The hormones secreted from the placenta are **placental gonadotrophin, human placental prolactin, estrogen, progesterone, relaxin.**

(i) **Placental gonadotrophin** : It is commonly known as **human chorionic gonadotrophin (HCG).** It stimulates the corpus luteum of ovary to maintain estrogen and progesterone secretion for preventing disintegration of uterine endometrium and maintaining the uterine bed for the foetus.

(ii) **Oestrogen and progesterone** : Within 2-3 months of pregnancy, the fully developed placenta itself begins to secrete oestrogen and progesterone to maintain the remaining part of pregnancy without the involvement of ovary.

(iii) **Placental prolactin** : It promotes the growth of the foetus as well as development of mammany gland of the mother and initiates milk formation.

(iv) **Relaxin** : It is a peptide hormone released at the end of pregnancy which helps to facilitate the smooth delivery of the baby by causing relaxation of the pelvic ligaments and cervix.

GASTRO-INTESTINAL HORMONES

The mucous membrane of stomach and intestine secretes some polypeptide hormones into the blood which regulate the secretion and movement of various parts of

Distinguish between Local Hormone and Trophic Hormone

Subject	Local Hormone	Trophic Hormone
1. Site of action	1. Those hormones which are released locally and have local effect are considered as local hormones, i.e., the hormones exert their actions at a site very close to their origin.	1. Those hormones which control the secretion of hormones by other endocrine glands are called trophic hormones, i.e., the hormones exert their actions on other endocrine glands.
2. Origin	2. They are not produced and secreted by typical endocrine glands. Examples : Prostaglandins, histamine, bradykinin, adrenaline, acetylcholine, etc.	2. They are produced and secreted by the adenohypophysis. Examples : FSH, LH, LTH, TSH, ACTH, etc.

digestive tract. These hormones are referred to as **local hormones** because they originate from the gastro-intestinal tract as well as act on it.

(a) **Gastric hormone :**

(i) **Gastrin** : The pyloric mucosa of stomach near the duodenum secretes a hormone, the **gastrin.** It is peptide in nature. It stimulates oxyntic glandular cells in the stomach wall to secrete gastric juice having pepsinogen, HCl, etc. It also stimulates gastric motility.

(b) **Intestinal hormone :**

(ii) **Secretin** : It is a protein hormone secreted by the duodenal mucosa in presence of chyme coming from the stomach. The secretin stimulates the secretion of bile from liver and it stimulates the secretion and release of sodium bicarbonate from the pancreas for the pancreatic juice. In additon, secretin decreases gastric acid secretion and causes contraction of pyloric sphincter.

(iii) **Serotonin :** This hormone is secreted from **enterochromatin cells** of the intestinal mucosa. It stimulates gastro intestinal motility and inhibits gastric secretion.

(iv) **Cholecystokinin–pancreozymin (CCK-PZ)** : These two hormones are chemically indifferent, i.e., the same peptide hormones perform stimulation of gall bladder contraction and enzyme-rich pancreatic juice secretion. These two hormones are now collectively called CCK-PZ. It may also inhibit gastric emptying and stimulate intestinal motility.

(v) **Enterogastrone** : This hormone is released from duodenal mucosa. It inhibits gastric motility and gastric secretion but it stimulates the gall bladder to contract and forces its accumulation of bile to pour into the duodenum.

Prostaglandin

Prostaglandin was the name given by **von Euler** in 1935 to a substance isolated from human seminal fluid and thought to be secreted by the prostate gland. Later it was shown that the PGs found in semen are secreted mainly by the seminal vesicles. Now it has been shown that PGs are synthesized in most and possibly all organs of the body from the polyunsaturated essential fatty acids, e.g., arachidonic acid, linoleic acid and linolenic acid.

The prostaglandins are a group of C_{20} unsaturated fatty acids that are biologically active as local hormones, i.e., they act mainly on the tissues from where they originate and also on some neighbouring tissue. So, they are of autocrine or paracrine nature. The PGs may be of different types that are divided into four main groups, viz., PGE, PGF, PGA and PGB—with each individual compound being designated by a subunit.

Functions : They exhibit multivarious actions of which some important ones are as follows :

1. **Prostaglandins in reproduction** :

(i) The PGs help in sperm transport in the female genital tract. PGs deposited in the vagina during coitus may act locally on the cervix and body of the uterus so as to assist in sperm transport.

(ii) Prostaglandin $F_2\alpha$ takes part in parturition as evident from high concertration $PGF_2\alpha$ in amniotic fluid during labour.

(iii) Prostaglandins play an important role in the regulation of female reproductive cycle. There is some evidence that PGE_2 and $PGF_2\alpha$ are related with the onset of menstruation.

(iv) As umbilical cord contains high concentration of prostaglandins, it is known that they may have some role in the regulation of placental blood flow.

2. Prostaglandins may act as **neuro-transmitters** in the central nervous system (CNS).

3. PGs prevent **lipolysis** in adipose tissue.

4. They inhibit gastric acid **secretion** and **formation** of peptic ulcers.

5. PGE_1 and PGE_2 do not inhibit the increased secretion of progesterone and dihydroprogesterone in response to gonadotrophins. PGE_2 potentiates the formation of dihydroprogesterone in response to gonadotrophins and thus, they help in **steriodogenesis.**

6. The PGs decrease blood pressure by causing **vasodilation** and they may influence the activity of various smooth muscles.

HORMONES

(Greek hormo = to stimulate)

In multicellular form, in course of evolution, special systems have been developed to perform various activities. Afterwards, in course of evolution, necessity arose to correlate the functions of the different systems so that they may act harmoniously as a unit. The internal environment of the animal body is maintained in steady state by **autonomic nervous system** and the **endocrine system.** The endocrine system brings about chemical coordination by complex organic compounds, called **hormones**. The word hormone is derived from the Greek word hormo, meaning "I impel" or "I arose to activity". The term 'hormone' was first proposed by **Hardy** but applied by two British animal physiologists, **Starling** and **Bayliss** in the year 1904 to denote a specific organic substance, effective in low concentrations, which is elaborated by cells in one part of an organism and transported through the blood stream or extracellular fluid to another part (target tissue) of an organism where it acts to bring about a specific physiological effect. Thus the hormones act like **chemical messengers** for coordination of the body functions. It is well established that inter-relationships exist between the nervous and endocrine systems. The nervous system palys an important role in regulating the release of many hormones and the hormones also influence the function of nervous system either directly or indirectly. Moreover, different parts of the nervous system release some hormones called **neurohormones.** Both the systems exhibit some sort of similarities and dissimilarities. The similarities are—(i) they regulate system of the body, (ii) they have chemical system of coordination and (iii) they maintain steady stable condition in homeostasis.

Distinguish between Nervous System and Endocrine System

Subject	Nervous system	Endocrine system
1. Nature	1. Physical coordination	1. Chemical corordination.
2. Pathway	2. Through nerve fibre.	2. Through body fluid (blood).
3. Mode of transmission	3. As electrochemical nerve impulse.	3. As chemical messengers.
4. Speed	4. Quick action, but its effects are short-lived.	4. Slow action, but its effects are more prolonged.
5. Direction of information	5. Unidirectional, i.e., towards a specific direction through one or a few nerve cells, gland cells or other neurons.	5. Towards target organs.
6. Fate	6. No change.	6. Destroyed after change.

Definition

Hormones are **chemical messengers** that control the biological processes in an organism. These are also considered as **information molecules**. These are secreted in response to changes in internal or external environment and transported by the blood stream or extracellular fluid to the target organs.

1. **Hormone is an organic substance, produced by cells in a minute quantity in one part of an orgnaism and transported to other parts to exert profound effects.**
2. **The chemical agent, which is secreted from a group of cells, directly passes into the blood stream and exert the activities of the selective target cells at distant places within the body is known as hormone (Bayliss and Starling, 1904).**
3. **Hormones are information-transferring molecules, which transfer information from one set of cells to another, for the good of the cell population as a whole (Huxley, 1933).**
4. **Hormones are organic substances produced in the body in minute amount by specialised tissues (endocrine tissues) and released into the blood stream or tissue fluid having some specific regulatory effects on the activity of certain organs, usually remote from the site of their origin (Thimann, 1948).**

Characteristics of animal hormones

1. Hormones are complex organic compounds of low molecular weight and with easy solubility.
2. Hormones are synthesised in specialised tissues or organs (endocrine glands) and are usually stored in them.
3. They are of low molecular weights which make them readily diffusible.
4. Hormones are produced in some organ and influence the functioning of some other organs.
5. Hormones are of low molecular weights which make them readily diffusible from blood to target tissues.
6. Hormones are effective in minute quantities as present in the blood.
7. More than one hormone may be released by the same gland; generally different kinds of cells found in a gland secrete separate hormones. Conversely, the same hormone may be secreted from more than one gland.
8. Hormone is destroyed and excreted as soon as its function is over.

9. It influences the activity of a process but cannot initiate a process.
10. The action of hormone is short-lived but not cumulative.
11. Hormones are highly specific in their action. Although all hormones reach every part of the body, but each one of them influences only a specific organ, called **target organ.** This is probably owing to the presence of specific **chemical receptors** in the cell membrane or cytoplasm or nucleus of target tissue to which the hormone is bound for exerting its action.
12. Hormones may be either stimulatory or inhibitory in nature. A physiological process may be stimulated by one hormone and inhibited by another. Moreover, the same hormone may produce stimulation in some case and inhibition in others.
13. Most physiological processes are regulated by the joint action of several hormones. Again, one hormone may produce many actions and several hormones may produce the same action.
14. The action of hormone may be specific or non-specific (widespread).
15. The hormone is not stored infinitely.

Classification of Animal Hormones

The secretions of endocrine glands are called hormones. Animal hormones can be grouped into three classes, such as : (A) according to their origin and site of action, (B) according to their chemical nature and (C) according to their solubility and receptor.

(A) According to their origin and site of action : Hormones can be classified mainly on the basis of origin and site of action. These are—

(1) **Ordinary hormones :** Hormones secreted from the classical endocrine glands belong to this group. These hormones exert their actions at sites remote from their orgin, e.g., thyroxine of thyroid galnd, estrogen and progesterone of ovary, androgens of testis, etc.

(2) **Trophic hormones :** Those hormones which control the secretion of hormones by other endocrine glands are called trophic hormones, e.g., TSH, FSH, LH, ACTH secreted by pituitary gland.

(3) **Local hormones :** Those hormones which are produced by certain tissues and act on nearby targets; for example, gastrin, secretin, etc., that are secreted by the mucous membrane of the gastro-intestinal tract and regulate the secretion of digestive glands.

(4) **Neuro-hormones :** These hormones are released by neurosecretory cells, transported to short distances by blood stream and have an inhibitory or stimulating effect on another endocrine gland. Example : neurohormones are secreted by hypothalamus.

(5) **Pheromones :** Pheromones are the chemicals which are secreted by one animal into the environment and affect the behaviour of other individual of the same species. Example : (i) Female silk moth releases bombykol to attract male silk moth. (ii) Tigers and lions are attracted for sexual reproducton by the pheromone liberated from their female counterparts. (iii) Again, the reproductive life of honey-bee is regulated by a pheromone liberated from the queen's mandibular gland.

The pheromones act as chemical agent which produce their effects in an animal on being percieved by olfaction or absorbed through the body surface. These pheromones play an important role in the maintenance of ecosystem and conservation of species. Hence, they are also known as **social hormones.**

(6) **Parahormones :** There are some blood borne chemical substances which do

not originate from specific endocrine cells. These chemical substances are known as **parahormones** or hormone-like substances as they cannot be called true hormones but they behave like hormones, e.g., erythropoietin, angiotensin, etc. are formed in the blood from the plasma proteins by the action of enzymes secreted by the kidney.

(B) Classification of hormones on the basis of chemical nature : Hormones are chemically diverse, they can be classified mainly into three classes, such as—protein or peptide hormones, amino acid or amine hormones and steroid hormones.

(1) **Protein or peptide hormones :** The hormones which are made up of many amino acids linked up by peptide bonds belong to this group. Proteins and peptides hormones consist of chains of amino acids, which may vary in size and form. These hormones are synthesised in the same manner that occur in normal protein synthesis. Examples : STH, ACTH, LTH of adenohypophysis, insulin and glucagon of islets of Langerhans, parathormone, etc. are simple proteins. TSH, FSH and LH of adenohypophysis are glycoproteins. ADH and oxytocin of neurohypophysis are smaller peptides.

(2) **Amino acid or Amine hormones :** Structurally these are the simplest hormone molecules. They are modified from the amino acid **tyrosin.** Examples of amines : thyroid hormones (tri-iodothyronine and tetra-iodothyronine) produced by the thyroid gland, epinephrine and norepinephrine together called catecholamines secreted by adrenal medulla, serotonin, melatonin, etc.

(3) **Steroid hormones :** These hormones are derived from cholesterol. Examples : aldosterone, cortisol and androgen secreted from the adrenal cortex; testosterone from testis; estrogen and progesterone from ovary, are all steroid hormones.

(C) Classification of hormones on the basis of solubility and location of receptors : Hormones may be classified into two kinds depending on their solubility and location of the receptors through which they act.

(1) **Water soluble hormones :** Some hormones which are water soluble cannot diffuse through the cell membrane of target cells. They work on the cell membrane bound receptors to exert their effects; e.g., peptides (such as glucagon, insulin, etc) and amines (such as adrenaline, noradrenaline etc).

(2) **Lipid soluble hormones :** Some hormones are lipid soluble and they can easily penetrate through the lipid matrix of the cell membrane of the target cells and invade into the cell. They exert their effects by acting through some intracellular receptors, e.g., thyroid hormones and steroid hormones.

Functions of animal hormones

The main function of hormone is to influence the activity of certain processes in the body, but do not appear to initiate such process. Hormones actually initiate quantitative change but not qualitative one. The effects produced by hormones can be summarised into general processes as follows :

(1) **Growth and development :** The growth of the body is controlled by hormones as cell proliferation is stimulated or inhibited by hormones. Early stages of development, such as cell division and differentiation of the zygotes or fertiliged eggs are under the control of hormones. Almost each hormone is involved either directly or indirectly with the growth of some or other organ of the body.

(2) **Reproductive activities :** Hormones secreted by gonads take part in reproduction

by regulating the development of sex organs. The hormones control the secondary sexual characters, gametogenesis, sex behaviours, etc. For example, androgen in male produces male characters and maturation of sperms. The progesterone acts jointly with estrogen to maintain growth of uterus and prevents the disintegration of uterine endometrium. Both estrogen and progesterone take part in the regulation of menstrual cycle. The progesterone controls female secondary sexual characters, maturation of the ovum, implantation of the fertilized egg, its retention to the uterine endometrium, etc. Again, estrogen helps in the maturation of graafian follicle in the ovary, in release of ovum from the mature follicle by causing a surge of L.H. secretion from the pituitary.

(3) **Metabolism** : The hormones have some metabolic activities that are mediated through their actions on enzymes. They regulate the overall metabolic functions of the body. The metabolism of carbohydrates, proteins and fats is greatly influenced by hormones. The production of heat in the body and calorigenesis is also affected by the intricate action of hormones, so as to provide energy for growth and development of the body.

(4) **Homeostasis** : Hormones regulate the function of different organs and tissues so as to adjust the life process according to the body's need. They also help to regulate the body temperature, water, ionic balance, blood glucose levels, etc., for maintaining the stability of the internal environment of the body.

(5) **Adaptations** : Adaptations to various external factors such as colour changes, visual adjustment to light intensities, etc. are regulated by certain hormones.

(6) **Animal behaviour** : Hormones regulate the behavioural patterns of animals such as aggressive behaviour, courtship behaviour, sexual display, parental care, mating, migration, housing, nest building, etc. Group behaviour of different animals specially the various insects are under the control of pheromones.

(7) **Regulation of other endocrine glands** : Hormones exert permissive effect on the actions of other hormones. A hormone may enhance the action of another hormone manifold. For example, the hormones, secreted by the pituitary gland, stimulate and control the secretion of hormones by the thyroid, gonad, etc.

(8) **Integument and hormones** : Hormones affect the integument as well as its derivatives. They affect mucus production, peeling, plumage, pigmentation and colour change. The secretion of sweat, sebum, milk, etc. is also controlled by hormones.

Somatotropin and Somatomedin : Somatotropin is a growth hormone secreted by the anterior lobe of pituitary gland; so somatomedin is a chemical produced within blood under the influence of somatotropin which helps the growth of bone.

Hormones and chemical signals in intercellular communication :

The coordination between cells is interacted through the chemical signals. They bind to their specific receptors found on the surface of the cell and trigger a sequence of intracellular changes that exert their physiological effects. The chemical signals are of the following categories (Fig 3.2).

(1) **Classical hormones** : Hormones act as chemical signals through which the coordination between various cells, tissues and organs of the body is achieved. The hormones secreted from typical endocrine glands are called **classical (endocrine) hormones.**

(2) **Paracrine hormone** : The chemical signals formed from certain cells of endocrine tissue diffuse in the extracellular fluid to affect neighbouring cells without being carried by the circulating blood. α-cell hormone, glucagon of Islets of Langerhans controls the secretion of the hormone insulin by β-cells. Gastrin secreted by G-cells of gastric mucosa controls secretion of HCl by parietal cells.

(3) **Autocrine hormone** : The chemical signals bind to receptors on the same cell

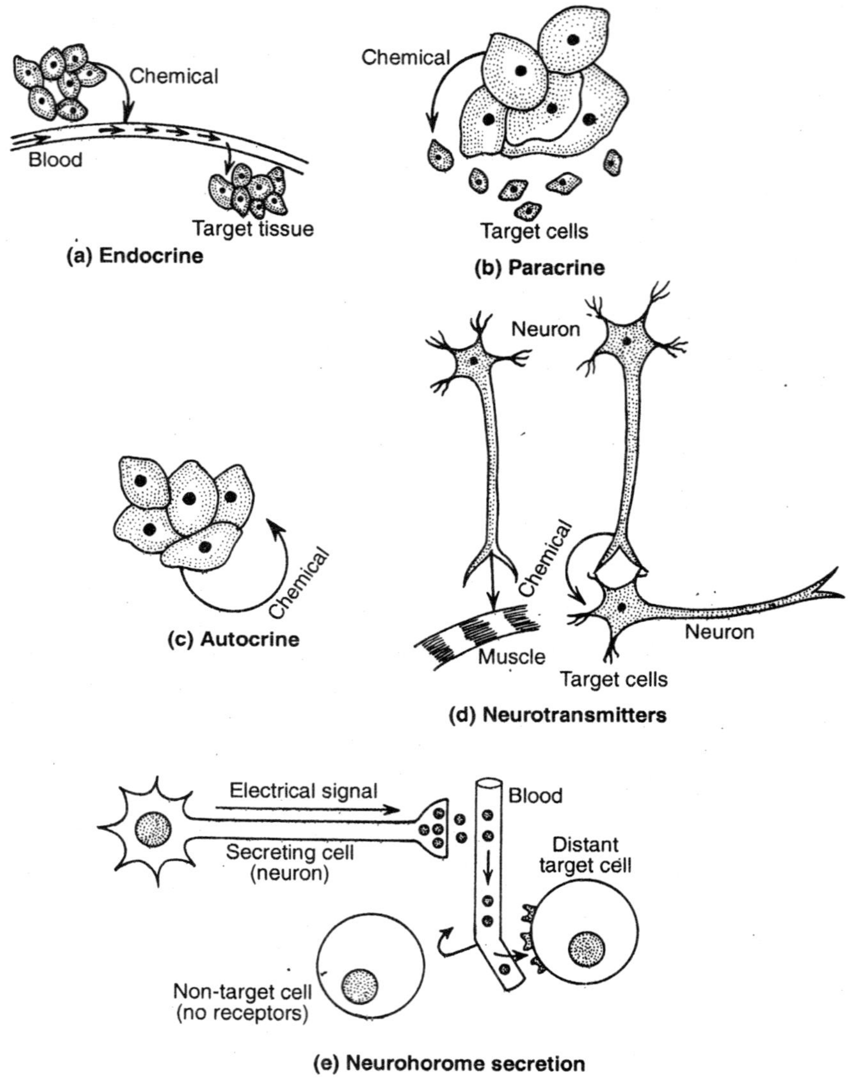

Fig. 3.2: Chemical messengers.

from which they are released. Example : platelet activating factor (PAF), a phospholipid secreted by platelets acts on the platelets to facilitate the aggregation of platelets during coagulation.

(4) **Neurotransmitters** : These are the chemicals secreted by nerve endings and act as neurotransmitters, e.g., acetylcholine, noradrenalin, dopamine, etc. They diffuse across the synaptic cleft through the extracellular fluid on a post-synaptic cell and do not enter the blood stream.

Difference between Neurohormone and Neurotransmitters : Chemicals that are produced within the nerve tissue but act as hormone are neurohormones, e.g., vasopressin. Chemicals that are produced at nerve endings and help in the transmission of nerve impulse are called neurotransmitter, e.g., acetylcholine, nor-adrenalin, etc.

Distinguish between Vitamins and Hormones

Particulars	Vitamins	Hormones
1. Source	1. These are not synthesised in the body and these are taken along with food.	1. These are produced within the body by the endocrine glands; hence, these are not dietary constituents.
2. Chemical nature	2. These are simple organic compounds such as organic acids, esters, etc.	2. These are amino acid derivatives, peptides, proteins or steroids.
3. Action	3. Vitamins act as co-enzymes; hence, they directly take part in metabolism.	3. Act as regulator of enzymes, thereby play an indirect role in the regulation of metabolism.
4. Excess and deficiency symptoms	4. Excess vitamins are excreted out. Their deficiency causes deficiency diseases (avitaminosis).	4. Both excess as well as deficiency symptoms cause functional disorders.

Distinguish between Hormone and Enzyme

Particulars	Hormones	Enzymes
1. Source.	1. Secreted from endocrine gland.	1. Produced in all living cells and generally act within the same cell. However, enzymes secreted by the exocrine glands act outside the gland.
2. Chemical nature	2. May be proteinaceous, amine or steroids.	2. Always proteinaceous.
3. Site of action	3. Carried by blood to a target organ.	3. Carried by some duct or act intracellularly.
4. Mode of action	4. Does not act as biocatalyst.	4. Act as biocatalyst.
5. Speed	5. Act slowly	5. Act very fast.
6. Effect of concentration	6. Deficiency and excess cause diseases and metabolic disorders.	6. Increase the reaction rate with increase in their concentration to a certain limit.

Distinguish between Somatostatin and Somatomedin

Particulars	Somatostatin	Somatomedin
1. Origin	1. Secreted from hypothalamus, gastrointestinal mucosa and δ-cells of pancreas.	1. Secreted mainly from liver and also from some other tissues.
2. Function	2. Retards growth by inhibiting the secretion of growth hormone from anterior pituitary.	2. Mediates the growth promoting action of growth hormone on target tissues; thus, it stimulates growth.
	3. Inhibits secretion of other gastrointestinal and pancreatic hormones.	3. Not concerned with regulation or secretion of gastrointestine and pancreatic hormones.

(5) **Neurohumours or neurohormones :** Higher animals with well-developed nervous system produce special type of hormones, the **neurohormones,** secreted by some modified nerve cells, the **neurosecretory** cells, having the morphological and functional characteristics of nerve cells and endocrine cells. The axons of neurosecretory cells do not form any synapse with other neurons but terminate at vascular spaces into which they release the **neurosecretion.** For example, the hypothalamus secretes the neurohormones. The hypothalamic releasing factors (CRH, TRH) stimulate the secretion of anterior pituitary hormones or store within the neurohypophysis (ADH, oxytocin), are secreted not by the pituitary itself but by neurosecretory cells of the hypothalamus.

Difference between Somatocrinine and Somatostatin : Somatocrinine is a chemical sectred from hypothalamus and helps secretion of STH, and somatostatin is a chemical that retards secretion of STH.

Control of secretion of hormones

The term hormone refers to any substance in an organism that carries a signal to generate some of alteration at the cellular levels. The hormones secreted by the endocrine glands represent one group of hormones that arise in one tissue, or gland and travel a considerable distance through the circulation to reach the target cell expressing cognate receptors.

Most of the physiological activities of the body are controlled by two mechanisms. The first is by the nervous system and the second is chemical coordination mediated through the secretions of the endocrine glands namely the hormones. Hormones can alter the rate of a physiological process but cannot initiate it. Thus, their effects are merely quantitative rather than qualitative. The molecular mechanism by which the hormones produce their effects at their target cells is very complicated. For every hormone there are some specific receptor sites on the cells of its target tissue.

Hormone or hormones secreted by one endocrine gland affect the functioning of some other endocrine gland and control the amount of hormone secreted by it. For example, hormones secreted by hypothalamus initiate or suppress the secretion of hormones by posterior pituitary gland. The hormones secreted by pituitary gland control the action of thyroid and adrenal glands of human body.

Secretion of hormones is controlled by the following ways :

(i) **Neural control :** The nerve impulses regulate some endocrine release. For instance, during stress and emotion, splanchnic nerve stimulates the release of catecholamines from adrenal medulla. The secretion of neurohypophyseal hormones and various secretions of hypothalamus are under this category. The act of suckling of baby reflexly stimulates adenohypophysis which secretes more prolactin. The release of prolactin appears to be an intrinsic property. The hypothalamus produces PIF (prolactin inhibitory factor) that prevents secretion of prolactin. Oestrogen stimulates lactation, lowers the concentration of PIF in hypothalamus and probably permits the prolactin secretion. During suckling the afferent impulses from the nipple reach the hypothalamus and then through the hypothalamohypophyseal tract, neurohypophysis discharges oxytocin and little vasopressin in the blood. The oxytocin circulates into the blood stream and causes contraction of the myoepithelial cells surrounding the alveoli of the gland and thus, ejection of the accumulated milk. So suckling produces both secretion and ejection of milk.

(ii) **Endocrine control** : Some endocrine glands regulate the secretion of other endocrine glands. For example, various releasing hormones of hypothalamus control the secretion of hormones of adenohypophysis. The secretion of adrenocortical, gonadal and thyroid hormones are stimulated respectively by adreno-corticotrophin, gonadotrophins and thyrotrophins that in turn are controlled by hypothalamic hypophysiotrophic hormones such as corticotrophin-releasing hormone, gonadotrophin-releasing hormone, thyrotrophin-releasing hormone, respectively.

(iii) **Feedback control or systems** : Feedback is the circumtance in which the response to a signal (e.g., of a cell to a hormonal stimulus) influences the source of the signal (in this case, the hormone-producing gland). Both hyper and hypoactivity of an endocrine gland produce structural or functional abnormalities or diseases. Therefore, normal functioning of endocrine glands and the level of hormones in the body need to be regulated. This is possible by feedback control. The release of hormone may be stimulated or inhibited by the feedback effect of some other hormone or metabolites [Fig 3.3(a)].

(a) In **positive feedback** the stimulus is amplified by the signals. This results in a larger subsequent response, which feeds back to produce an even greater stimulus, i.e., in positive feedback mechanisms, rising concentrations of a hormone cause another gland to release a second hormone which is then stimulatory to an increased output of the first hormone. A positive feedback system must have some mechanisms of shutting off release of the first hormone, otherwise the system would increase continuously in amplitude. In human, a gonadal estrogen increases the release of pituitary hormones, which in turn, stimulates ovarian estrogen production. Consequently, estrogen levels as well as gonadotrophin levels increase constantly. During the **follicular phase** of the menstrual cycle the secretion of FSH rises, whereas that of LH remains relatively low. On the 12th-13th day the estrogen production, enhanced by

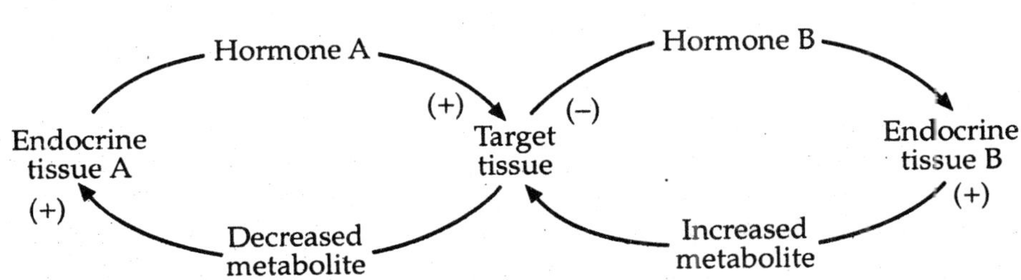

Fig. 3.3(a): General scheme of two hormone feedback systems.

the action of FSH, leads to stimulation of the release of FSH and LH, which in turn stimulates the release of estrogen via this positive feedback loop. A very high LH level in the blood is rapidly established and initiates **ovulation** on the 14th day. If this sudden rise in LH does not occur, or if it is too small, ovulation and, therefore, pregnancy cannot occur.

(b) In **negative feedback mechanism,** rising concentration of a hormone inhibits the release of second hormone from other gland, i.e., the stimulus is decreased by the response. Like most other regulatory mechanisms in the organism, hormonal action is mostly subject to negative feedback. For example, high levels of cortisol from adrenal cortex may inhibit the secretion of anterior pituitary corticotrophin and CRH from hypothalamus through long-loop feedback, all these lead to decline in cortisol secretion itself. High levels of trophic hormones sometimes inhibit the secretion of corresponding releasing factor from hypothalamus. Again, the RH from hypothalamus stimulates the anterior pituitary to secrete TSH. Now this TSH stimulates thyroid gland to produce hormone, thyroxin. If the level of thyroxin in the blood is high, it exerts a negative feedback effect on hypothalamus and adenohypophysis. Hypothalamus secretes less TRH (thyroxin releasing hormone) and in turn less TSH, respectively [Fig 3.3(b)].

Sometimes, blood level of some ions or metabolites also exhibits feedback control over hormone release. For example, a rise in serum Ca^{++} causes rectilinear fall in parathyroid hormone. Similarly, after a meal, glucose level of blood rises which stimulates secretion of insulin to act on it. With the fall in glucose level in blood, a decrease of insulin level takes place. In this way insulin maintains **blood glucose homeostasis.**

During blood glucose homeostasis the level of blood glucose may drop momentarily owing to muscular activity, especially if food intake is limited. The diminished level of blood glucose is recognised by α-cells of islets of Langerhans in pancreas. These cells then secrete glucagon hormone that acts on the hepatic cells of liver to cause the release of glucose. Thus, the blood glucose level becomes normal. The blood glucose level is elevated usually after a meal. Then the β-cells of islets of Langerhans release the hormone, insulin. This insulin induces the uptake of glucose from the blood into the liver and other cells. Thus, the glucose level of the blood is lowered to the normal circulating concentration. Lack of insulin, therefore, results in a serious inability to lower blood glucose, which results in diabetes mellitus.

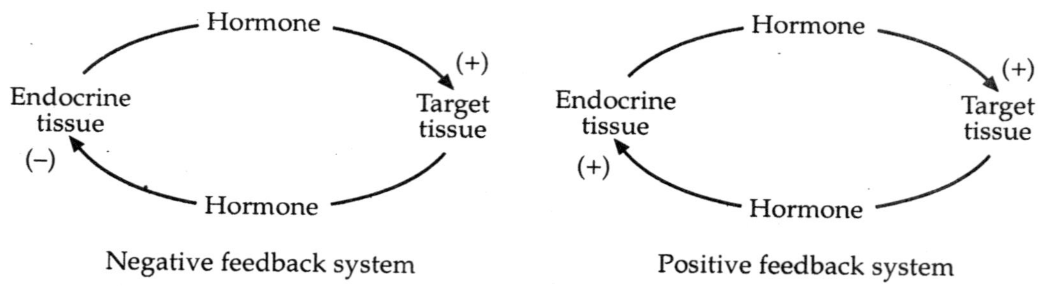

Fig. 3.3(b): Negative and positive feedback system.

(iv) **Long-loop and short-loop feedback mechanisms :** The mechanisms of feedback control of hypophysiotrophin and hypophysial hormone release are recognised. Peripheral target tissue hormones may exhibit feed back through a **long-loop system** to work at the level of the pituitary, at the level of the hypothalamus and even at higher brain centres.

In hormone feedback regulation mechanism, sometimes feedback control occurs at the level of hypothalamic hypophysiotrophic hormone secretion by a so-called **short-loop mechanism.** For example, the hormone inhibin secreted by the sertoli cells of testis may inhibit the anterior pituitary gland for the secretion of gonadal hormone. There is even evidence that secreted hypophysial hormones may show feed back on their cells of origin to inhibit their own secretion, referred to as **autoinhibition** or **autofeedback inhibition** (Fig 3.4).

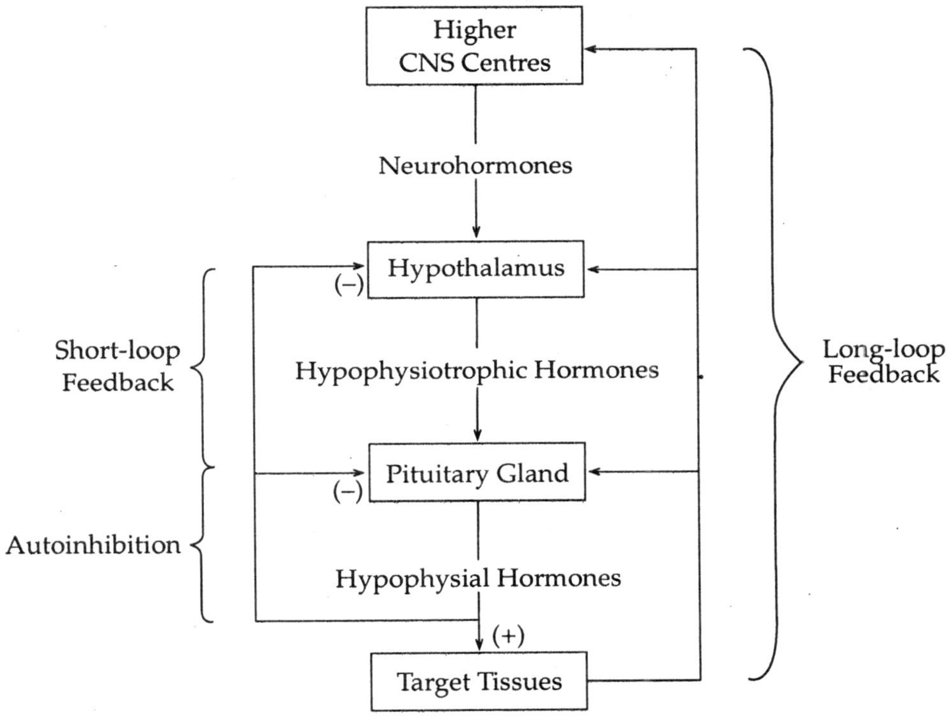

Fig 3.4: Model of long-loop and short-loop mechanisms in autoregulation of pituitary hormone secretion.

Differences between Protein Hormone and Steroid Hormone

Character	Protein Hormone	Steroid Hormone
1. Size	1. Larger in molecular sizes.	1. Smaller in molecular sizes.
2. Nature	2. Hydrophilic or lipophobic in nature.	2. Hydrophobic or lipophilic in nature.
3. Permeability	3. Cannot pass through plasma membrane.	3. Can pass through cell membrane.
4. Receptors for transportation	4. Extracellular receptors are required for transportation.	4. Intracellular receptors are required for transportation.
5. Requirement of messenger	5. Second messenger is needed.	5. Second messenger is not needed.
6. Examples	6. Insulin, glucagon, FSH, LH, etc.	6. Testosterone, progesterone, estrogen, etc.

Differences between Group I Hormone and Group II Hormone

Character	Group I Hormone	Group II Hormone
1. Nature	1. Lipophilic in nature.	1. Lipophobic in nature.
2. Transportation	2. Can carry proteins.	2. Cannot carry proteins.
3. Mode of action	3. Hormone action occurs through intracellular receptors.	3. Hormone action is occured via extracellular membrane receptors.
4. Half-life	4. Plasma half-life is lengthy, i.e., few hours to days.	4. Plasma half-life is short, i.e., few minutes.
5. Regulation of biological activities	5. Hormone receptor complex can mediate the biological activities.	5. Second messenger system regulates the biological action.
6. Example	6. Steroids, calcitriol, iodothyronines, etc.	6. Protein hormones, catecholamines, etc.

CHAPTER 4

Histology of Classical Endocrine Glands

(A) PITUITARY GLAND

The pituitary gland is the smallest endocrine gland of the body, weighs about 0.5 gm in adult. It is known as hypophysis (hypophysis—originated from Greek word 'hupophusis' meaning 'offshoot' i.e., thing develops from something else). It is a small sized, pink-coloured, pea-seed-shaped gland present below the hypothalamus. It is an unpaired gland. Secretions of pituitary gland controls the functions of other endocrine glands, for which pituitary gland is considered as **'master gland'.**

Position of pituitary gland

Pituitary gland is found at the base of the brain (forebrain), specially at the base of hypothalamus, so it is also called **hypothalamus cerebri.** It lies in the depression of the cavity of sphenoid bone—the sella turcica of the cranium of skull. It is connected to hypothalamus by an infundibular stalk formed of connective tissue with blood capillaries and nerve fibres. Fig 4(a).1.

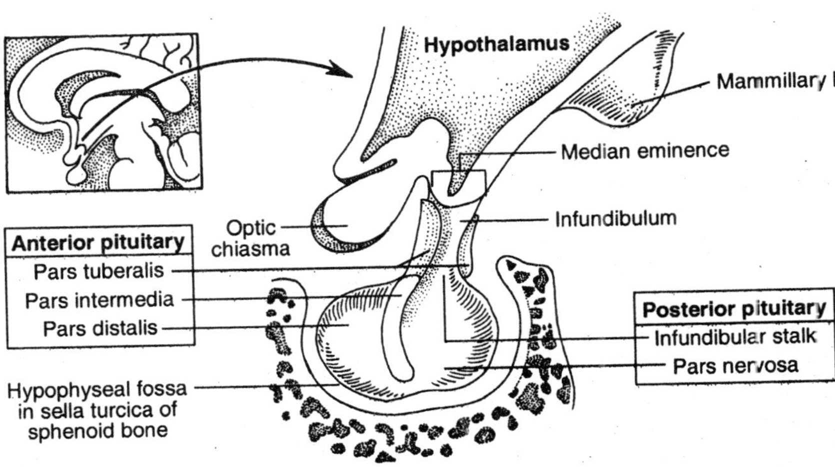

Fig. 4(a).1: Pituitary gland (position of pituitary gland).

Development of pituitary gland

The pituitary gland originates from dual embryonic structures. During the third week of development of the embryo, a hypophyseal pouch develops from the roof of the pharynx (upward), i.e., the part of oral ectoderm, first explained by Rathke, so it is called **Rathke's pouch.** The posterior part develops from the neuroectoderm of diencephalon as neurohypophyseal bud (downward). Gradually, by late in the second month of foetus, the hypophyseal pouch detaches from the roof of the pharynx and merges with the neurohypophyseal bud. Further development of both oral and neural ectodermal part of different histological origins unite to form a complete endocrine gland as pituitary.

During the fusion of anterior and posterior lobes of pituitary gland, part of posterior lobe called **infundibulum** remain connected permanently with base of hypothalamus, hence it is known as hypophysis. It is connected with the 3rd ventricle of diencephalon (Box 4.1).

Anatomy of pituitary gland

Blood supply of pituitary gland is very important. The blood supply derives from two groups of vessels coming off the internal carotid artery. The **superior hypophyseal arteries** supply the **median eminence** & the **infundibular stalk** and form a primary capillary network. The capillaries again join to form venules that branch again as a larger **secondary capillary network** in the **adenohypophysis**. The **inferior hypophyseal** arteries provide blood mainly for the **neurohypophysis** and a small supply to the stalk.

Capillaries of both networks are highly fenestrated and this is called hypothalamo-hypophyseal portal system. This system carries neuropeptides from the median eminence to the adenohypophysis, where they stimulate or inhibit hormone released by the endocrine cells.

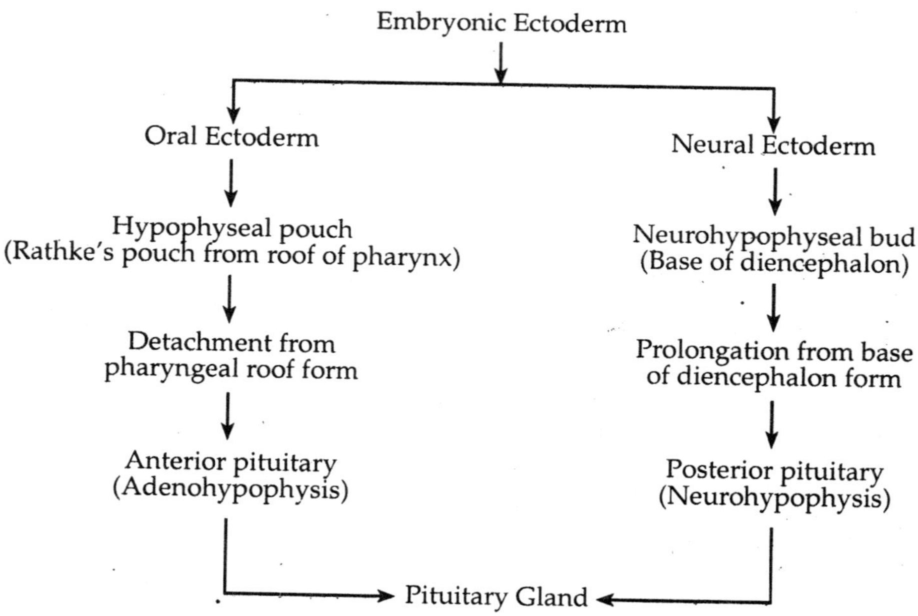

Box 4.1: Pituitary gland.

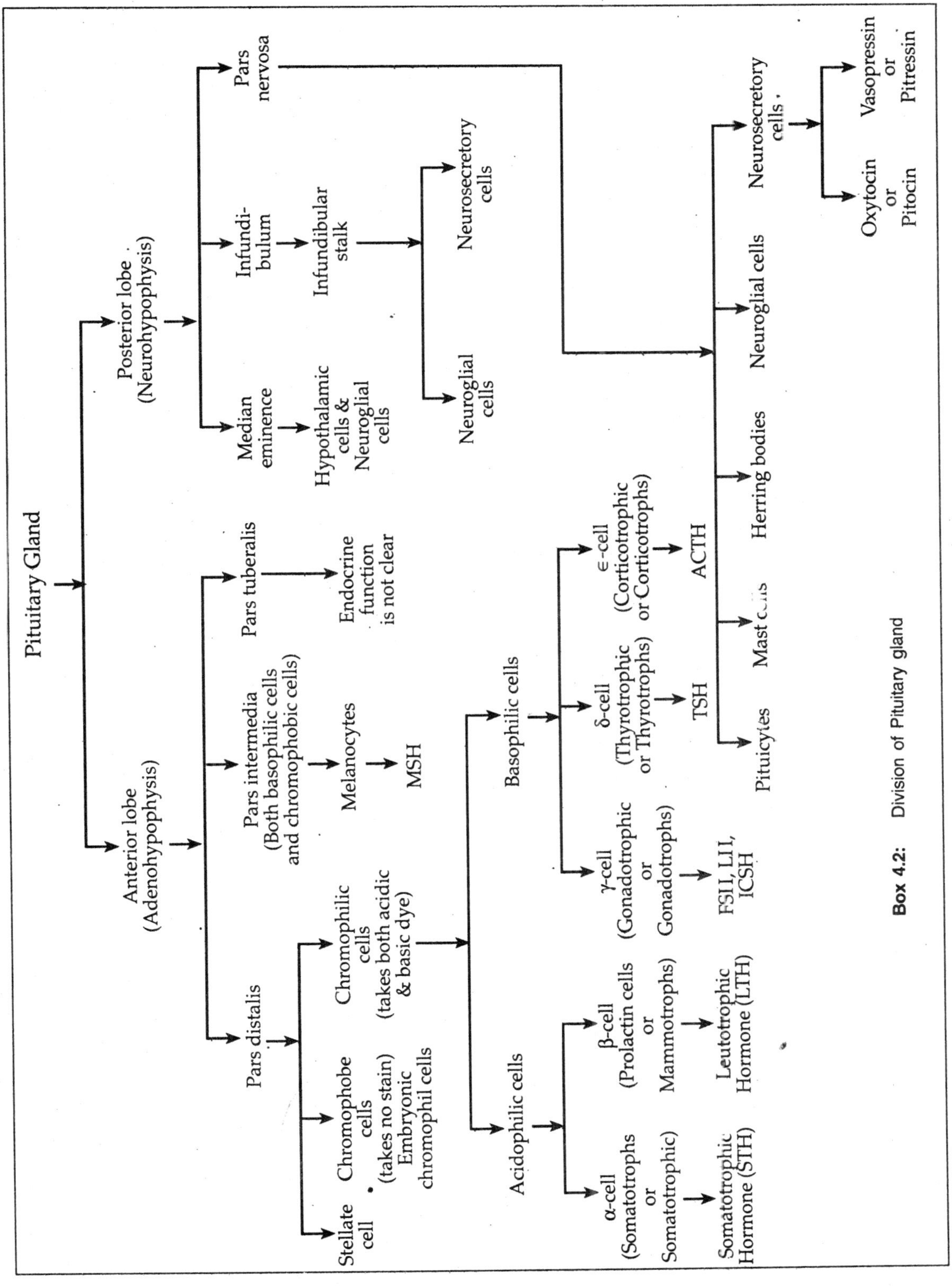

Box 4.2: Division of Pituitary gland

I. Adenohypophysis

Adenohypophysis (i.e., anterior lobe of the pituitary gland) is the glandular epithelial tissue. The anterior lobe of the pituitary gland consists of three derivatives of Rathke's pouch : **pars distalis, pars intermedia** and **pars tuberalis.**

Histological feature

A. Pars distalis

It is the main bulk of adenohypophysis and consists of irregular masses or columns of epithelioid cells with numerous blood sinuses and supported by loose framework of connective tissue.

Histological staining of pars distalis with Orange-G, Periodic acid—Schiff (PAS), Mallory's and Cleveland Wolfe Trichrome stains, etc. reveals two major kinds of gland cells like chromophobe cells and chromophil cells which constitute about 60 per cent cells of the pars distalis [Fig 4(a).2].

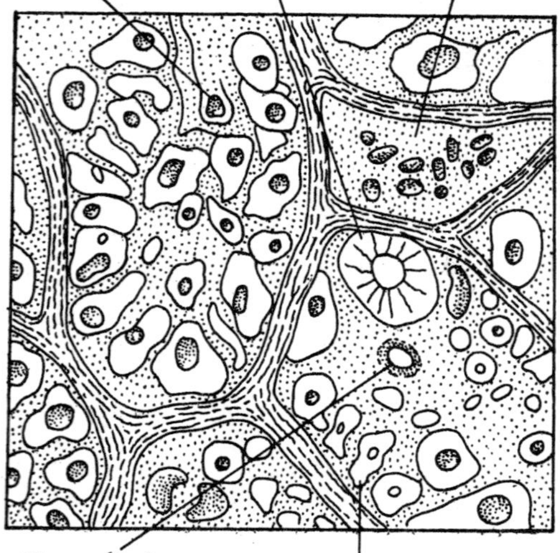

Fig. 4(a).2: T. S. of adenohypophysis (anterior pituitary).

(a) **Chromophobe cells :** These cells are so named because they are not stained with basic dyes or acid dyes and lack typical secretory granules. Chromophobe cells in general have got less cytoplasm than chromophils. EM structure shows that chromophobe cells contain very fine basophilic granules. Some believe that these cells are embryonic condition of chromophil cells. **Romeis** classified the chromophobes as gamma cells.

(b) **Chromophil cells :** Chromophil cells are those which take colour or stain. They take up both acid or basic dyes. Chromophilic cells again are of two types; acidophilic cells and basophilic cells. In human adenohypophysis contains 85 per cent acidophilic cells and 15 per cent basophilic cells [Fig 4(a).3].

1. **Acidophil cells :** Recent studies claim that acidophil cell secretes both growth hormone and lactogenic hormone. For the secretion of these two hormones there are two cell types—somatotrophic and lactotrophic cells.

(i) **Somatotrophic cell :** These cells are larger in size and oval or rounded in shape. Cells are acidophilic and take dark stain. These cells are packed with dense, round granules 350-400 mm in size. Nucleus is situated at the centre of the cell. Golgi bodies and ER are highly developed. These cells secrete somatotrophin or growth hormone or somatotrophic hormone (STH) for which they are named so.

(ii) **Lactotrophic cells or prolactin cells or mammotrophs or β-cells :** These types of acidophil cells are preferably stained with Azocarmine, Erythropsin or Acid fuchsin. Cells are either round or irregular in size. Granules of this type of cells are fewer and larger, ranging from 600-900 mm in size. Oval nucleus is situated at the periphery. Golgi complex is highly developed and ER remains spreaded throughout. They produce PRL (prolactin).

2. **Basophil cells :** There are different kinds of basophil cells secreting different types of trophic hormones like ACTH, TSH, FSH and LH. Differential staining methods

have been able to stain the different basophilic cell types.

(i) **Gonadotrophic cells or gonadotrophs or δ-cells :** The gonadotrophic cells are also positive with PA-Schiff stain. Cells that secrete FSH are larger and rounded cells whose secretory granules are spherical. The cells that secrete LH or are comparatively small and with scant cytoplasm. These cells also contain spherical secretory granules. Sizes of the gonadotrophic cell granules vary from 150-300 mm in diameter.

Highly evolved Golgi apparatus and sac-like ER are noticed within the cytoplasm of gonadotrophs. LH secretory cells are round or polygonal in shape and take light stain. Nucleus of those cells is wrinkled, whereas the FSH secretory cells are large round in shape. The nucleus is slightly wrinkled and the cells take dark stain.

(ii) **Thyrotrophic cells or thyrotrophs or δ-cells :** These cells are large polygonal having small nuclei. The nuclei are centrally placed. Cytoplasmic granules are fine and measured about 100-140 mm. These cells secrete TSH.

(iii) **Corticotrophic cells or corticotrophs ∈-cells (epsilon cells) :** The cells are oval or roundish and small in size. The nucleus is situated at the periphery of the cell. Cytoplasmic granules are very fine and comparatively low in number and measured about 100 mm. These cells secrete ACTH.

B. Pars intermedia

It is situated adjacent to pars distalis but remains separated from pars distalis by interglandular cleft. In man pars intermedia is reduced and it consists of both basophilic and chromophobic cells. It also includes melanocyte cells and fibrous tissue. The parenchymal cells of the pars intermedia surround colloid filled follicles. The cells lining these follicles appear to be derived from various secretory cells. TEM study reveals that these cells constitute apical junctional complexes and have vesicles larger than those present in the pars distalis.

Under EM the nucleus of melanocyte is round and central in position. Number of mitochondria, ER, Golgi bodies are well apparent in the cytoplasm. The cytoplasm is also filled up with secretory granules.

C. Pars tuberalis

It develops from the top of Rathke's pouch. Like the pars intermedia, the pars tuberalis is adjacent to and continuous with the pars distalis. It is separated from infundibulum by fibrous connective tissue. The main component of the pars tuberalis is a cuboidal-columnar cell which contains numerous small granules or fine colloid droplets. The mitochondria are short rod-like structures and small lipid and glycogen droplets are also found. Its epithelial cells contain undifferentiated and some small acidophilic and basophilic cells. Hence, they are Sudan black-B and PAS +ve. The actual function of pars tuberalis is not clear.

- **Rathke's pouch :** It is a glandular epithelium which grows upwards from the primitive buccal cavity (ectoderm) and meets a similar neural down growth from the floor of the third ventricle. The stalk of Rathke's pouch disappears. But that of the neural down growth persists and forms the pituitary stalk (infundibulum). From the anterior wall of Rathke's pouch arises the pars distalis; from the top originates the pars tuberalis and from the posterior wall develops the pars intermedia.

Cells of Rathke's pouch proliferate to give rise to the anterior pituitary. Accordingly, nerve fibers grow into the infundibulum from hypothalamus and give rise to the neurosecretory cells of posterior pituitary. The original cavity of Rathke's pouch forms the interglandular cleft.

- **Distinguish between chromophobes and chromophils :**

(i) Chromophobes have little or no affinity for either acidic or basic dyes while

chromophils can be subdivided into acidophils and basophils according to their affinities for dyes. The somatotrophs and mammotrophs represent the acidophils, and thyrotrophs and gonadotrophs are basophils.

(ii) Chromophobes are **agranular** and do not secrete any hormone. The function of these cells is not known and it is believed that they are mother cells from which other cells originate. But the chromophil cells are granular cells and they secrete hormones.

Hormones of Adenohypophysis

There are six (6) major anterior pituitary hormones whose biosynthesis, structure, function and secretory control have been well characterised which can be accurately measured in tissues and body fluids. These hormones are—ACTH, GH, TSH, LH and FSH. They may be classified into three groups : **Corticotropin** related peptides [ACTH, LPH (lipotropin), melanocyte—stimulating hormone (MSH), and endorphins], the **somatomammotropins** (GH and PRL) which are also peptides and the **glycoproteins** (LH, FSH and TSH).

(i) **Actions of somatotrophic hormones (STH) :** The chief function of STH is to help in the growth of the body; this is why it is also known as **growth-hormone.** It promotes the overall growth of the body and almost all visceral organs. STH produces the metabolic effects of protein, carbohydrate and fat.

(ii) **Action of ACTH :** The actions of ACTH can be described under two headings—adrenal actions and extra-adrenal actions.

The chief function of ACTH is to promote the growth of adrenal cortex and secretion of glucocorticoids hormones from it. ACTH can also produce some effects by acting directly on certain tissues. ACTH inhibits the catabolism and degradation of corticoid hormones in liver so as to prolong their activities in the body.

(iii) **Actions of TSH :** The main function of STH is to maintain the structure and function of thyroid gland. Under the influence of this hormone, the thyroid gland increases in size and becomes well organised.

(iv) **Functions of GTH :** The chief gonadotrophic hormones of adenohypophysis are FSH and LH. These hormones are called gonadotrophic because their prime function is to control the dovelopment of gonads (i.e., testis in male and ovary in female). Recently a third pituitary hormone prolactin (PRL) has been admitted to the class of GTH because of its gonadal effects. It helps to complete the development of mammary gland during pregnancy and initiates milk formation. After child birth, it promotes milk secretion.

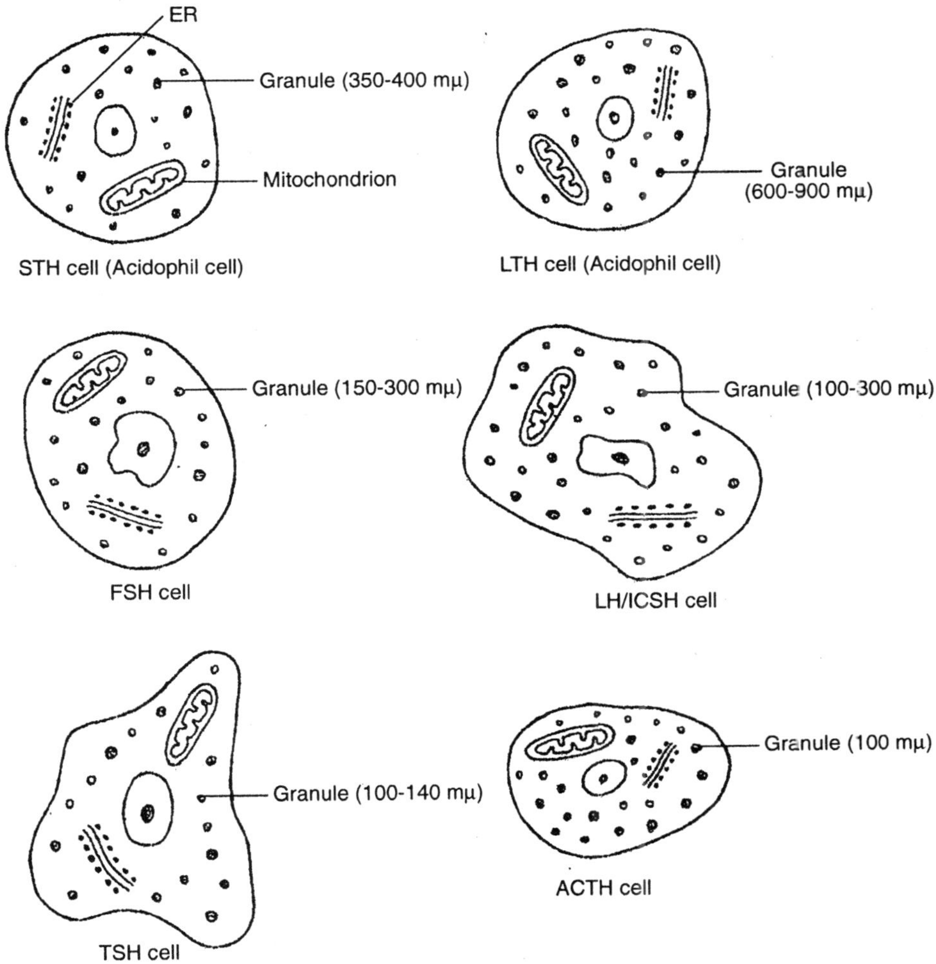

Fig. 4(a).3: Schematic representation of different types of chromophil cells.

II. Neurohypophysis or Posterior lobe of the pituitary gland

Neurohypophysis is an extension of the central nervous system (CNS) that stores and releases secretory products from the hypothalamus. Anatomically it includes **pars nervosa, median eminence** and **infundibulum.**

Histological feature

(a) **Pars nervosa :** Histologically the neurohypophysis commonly means the pars nervosa, which is the chief component, and the following elements are found :

(i) **Pituicytes :** These are the principal cells and contain fusiform or polygonal supporting **neuroglial cells** with delicate processes. They are large, branching, spindle-shaped cells with distinct cell bodies. Nucleus is round oval-shaped body with prominent chromatin material. Dendritic processes are absent. The axonic process is slightly elongated and terminal portion is comb-like in appearance. Golgi apparatus, mitochondria, ER, etc. are well recognised. EM structure reveals that three morphologically distinct **neurosecretory vesicles** are present in pars nervosa. Neurosecretory vesicle with diameters ranging between 10 and 30 mm accumulate in the axon terminals. Nerve terminals also consist of 30 nm vesicles that contain acetylcholine. Larger vesicles, ranging from 50 to 80 nm, resemble the dense core vesicles of the adrenal medulla, and adrenergic nerve endings are found in the same terminal. The pituicytes consist of adenopituicytes, micropituicytes, fibropituicytes and reticulopituicytes, and they do not secrete any hormone.

(ii) **Mast cells :** These are spherical or round cells with centrally placed nucleus.

(iii) **Herring bodies :** These are densely staining accumulations of stored neuosecretory substances, i.e., the membrane-bounded neurosecretory vesicles aggregate together to form Herring bodies that contain either **oxytocin** or **vasopressin** (antidiuretic hormone).

(iv) **Neuroglial cells :** These are fusiform or round cellls which are found in between the pituicytes.

(v) **Nerve and sinusoids** are well recognised within the pars nervosa.

(b) **Median eminence :** It is made up of hypothalamic cells, neuroglial cells and blood vessels.

(c) **Infundibulum :** It is the pituitary stalk which consists of clusters of numerous large sinusoidal vessels which are surrounded by neuroglial tissue. From the hypothalamus neurosecretory cells contain Nissl bodies and smaller neuro-secretory granules in the axons of the cells [Fig 4(a).4].

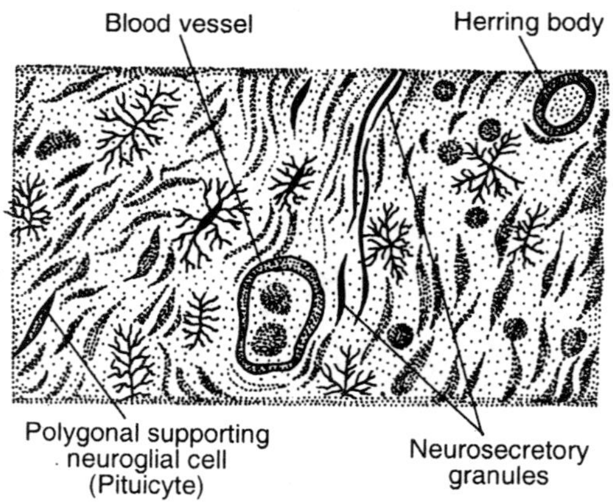

Fig. 4(a).4: T. S. of neurohypophysis.

Hormones of neurohypophysis i.e., of oxytocin and vasopressin

Oxytocin and **vasopressin** are the neurohormones which are found within the pars-nervosa of most mammals. They are localised within the axonal endings. Each hormone is a small peptide of nine amino acid residues. The two hormones differ in only two of these residues.

Each membrane-bounded neurosecretory vesicle of pars-nervosa contains either oxytocin or ADH. This vesicle also contains ATP and a neurophysin, a protein that bonds to the hormone by non-covalent bonds. Oxytocin and vasopressin are synthesized as part

Biological effects and origin of the hormones of Adenohypophysis, Pars-intermedia and Neurohypophysis

Hormone	Origin	Cellular origin	Chemical nature	Target cell or organ	Main functions	Disease/Disorder
1. Growth hormone (GH) or Somatotrophic hormone (STH)	Pars distalis	Acidophilic	Protein	Body cell	1. Develops bones and muscles. 2. Helps in anabolism of nitrogen. 3. Assists in metabolism of fat. 4. Helps to store glycogen in skeletal muscle and cardiac muscle.	**Hypersecretion** • Infant → Gigantism • Adult → Acromegaly **Hyposecretion** • Infant → Dwarfism • Adult → Acromicria
2. Prolactin (PRL) or Leutotrophic hormone (LTH)	Pars distalis	Acidophilic	Protein	Mammary gland	1. Development of mammary gland and control their secretion. 2. Prolongs the function of corpus luteum. 3. Helps to secrete progesterone.	Hyposecretion hampers the milk secretion.
3. Thyroid stimulating hormone (TSH)	Pars distalis	Basophilic	Glycoprotein	Thyroid gland	1. Controls the intake of iodine by thyroidal tissue. 2. Maintains the secretion of thyroid hormones.	**Hyposecretion** •Hypothyroidism **Hypersecretion** • Hyperthyroidism

Hormone	Origin	Cellular origin	Chemical nature	Target cell or organ	Main functions	Disease/Disorder
4. Leutinizing hormone (LH) or interstitial cell stimulating hormone (ICSH)	Pars distalis	Basophilic	Glycoprotein	Cells of corpus luteum of ovary & interstitial cells of Leydig	1. Helps to secrete androgen by stimulating Interstitial cells of Leydig of testes. 2. Maintains formation of corpus luteum in ovaries and secretion of progesterone.	Hyposecretion hampers ovum maturation and liberation, and also hampers sperm production.
5. Follicle stimulating hormone (FSH)	Pars distalis	Basophilic	Glycoprotein	Graafian follicle	1. Controls the growth of Graafian follicles within ovaries. 2. Maintains the secretion of oestrogen from Graafian follicles and ovulation with the joint effect of ICSH. 3. Probably maintains sperm production in males.	Hyposecretion gradually incorporates sterility by degrading the rate of development and maturation of sperm and ovum.
6. Adrenocorticotrophic hormone (ACTH)	Pars distalis	Basophilic	Polypeptide	Cortical cells of adrenal gland.	1. Helps to secrete different hormones from adrenal cortex, called aldosterone, deoxycorticosterone, cortisone, cortisol, corticosterone.	**Hypersecretion** • Cushing syndrome, polycythemia and glycosuria, etc.

Hormone	Origin	Cellular origin	Chemical nature	Target cell or organ	Main functions	Disease/Disorder
7. Melanocyte stimulating hormone (MSH)	Pars Intermedia	Basophilic & Acidophilic	Polypeptide	Melanocyte cell of skin	1. Helps to secrete melanin by stimulating the melanoblast cells.	**Hyposecretion** ● Degradation of melanin formation.
8. Vasopressin or Antidiuretic hormone (ADH) or Arginine vasopressin (AVP) or Pitreccin.	Pars Nervosa	Hypothalamic supraoptical & paraventricular nucleus	Polypeptide	Kidney & blood vessels.	1. Increases blood pressure by contraction of arterioles. 2. Helps in reabsorption of excess amount of water from distal convoluted tubules of nephron.	**Hyposecretion** ● Polyurea or diabetes incipidus.
9. Oxytocin or pitocin	Pars Nervosa	Hypothalamic periventricular nucleus	Polypeptide	Uterus, mammary gland.	1. Helps to secrete milk by contracting the involuntary muscles of mammary gland. 2. Helps to relax uterine muscles during parturition. 3. During fertilization, helps to enter sperm within the female reproductive tract.	**Hyposecretion** ● Hampers milk secretion. ● Hampers uterine contraction, so disturbance created during parturition.

of a large molecule that includes the hormone and its specific neurophysin. The large molecule is proteolytically cleaved into the hormone and neurophysin as it travels from the perikaryon to the axon terminal. Immunocytochemical staining procedure reveals that oxytocin and vasopressin are secreted by different cells in the hypothalamic nuclei and then carried through the nerve fibres to the posterior pituitary where they are stored. From here the hormones are released into blood according to the need of the body. Since the posterior pituitary hormones are produced by the nerve cells, these are also called **neurohormones.**

Actions of vasopressin

(1) **Antidiuretic action :** Vasopressin stimulates reabsorption of water by the distal convoluted and the collecting renal tubules and thus regulates urine volume. The action of vasopressin may be owing to the increase in the enzyme is hyaluronidase in the renal tubules and thus, increases the permeability of the renal tubules and thereby helps to conserve water by reducing excretion through urine. Conversely, when the blood becomes dilute due to the presence of excess water in it, the release of vasopressin is suppressed to excrete the excess water through urine because it prevents **diuresis** (i.e., excretion of dilute urine). Due to lack of vasopressin, large quantities of dilute urine is excreted. Vasopressin decreases urine volume by increasing reabsorption of water by renal tubules; hence, this hormone is also known as antidiuretic hormone (ADH).

(2) **Vasoconstriction :** Antidiuretic hormone (ADH) causes profound vasoconstriction and increases blood pressure by stimulating contractions of the smooth muscle cells in the wall of the arterioles. For this reason the ADH is known as vasopressin. The exact physiologic importance of the action of ADH is not clear. It is believed that a rise of ADH release after haemorrhage may assist to prevent the fall of blood pressure.

(3) **On heart :** Vasopressin reduces the heart beat.

(4) **On plain muscles :** The muscular walls of the urinary bladder and ureter are stimulated by the action of vasopressin.

(5) **On respiration :** Hyperpnoea with occasional apnoea is noticed with a high dose level of vasopressin. This is owing to changes in blood pressure which reflexly acts on the respiratory centre.

(6) **On metabolism :** Vasopressin produces glycogenolysis, hyperglycaemia and glycosuria. Sugar tolerance is reduced. This effect is only a secondary one.

(7) The intestinal muscles contract and movements of stomach, small and large intestines are increased by the actions of high dose level of vasopressin.

Actions of oxytocin

(1) **On milk ejection :** Oxytocin helps in milk ejection during suckling by contracting the smooth muscles of the mammary gland. The new mother, when nurses her baby, secretes her own oxytocin which helps lactation by the contraction of the myoepithelial cells around the mammary gland's alveoli.

(2) **On uterine contraction :** During parturition oxytocin stimulates the contraction of uterine smooth muscles for expulsion of the foetus. In deficiency of oxytocin secretion normal delivery of the child is not possible.

(3) **On fertilization :** This hormone is secreted during coitus and facilitates fertilization by the contraction of the female genital tract.

(4) **On sperm transport :** During coitus, it produces movements of female genital tract for transport of sperms from vagina to fallopian tube through the uterus.

(5) **On metabolism :** Oxytocin produces hyperglycaemia in large doses. The hormone given in large doses and in abundant fluid volumes may cause water intoxication owing to antidiuretic effect of oxytocin on the nephron.

(6) Another action of oxytocin is to stimulate contraction of gall bladder, intestine and urinary bladder.

(7) It may regulate the feeding behaviour.

Differences between Oxytocin and Vasopressin

Biological effects	Oxytocin	Vasopressin
1. Action	1. It is physiologically active in females only.	1. It is physiologically active in both males and females.
2. Water diuresis	2. It has no effect.	2. Its main function is to promote water reabsorption from renal tubules and vasoconstriction (i.e., inhibits water diuresis).
3. Lactation	3. It stimulates myoepithelial cells of mammary gland for secretion of milk.	3. It has no effect.
4. Potency in raising blood pressure	4. It is less potent in raising blood pressure.	4. It is more potent in raising blood pressure.
5. Parturition	5. During parturition it stimulates the contraction of uterine smooth muscles to facilitate the child birth.	5. No effect
6. Intestinal contraction	6. No effect.	6. Stimulates.

(B) THYROID GLAND

In human the thyroid gland is one of the important endocrine glands. It is a bilobed endocrine gland situated at the root of the thorax, antero-lateral to the larynx and upper trachea. It consists of two lateral lobes arranged on either side of the trachea. These two lobes are joined by a thin portion of thyroid tissue, called the **isthmus,** crossing in front of the second, third and fourth tracheal rings. As a normal variant the left lobe is often smaller than the right lobe. Secretory follicles of this gland constitute the structural and functional units. The thyroid gland is the main iodine functioning organ in the body and it produces the following three hormones; **thyroxine (T_4 or tetraiodothyronine), triiodothyronine (T_3)** and **calcitonin** or **thyrocalcitonin,** each of which is essential to normal metabolism and homeostasis.

Development

In the human embryo the thyroid gland develops from the primitive foregut. This gland originates from the endoderm of the cephalic portion of alimentary canal of embryo. A sac-like outgrowth first develops in the midventral surface of the pharynx at the level of second pair of pharyngeal pouches. In adult this outgrowth (diverticulum) expands and remains attached with the pharynx by a narrow solid duct, **Thyroglossal stalk.** Later the stalk atrophies and the gland remains free. With the changes in structure the thyroid develops its capacity to secrete thyroid hormone. The functional capacity of this gland appears in a stepwise fashion, the ability to accumulate iodine being followed by the development of other stages of thyroid hormone synthesis.

Anatomy

In mammals, the thyroid gland is lobed in nature and located in the neck, anterolateral to the larynx and upper trachea. In man, the thyroid is a bilobed endocrine gland and both the lobes are joined near their lower poles by an **isthmus bridge** crossing in front of the lower larynx. The gland is oval or pear-shaped in structure. This gland is pink in colour and is enclosed in a thin collagenous fibrous **capsule** from which internal **septa** penetrate the parenchyma, dividing it into irregular **lobules.** In human, the gland measures about 2.5-4 cm in length and 1.5-2 cm in width and 1-1.5 cm in thickness. The adult human thyroid gland weighs 15-20 gm but is influenced by age, sex, reproductive state and diet. The thyroid gland is well vascularised by paired superior and inferior thyroid arteries and is innervated by sympathetic nerve fibres from cervical region of spinal cord of CNS [Fig 4(b).1].

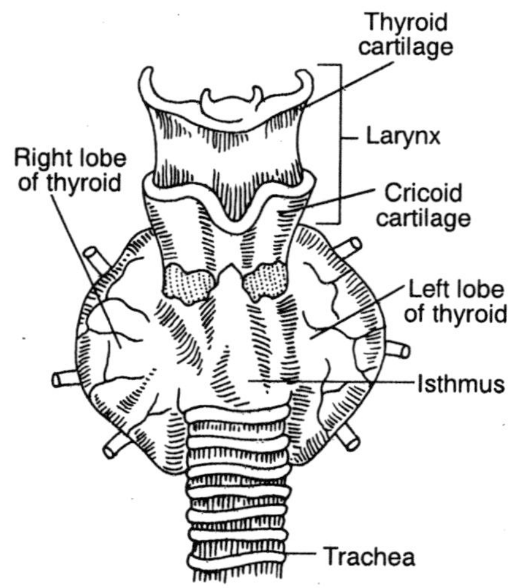

Fig. 4(b).1: Location and anatomy of thyroid gland (ventral view).

Histological structures

Thyroid gland is formed of **follicles** or **sacs** or **acini.** Each follicle is a roughly spheroidal cyst-like compartment with a wall formed by a simple cuboidal or columnar epithelium, called **follicular epithelium.** The cavity of the follicle is filled up with colloid. The colloid is homogeneous material which is eosinophilic in nature after **H-E stain.** Colloid is protein in nature, secreted by epithelial cells. Under **light microscope** this gland is invested by outer capsule which is made up of white fibrous connective tissue. The follicles are of various sizes which vary from 15-150 µm in diameter. Large follicles are usually distributed towards the periphery and the smaller ones are found near the centre.

The entire structural component of the gland is known as parenchyma. In between the parenchyma connective tissue intervenes to form the **septa.** These septa extend up to the follicle but the septum is very thin near the follicle. One follicle is separated from the other by reticulum fibre. Thyroid follicles are separated by connective tissue. Within the meshes of connective tissue few lymphocytes, histocytes, sections of blood vessels and nerves are noticed.

On the basis of regional distribution and function, follicles are distinguished into two categories—large and small follicles. Large follicles are formed of cuboidal epithelial cells, and the cavities of these follicles are filled up with densely stained colloid substances. The smaller follicles are small and lined by simple cuboidal epithelium. The quantity of colloid substances is very less and very lightly stained. Under electron microscope the follicular cells are found to contain Golgi apparatus near the luminal end. Mitochondria, ER and lysosomes are scattered throughout the cytoplasm. Nucleus is well recognised at the centre of the cell. There are few terminal bars at the apical side of the follicular cells, and the cells are held together with the help of terminal bars. Each cell has well-developed microvilli. In the periphery of the cell many phagosomes are found. Histochemically lipid droplets, different proteins, laden granules are noticed.

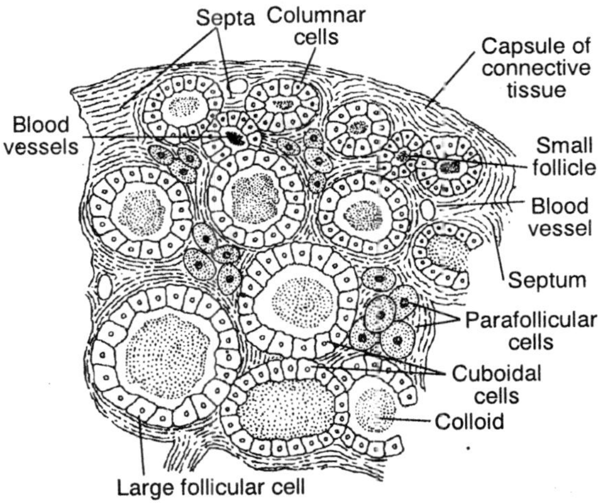

Fig. 4(b).2: T.S. of thyroid under light compound microscope.

Using **electron microscopic** and **histochemical methods,** two types of cells have been identified in the thyroid vesicle—(i) the numerous **principal** or **chief follicular cells** have lesser number of mitochondria containing the different proteolytic and oxidative enzymes which are responsible for the synthesis of thyroid hormones. (ii) A lesser number of **mitochondrial rich,** high cuboidal cells are also present in between the follicular cells. These are known as **para-follicular cells (C-cells).** These cells secrete many granules containing hormone, known as **calcitonin.** Principal follicular cells are the main constituent of follicular epithelium. Parafollicular cells may occur within the follicular epithelium or in the regions between or adjacent to the follicles [Fig 4(b).2 and 3].

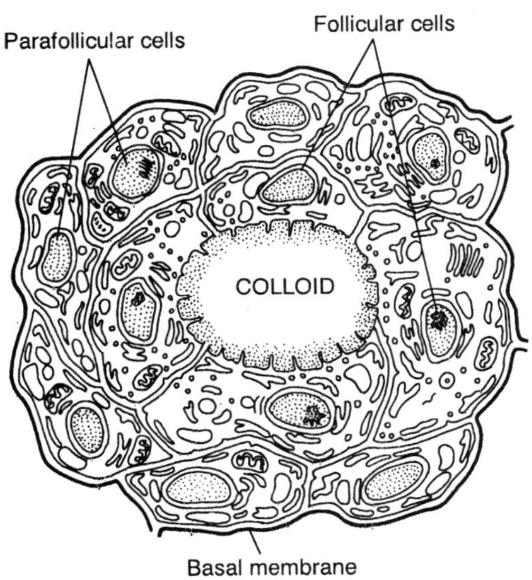

Fig. 4(b).3: Diagrammatic representation of the parafollicular cells of the mammalian thyroid gland.

Differences between Cheif Follicular Cells and Parafollicular Cells

Subject index	Chief Follicular Cells	Parafollicular Cells
1. Number	1. Comparatively large in number.	1. Comparatively small in number.
2. Shape of nucleus	2. Nucleus is round in shape.	2. Nucleus is irregular in outline.
3. No. of mitochondria	3. Have a lesser number of mitochondria.	3. Have a lesser number of mitochondrial-rich.
4. Presence of oxidative enzyme	4. Have different oxidative and proteolytic enzymes.	4. Have high concentration of oxidative enzyme.
5. Presence of microvilli	5. Have well-developed microvilli.	5. Absence of microvilli.
6. ER	6. ER larger in diameter.	6. Comparatively less in diameter.
7. Golgi-apparatus	7. Contain Golgi-apparatus near the luminar end.	7. Golgi-apparatus is prominent.
8. Cytology	8. Cytology is not altered by high blood calcium level.	8. Degranulation is due to high blood calcium level.
9. Secretion	9. Secrete triiodothyronine (T_3) and thyroxine (T_4).	9. Secrete calcitonin.
10. Binding of antibody	10. Bind antibody to thyroglobulin.	10. Bind antibody to calcitonin.

• Thyroid glands at abnormal conditions

In **hyperactive conditions** of thyroid, cells may become more columnar. The lining epithelium increases and becomes folded. The mitochondria increase in number and the Golgi-apparatus enlarges and colloid apparatus appear near it. The vesicles become irregular—some hyperdistended and others collapsed and they are basophilic in staining reaction. In **hypoactivity** condition the epithelium becomes flat on squamous type and the staining reaction of the vesicles becomes acidophilic. After puberty colloid store increases and as suggested by the histological changes, activity slowly decreases. This explains decrease in BMR and susceptibility to cold in old age [Fig 4(b).4].

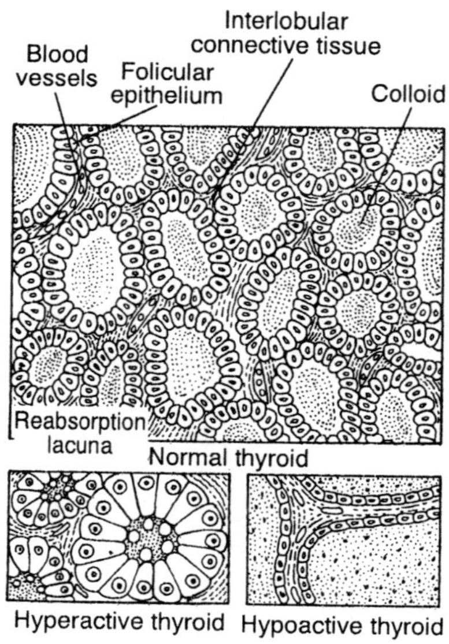

Fig. 4(b).4: Histological structure of thyroid gland showing normal, hyperactive, hypoactive thyroid cells.

In early foetal life, thyroid comprises a solid clump of cells. Vesicles start appearing at the fourth month. Each group of cells secrete colloid substances at a common centre and in this way the rudimentary vesicles form.

Functions of thyroid hormones

A. Functions of Thyroxine (T_4) and Triiodothyronine (T_3) :

These two hormones have the same functions. T_4 is considered as the principal hormone of thyroid gland and T_3 is more potent. The actions of T_4 and T_3 in the body are as follows :

(a) **Metabolic actions**

(1) **On carbohydrate metabolism :**

(i) Thyroid hormones raise the blood sugar level by increasing food intake, absorption of glucose from intestine, glycogenolysis, neoglucogenesis, etc.

(ii) These hormones also increase the oxidation of glucose in tissues.

(iii) Promote neoglucogenesis in liver by enhancing the activities of phospho enol pyruvate carboxykinase (PEPCK) and pyruvate carboxylase.

(2) **On protein metabolism :**

(i) Under normal conditions (i.e., when the blood levels of T_4 and T_3 are within normal range), they help in protein synthesis but when secreted in excess, they cause protein breakdown.

(ii) In hyperthyroidis, excessive protein catabolism leading to body wasting are noticed as evidenced by excessive nitrogen excretion in the urine.

(3) **On fat metabolism :**

(i) T_3 and T_4 stimulate the catabolism of fat by activating the enzyme lipase present in the tissues.

(ii) Increase the oxidation of fatty acids.

(iii) It is to be noted that concentration of cholesterol in blood is inversely proportional with the level of thyroid activity.

(4) **BMR and calorigenesis :**

T_3 and T_4 increase the BMR by stimulating oxidation of food stuff in the tissues and therefore they are also called 'calorigenic hormones. During cold the secretion of thyroid hormones is increased which by stimulating calorigenesis help in thermoregulation and prevent fall of body temperature.

(5) **Vitamin metabolism :**

(i) Assist in conversion of carotene to vit. A and vit. A to retinol.

(ii) Increase the requirement of vit. B_6, vit. B_{12} and vit. C.

(iii) Hyperthyroidism may cause vit. D deficiency.

(6) **On calcium and phosphorus metabolism :**

Remove Ca and P from the bones leading to osteoporosis. This action differs from that of parathyroid in causing no rise of serum Ca, and increasing Ca loss both in faeces and urine.

(b) **Growth and differentiation**

(i) Thyroid hormones assist in growth by synthesis of phosphocreatine.

(ii) T_4 and T_3 stimulate differentiation of tissues which indirectly help in growth by facilitating the action of STH.

(iii) Thyroid hormones play an essential role in mental growth and development of central nervous system. Deficiency of these hormones help to become mentally retarded.

(c) **Action on circulatory system**

Thyroid hormones increase absorption of vit. B_{12} from the intestine which is required for the synthesis of haemoglobin and thereby erythropoiesis (formation and maturation of RBC). T_3 and T_4 increase the activity of heart.

(d) **Action on digestive system**

T_4 and T_3 promote hunger, appetite,

movement of gastrointestinal tract and absorption of various substances from the intestine.

(e) **Action on reproductive system**

(i) The activity of the thyroid varies mostly at different ages specially in the female. Thyroid hormones control the normal function of gonad and development of secondary sex characters. T_4 and T_3 show increased activity at puberty, during menstruation, pregnancy and lactation; after the menopause it tends to atrophy.

(ii) Less amount of these hormone secretion delays onset of puberty.

(iii) Increase the output and fat content of milk.

(f) **On temperature regulation**

(i) Thyroid maintains the regulation of normal body temperature.

(ii) Heat induces inactivity of the thyroid, the mitochondria and Golgi complex shrink, and the colloid material accumulates.

(iii) Hypothyroidism increases susceptibility to moderate cold.

B. Functions of thyrocalcitonin (TCT) or calcitonin (CT)

(a) **Action on kidneys**

(i) CT reduces the reabsorption of Ca^{++} and inorganic phosphate from Henle's loop and distal convoluted tubule.

(ii) CT enhances Ca^{++} loss through urine.

(b) **Action on bone**

(i) CT helps to decrease the blood calcium level by preventing reabsorption of bone (i.e., release of calcium from bones).

(ii) CT stimulates the growth of osteoblast.

(c) **Action on vit. D metabolism**

CT in lungs and kidneys converts 25 hydroxycholecalciferol to 24, 25-dihydroxycholecalciferol in association with vit. D metabolite which may influence ca^{++} metabolism.

Differences between Thyrotrophin and Thyroxine

Subject	Thyrotrophin	Thyroxine
1. Origin	1. Basophil cells, called thyrotrophs of adenohypophysis.	1. Follicular cells of thyroid gland.
2. Chemical nature	2. It is glycoprotcin in nature.	2. It is a modified amino-acid.
3. Function	3. (i) It maintains the structure and function of thyroid gland and thereby affects the tissue metabolism indirectly. (ii) It functions through cell membrane receptors and cAMP.	3. (i) It regulates the tissue metabolism directly by modifying the enzymes in various tissues. (ii) It functions through intracellular receptors and modulation of genes for protein synthesis.

(C) PARATHYROID GLAND

Anatomically parathyroid gland is associated with thyroid gland. In mammals they are well developed and they are responsible for calcium and phosphorus metabolism. The description of this gland was given by **Sand Storm** (1880). In man, there are two pairs of small oval parathyroid glands that remain embedded in the posterior (dorsal) surface of the thyroid gland. Each lobe of thyroid contains a pair of parathyroids arranged vertically (i.e., one above the other).

Development

Parathyroid gland is derived from pharyngeal endoderm in association with 3rd and 4th branchial pouches of mammals.

Anatomy

In man, there are two pairs of small oval parathyroid glands ($6 \times 3 \times 2$ mm) that remain embedded in the posterior surface of the thyroid gland. Each lobe of thyroid contains a pair of parathyroids arranged vertically behind each lobe. Total weight is about 140 mg. This parathyroid gland is well vascularised by paired superior and inferior thyroid arteries. The gland is innervated by nerve supply same as the thyroid, probably purely vasomotor. Accessory parathyroids may be found in the thyroid, thymus or near the arch of aorta [Fig 4(c).1].

Histological structures

Each parathyroid gland is made up of masses or columns of epitheloid cells and numerous blood sinuses in between them. Two types of cells are present in it—**Chief cells** or **Principal cells** and **Oxyphil** or **Eosinophil cells.**

Chief cells are more numerous and comprise about 99% of the parathyroid's cellular population which remain throughout the life. These are small faintly staining agranular cells and contain completely clear cytoplasm. The cells are provided with comparatively large vesicular nucleus. This nucleus is round and centrally placed. The cytoplasm contains Golgi-complex, ER or mitochondria. The cells contain glycogen molecules. Chief cell comprises β-androgenic receptors as well as glucocorticoid receptors. Sometimes these cells enlarge and possess numerous cytoplasmic vacuoles; they are then called **water-clear cells**. Chief cells persist up to 10th year of life in human beings.

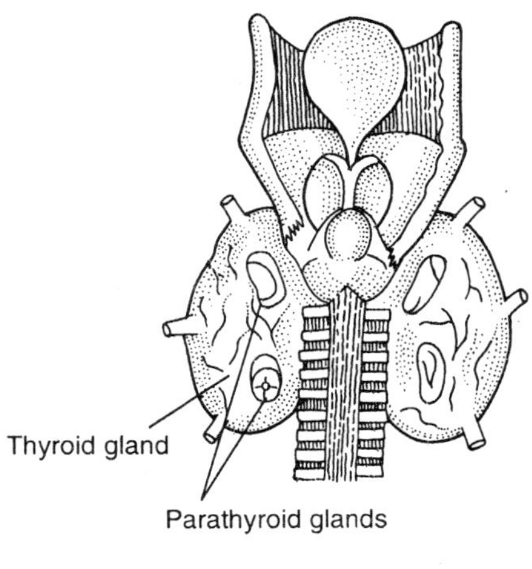

Fig. 4(c).1: Location of thyroid and parathyroid in dorsal view of trachea.

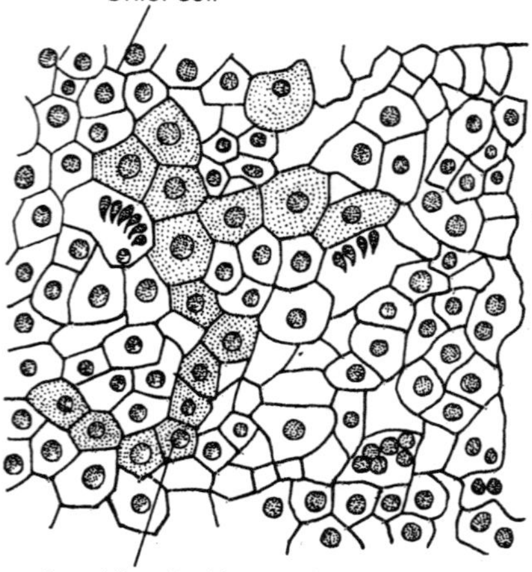

Fig. 4(c).2: Diagrammatic representation of histological structure of parathyroid gland.

The **oxyphil.cells** or **eosinophil cells** are few in number and represent only about 1% of the total parathyroid cellular population. These are large polyhedral granular cells containing acidophilic cytoplasm. Granules of oxyphil cells stain with eosin and other acid dyes. These cells are eosinophilic cells rich in mitochondria.

Both cell types contain fatty granules or minute spherical globules. Small colloidal vesicles (like those of thyroid) without any iodine and variable amounts of adipose tissue may be found within the gland [Fig 4(c).2].

Functions of hormones of parathyroid gland

The hormone of parathyroid gland is called **parathormone** (PTH). This is a polypeptide hormone. The chief function of PTH is to regulate blood level of calcium and phosphorus. The physiological effects of PTH are as follows :

1. **On kidney :** PTH regulates the excretion of inorganic phosphate in the urine. After injection of PTH there is increased phosphate excretion in the urine and serum phosphate level falls. Again, this hormone increases renal tubular reabsorption of Ca^{++}. Parathyroidectomy leads to increase in renal Ca^{++} output which can be inhibited immediately by the administration of PTH.

2. **On bone :** PTH acts in response to a lowering of blood calcium by stimulating the osteoclasts to reabsorb bone and free calcium ions from the reserve skeletal depots. After introduction of this hormone, blood calcium level rises due to mobilisation of calcium from the bones.

3. **On intestine :** It stimulates intestinal absorption of dietary Ca^{++} and phosphates.

4. **On blood corpuscles :** PTH is essential to accelerate the mitotic rate of red cell progenitors and thymic lymphocytes.

5. **On calcium level in the body :** PTH is essential for the regulation and concentration of calcium ions in the body fluids. After parathyroidectomy it was found that the blood calcium level falls and causes a neuromuscular irritability—the **tetany**.

6. **On vitamin D metabolism : DeLuca** (1968) has opined that vit. D is not metabolised to its functional form in absence of PTH. He provides a new light in the interrelationship between vit. D and PTH. According to him PTH stimulates vit. D_3 biosynthesis from vit. D precursors by the kidney and this vit. D_3 in turn enhances intestinal Ca^{++} uptake.

(D) THYMUS GLAND

Thymus is partly an endocrine gland and partly a lymphoid structure. It is housed in the anterior and superior mediastina of the thorax behind the sternum. The thymus is quite large in the young animal, but as the animal grows, it undergoes gradual and continuous involution. This gland extends from the pericardium up into the neck to the lower border of the thyroid gland. The thymus consists of two fused asymmetrical, elongated and flask-shaped lobes. The left lobe is smaller than the right. The immunological function of this gland was first studied by **Miller** (1961). The histological structure and the endocrine functions of thymus gland was recognised by **Good (1964)**, **Cooper (1976)**, **Kendeu (1990)**, **Ritter** and **Crispe (1992)**, etc [Fig 4(d).1].

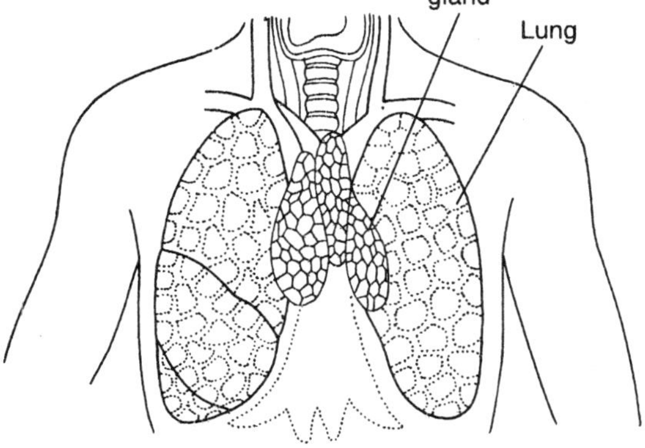

Fig. 4(d).1: Location of human's thymus gland.

Development

Thymus gland develops from the endoderm of the third and probably of the fourth branchial clefts on both sides and in mammalian embryos it is the primordial lymphoid organ. The outgrowths coalesce to form a single mass in the midline. This thymic mass subsequently becomes separated from the pouches and remains as a separate gland. The thymus is probably the main source of lymphocyte production in mammalian embryonic life; the rudimentary spleen, for example, does not contain the primordial cells necessary for lymphoid differentiation. At birth, when the spleen and lymph nodes are still poorly developed, the thymus is already a prominent lymphoid organ.

Morphology

Thymus is a bilobed flattened organ and lies between the posterior part of the thyroid gland and anterior to heart. The thymus consists of two asymmetrical, elongated and flask-shaped lobes. Each lobe is composed of innumerable lobules and the lobule is made up of small follicles of about 1 mm in diameter. Thymus is the largest relative to body weight in the foetus and in childhood up to the age of puberty, after which it undergoes gradual and continuous involution. During regression the thymic tissue is generally replaced by fat and connective tissue.

Thymus gland is well vascularised by blood vessels and lymph vessels and it is innervated by vagus nerve and cervical sympathetic nerves [Fig 4(d).2].

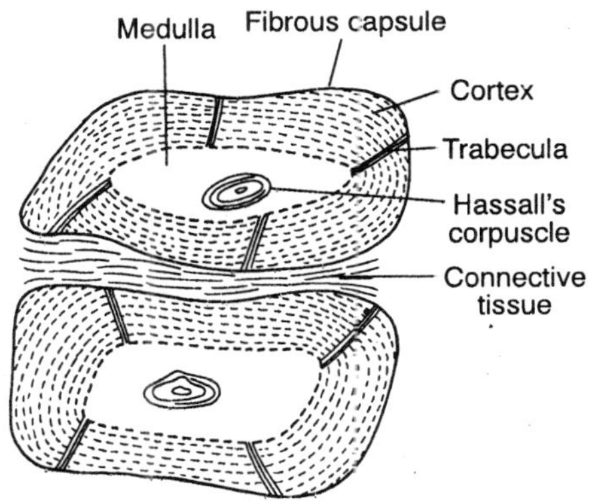

Fig. 4(d).2: Schematic representation of thymus lobules.

Histological structure

The thymus is the only lobulated organ and it consists of three parts, i.e., capsule, cortex and medulla.

(a) **Capsule :** Thymus gland is invested by a thin external dense connective tissue variably rich in **collagenous fibres, fibroblasts, plasma cells, granulocytes, lymphocytes, mast cells, fat cells** and **macrophages.** From this capsule connective tissue **septa** enter the gland and helps in the development of thymic lobules. Within the gland septa and trabeculae are formed by the connective tissue capsule extensions. The capsule and trabeculae also contain blood vessels, efferent lymphatic vessels and nerves.

(b) **Cortex :** It looks very similar to the lymphoid tissue of the ordinary lymphatic nodes, but lack of primary follicles. The cortex consists of densely packed masses of cells that morphologically look like lymphocytes. Cells are of various kinds—

(i) The **reticular cells are** elongated and have protoplasmic processes. EM study reveals that these processes are joined by desmosomes. The cells are acidophilic in nature possessing pale oval nucleus with one or two nucleoli. The cell cytoplasm is provided with mitochondria, Golgi apparatus, ER, ribosomes, etc. Scattered among these cytoplasmic organelles within the reticular cells few vesicles are noticed. The vesicles are supposed to be lysosomes.

(ii) **Lymphocytes** are of medium (7 to 10 μm in diameter), large (11 μm in diameter) and small (less than 7 μm in diameter) types. These are densely packed masses of cells within the cortex. They are supposed to be modified thymocytes. The cortex of thymus is highly basophilic due to presence of numerous closely packed small lymphocytes with deeply staining nuclei. They are more abundant than large lymphocytes. Small lymphocytes have dense round nucleus and the cytoplasm of these cells contains few ribosomes, mitochondria and GER.

Some large lymphocytes are present close to the capsule and the cytoplasm contains polyribosome, few mitochondria, GER, vesicles and lipid droplets. Cortical lymphocytes are distributed in a clear random manner between the epithelioreticular cells.

(iii) Numerous **macrophages** are also present in the cortex of thymus for phagocytosis of degenerating (rejected) lymphocytes. Macrophages which are heavily laden with lysosomes can be demonstrated with PAS reaction; they are called PAS cells.

(iv) A few **plasma cells** are also observed.

(v) At the peripheral region of cortex and near the blood capillaries, the protoplasmic processes of reticulocytes produce a continuous thin partitions to separate the

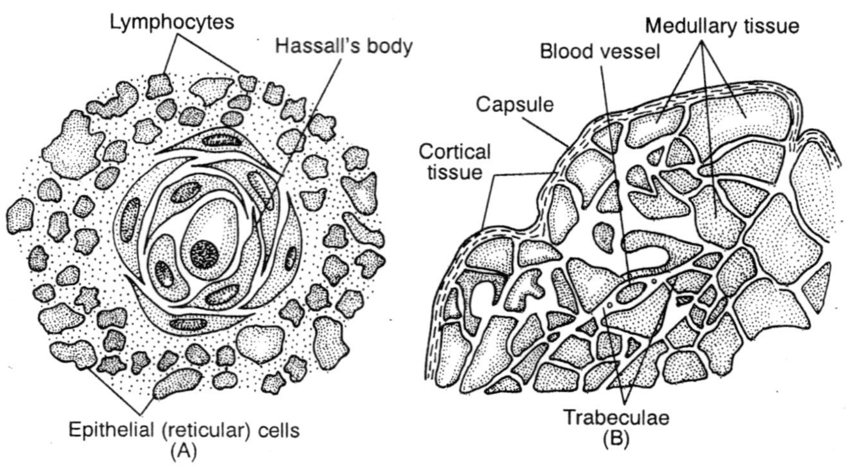

Fig. 4(d).3: Thymus Gland : (A) Diagram shows thymic medullary tissue. (B) Diagrammatic representation of histological structure of the thymus.

parenchyma from blood capillaries, called **blood thymus barrier.**

The stroma resembles reticular connective tissue but **reticular fibres are absent** [Fig 4(d).3].

(c) **Medulla :** It is a broad and branched band of thymic tissue. The medulla is filled up with reticular cells like those in the cortex. These cells are easily visible due to much less number of lymphocytes than in the cortex. There are variable numbers of plasma cells, mast cells, eosinophil cells and very few macrophages. Reticulocytes are of various shapes and sizes. Some are provided with small cytoplasmic or large cytoplasmic filaments. **Hassall's concentric corpuscles** or **thymic corpuscles** are organisation of flattened epithelial (reticular) cells and are the characteristic feature of the thymus. Macrophages are rarely observed and plasma cells are absent. The central cells are larger and show signs of degeneration and hyalinizaton. They may degenerate completely and cysts or calcareous deposits appear in them. According to **Blau** (1967), the Hassall's corpuscles may be actively phagocytic structures. **Ritter** and **Crispe** (1992) found that thymus secretes a number of hormones—Thymosin (α_1 and β_4), thymosterin lymphocyte stimulating hormone (LSH), Homeostatic thymic hormone (HTH) and thymopoietin.

Arteries enter along the medullary axis and distribute largely to the cortex. The **venous drainage** from the cortex is by interlobular veins, medullary veins and return the blood from medulla [Fig 4(d).4].

In humans, thymus is fully formed and functional at birth. The characteristic feature of thymic structure persists until about the time of puberty. After that lymphocytes processing and proliferation are abruptly reduced and the lymphatic tissue is largely replaced by adipose tissue. This is known as **involution**. By the old age thymus is degenerated to a quite

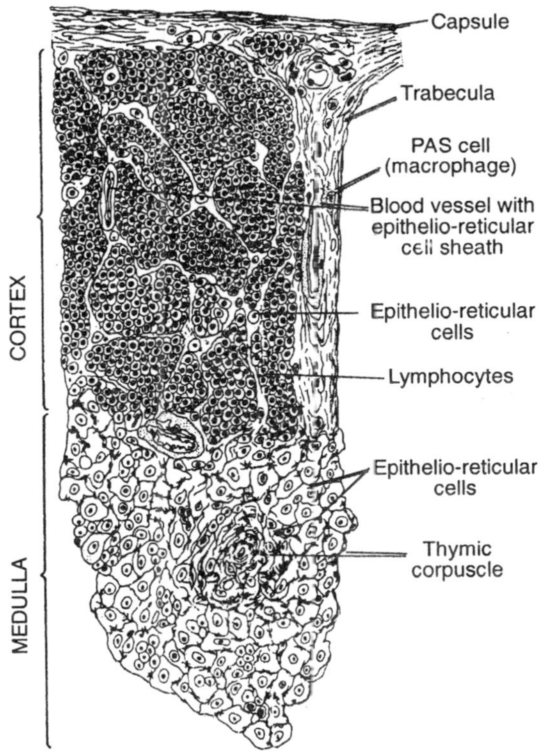

Fig. 4(d).4: Diagram showing histolcgical details of a portion of a thymic lobule.

thin chord of tissue which, however, remains in active state. This is recognised as **immunity theory of ageing.** Despite progressive decrease in their number with involution, thymic lymphocytes continue to differentiate and proliferate and thus, maintain a continuing supply of T-cells throughout life.

Function of hormones of thymus gland

Like other endocrine glands the endocrine function of thymus gland is not well recognised. A number of biologically active substances have been extracted from this gland which act as **thymic hormones** so that thyroid gland secretes a number of hormones like **thymosin α_1 and thymosin β_4, thymosterin, lymphocyte stimulating hormone (LSH), homeostatic thymic hormone (HTH)** and **thymopoietin.**

1. Thymosin : It is of two kinds.

(a) **Thymosin α_1** : It is a polypeptide hormone which helps in antibody production. It also depresses neuromuscular transmission (by regulating the amount of acetylcholine at the neuromuscular junction of skeletal muscles). An excess production of thymosin α_1 or thymin by the abnormal thymus results in a disease, **myasthenia gravis** in which the skeletal muscles are weak and there is a derangement of neuromuscular transmissions.

(b) **Thymosin β_4** : It is a large protein hormone which assists in differentiation of T-lymphocytes and also stimulates mitosis of T-lymphocytes.

2. Thymosterin : It is a steroid derivative hormone which inhibits tumour growth and stimulates antibody synthesis.

3. Lymphocyte stimulating hormone (LSH) : It is a small heat labile protein hormone which is essential for the normal process of lymphopoesis in the body. In infant mammal it secretes a humoral factor which stimulates lymph nodes to form lymphocytes and plasma cells which produce antibodies. In this way, it keeps the owner immune from certain diseases by providing a normal immunological response to foreign antigens. Consequently thymus removal at birth results in lymphocyte deficiency and lack of immunity. In adults, however, the thymus is not essential to life.

4. Homeostatic thymic hormone (HTH) : It is a small protein molecule which is made up of amino acids, amino sugar and a nucleotide. It is immunologically active.

5. Thymopoietin : It is also a protein hormone which stimulates the bone marrow to produce thymic lymphocytes.

(E) PINEAL GLAND

The pineal gland is a neuroendocrine gland that regulates daily body rhythm. The adult human pineal (epiphysis) is a pinecone-shaped organ, a shape that suggested the organ's name. This gland receives its stimuli through vision; hence, it is also called **third eye.** This gland was first discovered by **Herophilus**. The philosopher **Descartes** considered pineal gland as the 'seat of soul' and receives stimuli through this "third eye". **Larner** (1948) first established the biological activities of the gland. The pineal is innervated by postganglionic fibres originating from the superior cervical ganglia; the pineal is, therefore, an effector organ of the autonomic nervous system.

Development

The human pineal gland arises as a median evagination of the diencephalic roof of the embryonic brain; i.e., it develops from neuroectoderm of the posterior portion of the roof of the diencephalon and remains attached to the brain by a short stalk.

Anatomy

The human pineal gland is a somewhat flattened, cone-shaped, grey body measuring about 5-8 mm in length and 3-5 mm in breadth. It is located at the posterior wall of the third ventricle near the centre of the brain by a short hollow stalk. Pia-mater covers the body and gives rise to connective tissue septa that carry a number of blood capillaries into the organ. These septa separate cellular element into cords [Fig 4(e).1].

Histology

The pineal gland is a flattened and pine cone-shaped structure which consists of two types of major cells—pinealocytes and interstitial (glial) cells. The cells of the pineal are neural in origin, but bear little resemblance to nerve cells when fully differentiated. Besides these connective tissue cells, mast

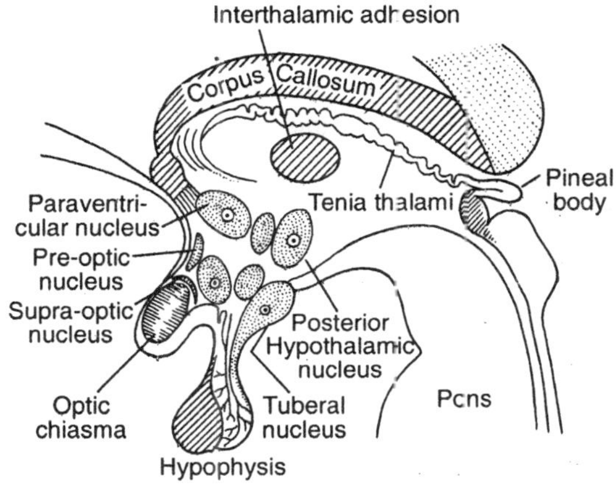

Fig. 4(e).1: Segittal section of human brain stem showing the anatomical position of pineal body.

cells, Schwan cells and axons of autonomic nerves are also present in the pineal gland [Fig 4(e).2].

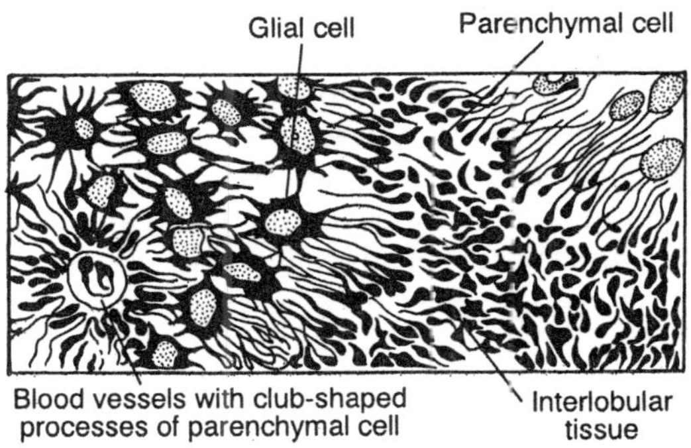

Fig. 4(e).2: Semidiagrammatic representation of an adult human pineal body showing two lobules.

(i) **Pinealocytes or parenchymal cells :** Pinealocytes are the chief cells of the pineal gland. They are arranged in clumps or cords within lobules formed by connective tissue septa that extend into the gland from the pia mater that covers its surface. Pinealocytes have a large deeply infolded nucleus with one or more prominent nucleoli and contain lipid droplets within their cytoplasm. E.M. studies reveal that they show typical cytoplasmic organelles along with numerous dense cord, membrane bounded vesicles in their elaborate and elongated cytoplasmic processes. The processes also contain numerous parallel bundles of microtubules. The expanded, club-like endings of the processes are associated with the blood capillaries. A moderately well-developed ER and Golgi apparatus and dense membrane bounded vesicles also typify these cells. In spite of lipid droplets, lipochrome pigment droplets and lysosome-like structures are often present. Histochemically the parenchymal cells contain acid phosphatase, succinic dehydrogenase, and some non-specific esterase and lipase.

(ii) **Interstitial (glial) or supportive cells :** They constitute about 5% of the cells in the gland. These cells have staining and ultrastructural features that closely resemble those of **astrocytes** and are reminiscent of the **pituicytes** of the posterior lobe of the pituitary gland. Pineal interstitial cells are markedly stellate in appearance and lie between the clusters of pinealocytes and in perivascular spaces. The cytoplasm is somewhat more basophilic. These cells have a dense nucleus, fewer mitochondria, granular reticulum and free ribosomes. There are occasional deposits of glycogen [Fig 4(e).3].

• The human pineal body is characterised by the presence of calcified concretions, called **corpora arenacea** or **brain sand.** These concretions are composed of a mineralised organic matrix and usually appear in the capsule and septa. These laminated calcareous nodules consist of calcium phosphate and carbonates. Function of these concretions is not clear (**Wood**, 1981).

Functions of pineal hormone

The pineal gland is secretory in nature which secretes the **melatonin** hormone.

1. **On gonads :** The ability of melatonin to modify gonadal function suggests that its secretion is associated with the timing of estrous and menstrual cycles, probably mediated through the decrease in gonadotrophic releasing factor of the hypothalamus.

2. **On photoperiodism :** The pineal gland is a photosensitive organ and an important time-keeper and regulator of the day/night cycle (circadian rhythm). During the day, light impulses inhibit the production of the melatonin hormone. So, pineal function, as

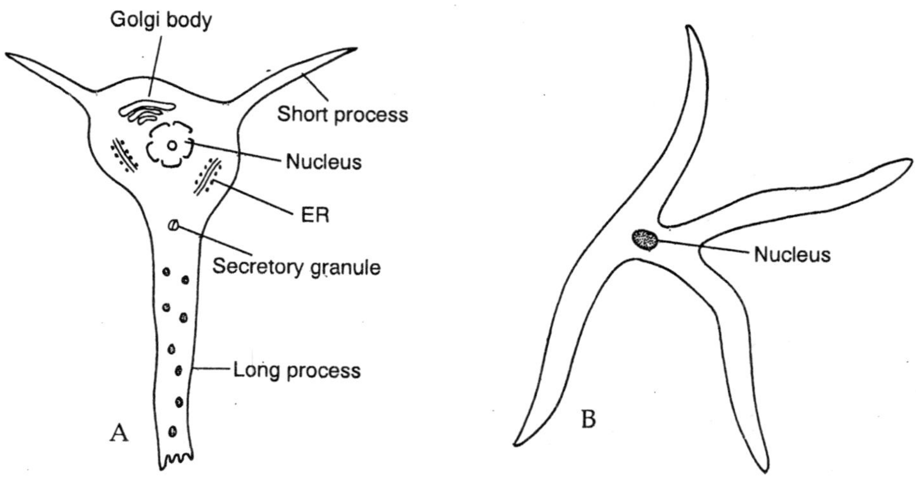

Fig. 4(e).3: Pineal body (A) Pinealocyte (E. M. structure), (B) Astrocyte (Supportive or glial cell).

measured by changes in the plasma level of melatonin, increases during darkness and decreases during light. These circadian changes of melatonin secretion play an important role in regulating daily body rhythms in human.

3. **On neuroendocrine function :** The pineal gland seems to participate in the regulation of the rhythmic activity of the endocrine system, by the elaboration of specific hormone or compounds such as methoxyindoles. The prime stimulus for this secretion may well be mediated by visual reflexes.

4. **On immunity :**

(i) Melatonin appears to enhance the functioning of the immune system and decreases the incidence of cancer.

(ii) Pineal gland is a source of a compound that cures schizophrenia.

5. **On other functions :**

(i) The pineal body shows a quick phosphorus metabolism as measured by the uptake of radioactive phosphorus.

(ii) Melaton in influences the sleeping centre and causes sleeping.

(iii) Melatonin induces to decrease the tropic hormones like TSH, LTH, ACTH, etc.

(iv) In young goats the pineal body displays a high rate of glucose utilisation being employed information of amino-acids. But this capacity diminishes with advancing age.

(F) ADRENAL (SUPRA RENAL) GLAND

Adrenal gland is considered to be essential gland in vertebrates. This gland secretes both steroid hormone and catecholamines. The adrenal glands are small, two in number, triangular in shape and are embedded in the peri-renal fat at the superior poles of the kidneys. The right gland is smaller and looks like a cocked hat, and the left one is roughly crescentic and usually larger. Each gland in the adult usually is about 5-9 gm.

This gland is covered with a thick connective tissue capsule from which trabeculae extend into the parenchyma, carrying blood vessels and nerves [Fig 4(f).1].

Anatomy

The adrenal gland is roughly triangular in shape and looks like a cap on the kidney. The adrenal gland combines with two distinct neuroendocrine systems, namely **cortex** and **medulla** into one organ, i.e., the secretory parenchymal tissue is organised into **cortical** and **medullary** regions. The **cortex** is the steroid secreting portion. It is housed beneath the capsule and constitutes nearly 90% of the gland by weight. The **medulla** is the catecholamine-secreting portion which lies deep to the cortex and forms the centre of the gland. The whole gland is covered by a well-developed capsule. The two parts are structurally, functionally and embryologically different. Histologically adrenal gland consists of **outer cortex (adrenal cortex)** and **inner medulla** [Fig 4(f).2].

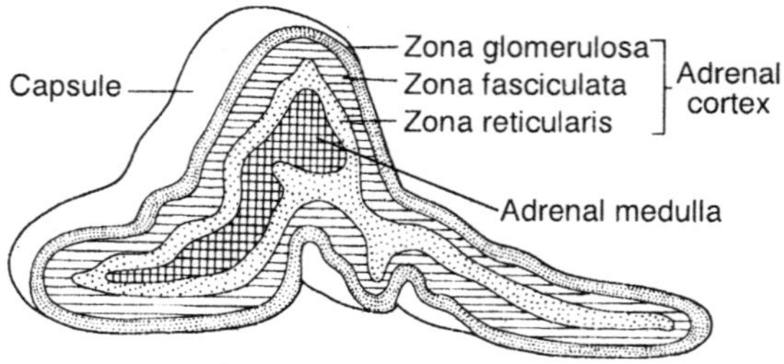

Fig. 4(f).2: It shows section through adrenal (ad = to) gland.

Development

The cortex and medullary components of supra-renal gland originate from different embryonic primordia. Embryologically, the cortical cells originate from mesodermal mesenchyme, whereas the medulla originates

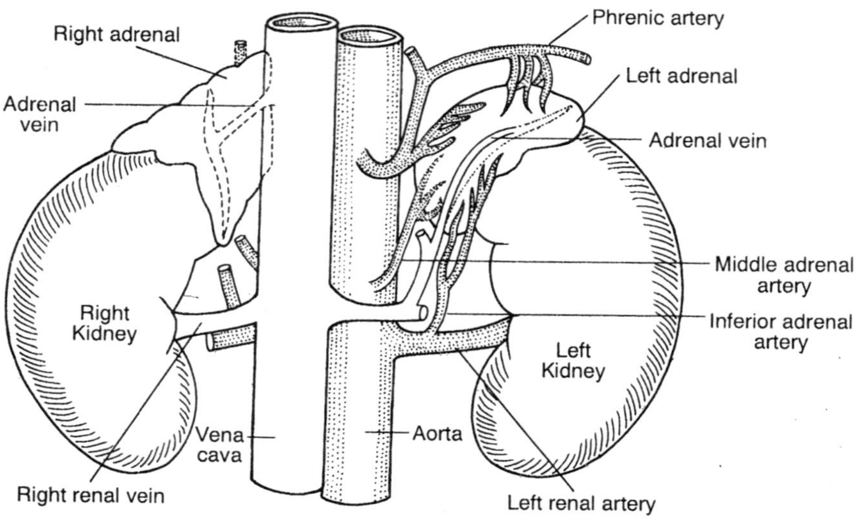

Fig. 4(f).1: It shows major arterial supply and venous drainage of the human adrenal gland.

from neural crest cells that migrate into developing gland. The parenchymal cells of the adrenal cortex are controlled by the anterior lobe of the pituitary gland and function in regulating metabolism and maintaining electrolyte balance. But the medullary secretion is controlled by nervous stimulus.

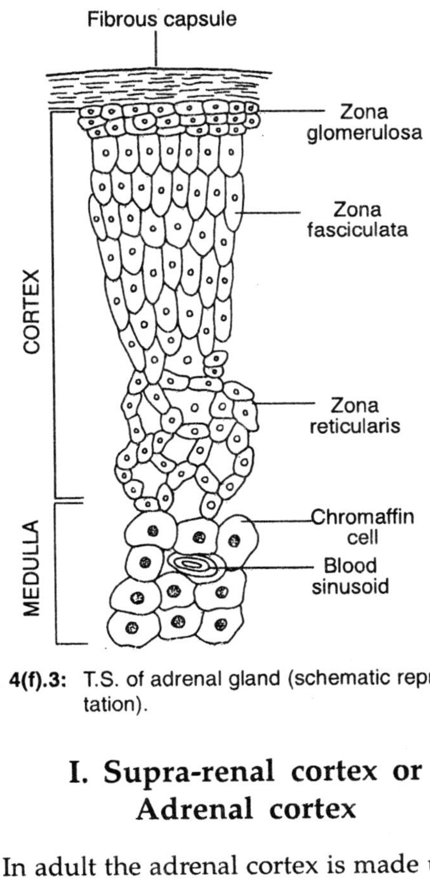

Fig. 4(f).3: T.S. of adrenal gland (schematic representation).

I. Supra-renal cortex or Adrenal cortex

In adult the adrenal cortex is made up of polyhedral èpithelial cells arranged in cords, generally two cells thick, that run radially from capsule to medulla. The cells contain well-defined nucleus, typical mitochondria, Golgi apparatus and numerous doubly refractile lipid granules in the cytoplasm. The adrenal cortex is invested by a capsule from which trabeculae pass into the gland, carrying blood vessels and nerves. The cells are arranged in the following three layers from outside inwards.

(a) **Zona glomerulosa** : It is the narrow outer zone which lies under a fibrous capsule. The cells of this zone are arranged in closely ovoid clusters just like bunch of grapes and curved columns that are continuous with cellular cords in the zona fasciculata. In humans some areas of the cortex may lack a recognizable zona glomerulosa. A rich network of fenestrated sinusoidal capillaries surrounds each cell cluster. The cells of this layer have abundant smooth surface ER, multiple Golgi complexes, large mitochondria with shelf-like cristae, free ribosomes and rough surface ER. Lipid droplets are sparse. This layer is made up of group of small columnar cells and this zone is light bluish in colour after H.E. stain owing to the presence of basophilic granules. Cells of zona glomerulosa synthesize and secrete mineralocorticoids mainly aldosterone and deoxy-corticosterone. Aldosterone acts in the control of blood pressure.

(b) **Zona fasciculata :** The thick middle zone of cortex that constitutes about 80 per cent of the cortical volume. The cells of this zone are large and polyhedral. They are arranged in long straight cords, one or two cells thick, that are separated by sinusoidal capillaries. The cells of this layer have a lightly staining spherical nucleus. Binucleate cells are common in this zone. Nuclei are larger and less dense. TEM studies reveal characteristics, typical steroid secreting cells, i.e., a highly developed smooth surface ER and mitochondria with tubular cristae. They are also provided with a well-developed Golgi-apparatus and numerous profiles of rough surface ER. Cytoplasm under H and E-staining shows extensively vacuolated indicating presence of lipid droplets in life. The cells of zona glomerulosa are so pronounced that sometimes these are called as **spongiocytes.** The zona fasciculata secretes glucocorticoids, so called because of their role in regulating gluconeogenesis and glycogenesis. The main glucocorticoids are hydrocortisone (cortisol) and corticosterone [Fig 4(f).4].

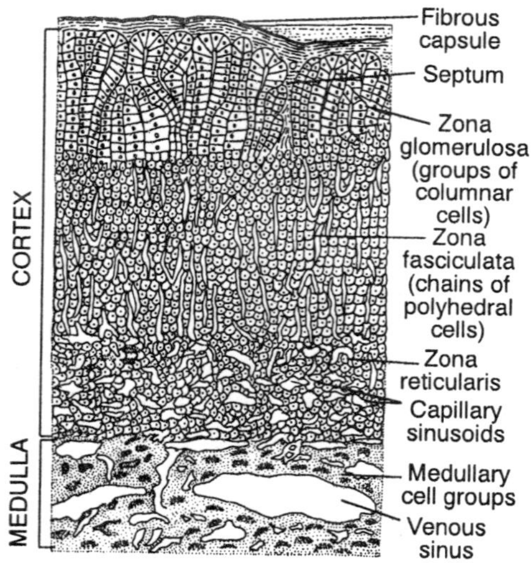

Fig. 4(f).4: Diagrammatic representation of section of adrenal (suprarenal) gland showing arrangement of cells in three layers of the cortex and part of medulla at the bottom.

(c) **Zona reticularis :** The cells of this zone are noticeably smaller than those of the zona fasciculata. The cells and their nuclei are more deeply stained. They are arranged in anastomosing cords separated by fenestrated capillaries. The cells have few lipid droplets. Both light and dark cells are noticed. Dark cells have abundant large lipofuscin pigment granules, and deeply staining nuclei are evident. The cells of zona reticularis are small, because they contain less cytoplasm than the cells in the zona fasciculata. Thus, the nuclei appear more closely packed. They have a well-developed smooth surface ER and numerous elongated mitochondria with tubular cristae but they have little rough surface ER.

Zona reticularis secretes sex hormones and a small amount of glucocorticoids but no aldosterone [Fig 4(f).5 and 6].

Functions of adrenocortical hormones

The sterol compounds of adrenal cortex is known as cortin that contain a number of steroids. It is broadly of two groups—(a) **Adrenal corticoids** and (b) **Sex steroids.**

(a) **Adrenal corticoids** are the following :

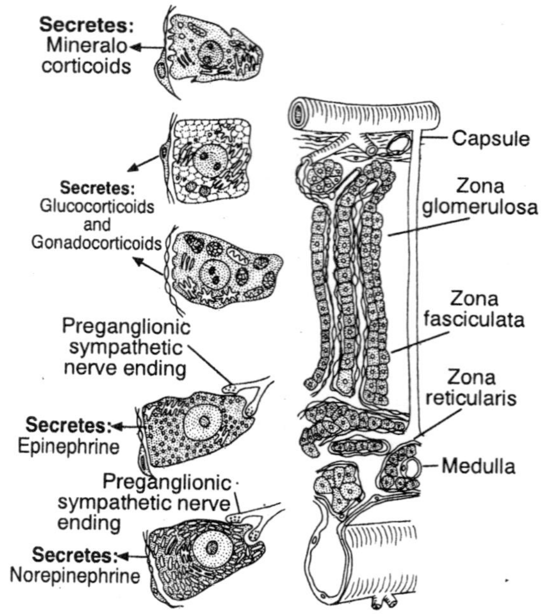

Fig. 4(f).5: Diagram illustrating the organization of the cells within the adrenal gland and their relationship to the blood vessels.

1. **Glucocorticoids :**

(i) 17-Hydroxy-corticosterone or cortisol or Kendall F-compound;

(ii) Cortisone or Kendall E compound or 17-Hydroxy-11-dehydroxy corticosterone;

(iii) Corticosterone or Kendall B compound;

(iv) 11-Dehydrocorticosterone or Kendall A compound.

2. **Mineralo corticoids :**

(i) Aldosterone or Electrocortin or 18-A idocorticosterone;

(ii) Deoxycorticosterone or Deoxycortone or 11-Deoxycorticosterone;

(iii) 17-Hydroxy 11-deoxycorticosterone or Reichstein (S compound)

(b) **Sex corticoids :** (i) Androgen (ii) Dehydroepiandrosterone (iii) Oestrogen and progesteron.

The hormones of supra-renal cortex are grouped into **glucocorticoids** that are concerned in carbohydrate metabolism;

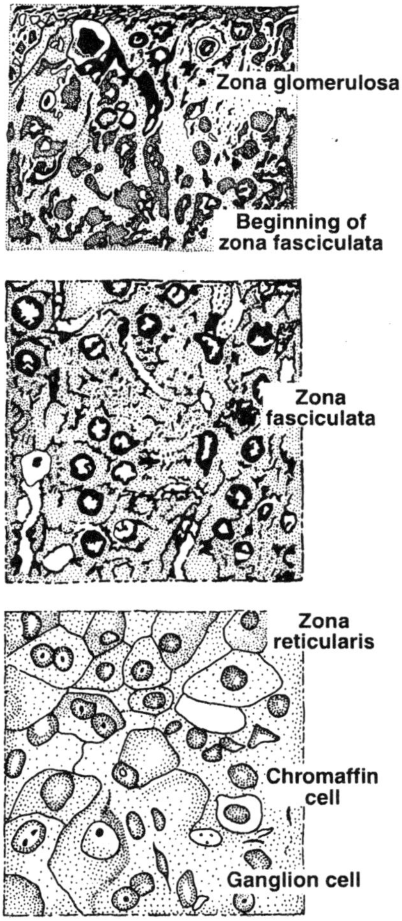

Fig. 4(f).6: Diagrammatic representation of histological structure (magnified) of zona glomerulosa, zona fasciculata and zona reticularis of cortex of the adrenal gland.

mineralo-corticoids that are concerned in mineral metabolism and **sex corticoids** that are responsible for sex functions.

Functions of glucocorticoids

(a) **On carbohydrate metabolism :**

(i) These hormones increase glycogen synthesis (glycogenesis) and storage in liver and muscles.

(ii) Reduce oxidation of glucose in tissues.

(iii) Stimulate formation of glucose from protein and fat (i.e., neoglucogenesis) in liver.

As a resullt of these actions glucocorticoids raise the blood sugar and urinary urea levels.

(b) **On blood :**

(i) Glucocorticoid hormones help in the destruction of leucocytes like eosinophils and lymphocytes and formation and maturation of RBC (i.e., erythropoiesis).

(ii) Increase the red blood corpuscles count.

(c) **On antistress action :** These hormones help the body to combat against stressful conditions. In deficiency of these hormones, a person cannot withstand stress.

(d) **On anti-inflammatory action :**

(i) These hormones protect the body from inflammations and allergic reactions.

(ii) Reduce the number of circulating monocytes, eosinophils and lymphocytes.

(iii) Prevent histamine release from mast cells.

(e) **On immunologic effects :** Glucocorticoids decrease the formation of antibodies and thereby assist to reduce the detrimental effects of antigen-antibody reactions.

(f) **On food intake :** Glucocorticoids help to maintain appetite and food intake. In deficiency of these hormones food intake is reduced owing to loss of appetite.

(g) **On cardiovascular system :**

(i) These hormones stimulate cardiac output.

(ii) Increase blood pressure by enhancing the action of catecholamines.

(iii) Inhibit capillary permeability.

(h) **On GI system :**

(i) These hormones help to maintain proper functioning of GI system.

(ii) Stimulate secretion of trypsinogen and pepsinogen.

(i) **On fat metabolism :**

(a) Glucocorticoids stimulate lipid absorption from the intestine.

(b) These hormones accelerate mobilisation of fattyacids and glycerol from the depots and its disintegration in the liver to form ketone bodies through their ability to mobilise free fatty acids.

(c) Depress the synthesis of lipid from carbohydrate.

Functions of mineralo-corticoids

This hormone is mainly released from zona glomerulosa.

I. Primary or direct action :

(a) **On mineral metabolism :**

(i) The principal function of these hormones is to regulate the reabsorption of Na^+, Cl^-, etc. and water from the renal tubules so as to maintain the blood levels of these materials.

(ii) These hormones increase the reabsorption of Na^+ and Cl^- but reduce that of K^+. With the retention of Na^+ and Cl^- the reabsorption of water is spontaneously facilitated. Thus, these hormones assist to conserve sodium salts and water in the body along with excretion of K^+ in urine.

II. Secondary or direct actions :

(a) **On water metabolism :**

(i) Mineralocorticoids stimulate in the absorption of water from renal tubules to maintain the water balance.

(b) **On blood :**

(i) Help to increase the haemoglobin and plasma protein in blood.

(ii) Stimulate in the maintenance of acid-base balance of the blood.

(c) **On cardiovascular system :**

(i) Hypersecretion of mineralocorticoids increases the cardiac output and hyposecretion inhibits cardiac output.

(ii) These hormones are responsible for the maintenance of excitability of heart.

(d) **On carbohydrate and protein metabolism :** Action is much but less than gluco-corticoids.

(e) **On fluid volume :**

(i) Stimulatė the thirst centre and as a result persons show thirsty.

(f) **On renal system :** Mineralocorticoids regulate renal function.

(g) **On stress effect :** More effective in protection against stress. Mineralocorticoids are essential for life because their absence cause salt imbalance and death.

Functions of adrenal sex steroids

These hormones are secreted from zona reticularis. The chief functions are given below. The hormones are androgen, estrogen and progesterone.

Effects in males :

(i) Androgen stimulates spermatogenesis jointly with FSH. Normally, androgen stimulates spermatogenesis in a paracrine fashion by diffusing into the seminiferous tubules directly from the sertoli cells. Both FSH and androgen stimulate the sertoli cells to release a protein, called androgen binding protein in the lumen of the seminiferous tubules. This maintains a high stable supply of androgen in the tubular fluid which enables the androgen to promote spermatogenesis.

(ii) Androgen hormone helps to develop the accessory sex organs and secondary sex characters.

(iii) The function of androgens is to develop masculine features in males. At the time of onset of puberty, the adenohypophysis begins to secrete ICSH (LH) which triggers the secretion of androgens from the testis. The androgens in turn bring forth the pubertal changes in the male.

• **Name the cell layers of adrenal cortex and the principal hormones secreted from them.**

	Name of layers	Hormones
(i)	**Zona glomerulosa**	Aldosterone, Deoxycorticosterone
(ii)	**Zona fasciculata**	Cortisol, Cortisone, Corticosterone, etc.
(iii)	**Zona reticularis**	Sex corticoids (Androgen, Estrogen, Progesteron)

• **What is aldosterone escape?**

Aldosterone increases Na^+ absorption in kidney but there is a limit of this reabsorption, beyond which an increase in aldosterone level cannot increase Na^+ absorption. Thus, even in presence of sufficient aldosterone level, Na^+ drains out through urine; this is known as **aldosterone escape**. This phenomenon reveals that in addition to aldosterone, there must be some other factors which control Na^+ reabsorption.

(iv) Increases BMR.

(v) Stimulates the growth of bones and muscles.

(vi) Androgen stimulates erythropoiesis.

Effects in females :

(i) Estrogen and progesterone jointly help in growth and development of the reproductive system.

(ii) Estrogen is responsible for development of secondary sex characters and pubertal changes in female.

(iii) Progesterone acts jointly with estrogen to maintain growth of uterus.

(iv) Progesterone acts synergistically with estrogen to facilitate the proliferation and development of mammary glands.

(v) Estrogen causes calcification and growth of bones.

(vi) Estrogen stimulates the synthesis of protein and fat in the body.

• **Functional divsions of adronal cortex with respect to steroid secretion :**

The **zona glomerulosa** secretes aldosterone. Its major function is the regulation of body sodium and potassium ion levels by stimulating the sodium pump of cell-membranes particularly in the renal tubules. It also participates in blood pressure control through rennin-angiotensin system. Aldosterone secretion is largely ACTH independent. The **zona fasciculata** secretes glucocorticoid hormones, principally cortisol which has numerous wide-ranging metabolic effects. Its important function is raising blood glucose levels and increase cellular synthesis of glycogen. Its secretion is controlled by ACTH. The **zona reticularis** is probably responsible for the secretion of small quantities of androgens and glucocorticoids.

II. Adrenal Medulla

Histological structure

The central portion of the adrenal gland, the **medulla** is composed of a parenchyma of large, pale staining epithelial cells called **chromaffin cells (medullary cells).** These cells are irregular masses of polyhedral granular cells, surrounded by numerous sinusoidal blood capillaries. Large distinct nucleus is present in each cell. The chromaffin cells are, in effect, modified neurons. Numerous myelinated, preganglionic nerve fibres pass directly to the chromaffin cells of the medulla. When nerve impulses carried by the sympathetic fibres reach the catecholamine secreting chromaffin cells, they release their secretory products. Therefore, those cells are considered the equivalent of postganglionic neurons. However, they lack axonal processes. These cells stain black with osmic acid, green with iron salts and brown with chromic acid. For the last property, the medullary cells are called chromaffin cells.

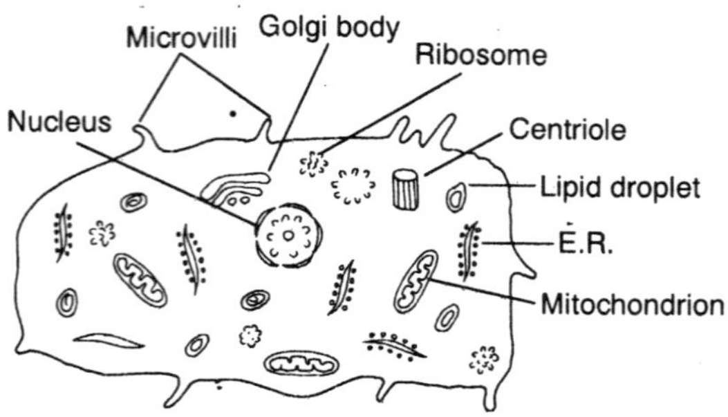

Fig. 4(f).7a: Ultra-structure of cortical cell.

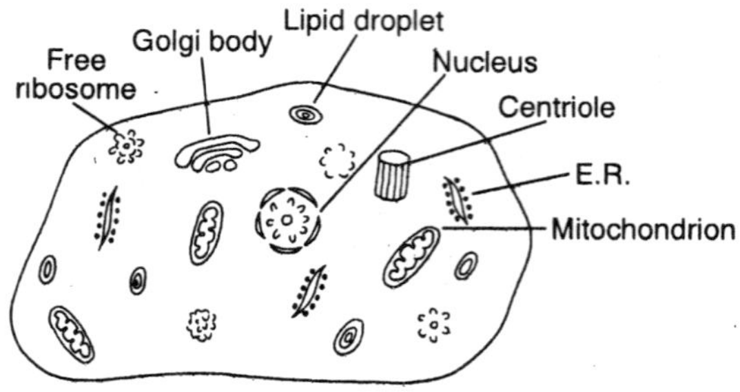

Fig. 4(f).7b: Ultra-structure of medullary cell.

Ganglion cells are also present in the medulla. These are small lymphocyte-like cells having dark nucleus with scanty cytoplasm. Staining reactions help to determine the limit between cortex and medulla. The axons of ganglion cells extend peripherally to the parenchyma of the adrenal cortex to modulate its secretory activity and innervate blood vessels.

E. M. structure of adrenal medullary cells : Chromaffin cells are organised in ovoid clusters and short interconnecting cords. The blood capillaries are arranged in intimate relation to the parenchyma. The medullary cells show dark granules. Each granule is enclosed by a smooth surfaced membrane and is dense in its core than in its periphery. Average diameter of the granules are about 200 μm. Ultrastructurally the chromaffin cells are characterised by numerous secretory vesicle, profiles of rough surfaced ER, distinct mitochondria and a well-developed Golgi apparatus. Cells have smooth plasma membrane. Microvilli are absent in those cells. The medullary cells do not have many rough surfaced vesicles. Moderate content of free ribosomes is also present. The TEM also reveals two populations of chromaffin cells distinguished by the nature of their membrane bounded vesicles—one population of cells contains only large **dense core vesicles.** These cells secrete **norepinephrine**. The other population of cells contain vesicles that are smaller, more homogeneous and less dense. These cells secrete **epinephrine** [Fig 4(f).7b].

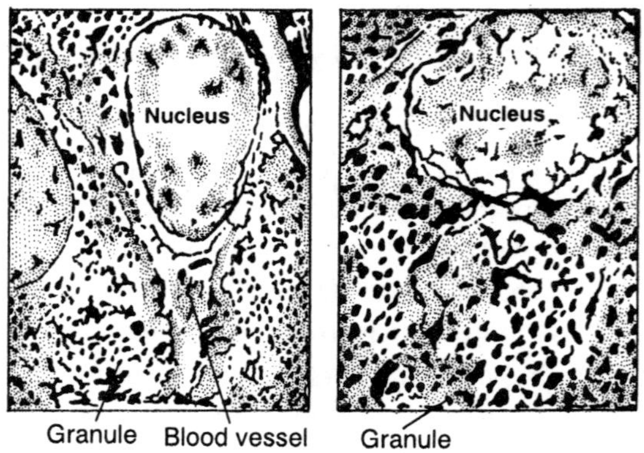

Fig. 4(f).8: Diagrammatic representation of electron micrographs of adrenal medullary cells showing abundant membrane-limited dense granules which are sites of storage of catecholamines.

Catecholamines : Catecholamines are amine derivatives of catechol compounds derived from the phenolic amino acid tyrosine. They include adrenalin (or epinephrin), noradrenalin (or norepinephrine) and dopamine which act as neurotransmitters or neurohormones. Catecholamines are housed in adrenal medulla and some nerve endings.

Functions of adrenal medullary hormones

Adrenal medulla secrete two hormones of catecholamine group, mainly **adrenalin** or **epinephrine** and to a smaller extent **noradrenalin** or **norepinephrine**. These hormones exert the following actions in the body.

(a) **Function of adrenalin (epinephrine)**

1. **On carbohydrate metabolism :**

(i) Blood sugar is raised due to breakdown of glycogen (i.e., glycogenolysis) in liver and muscles through **cori cycle.** This hormone activates phosphorylase in liver and skeletal muscles and hence blood sugar rises.

(ii) This hormone stimlates neoglucogenesis in liver by acting as an inducer like pyruvate carboxylase, glucose-6-phosphatase, etc.

(iii) Increases glycolysis (i.e., breakdown of glycogen to pyruvic acid or lactic acid) in muscles.

2. **On fat metabolism :**

(i) Epinephrine increases breakdown of fat into fatty acid and glycerol (i.e., lipolysis) in adipose tissues.

(ii) It helps in mobilization of free fatty acids from adipose tissue by enhancing lipase action.

(iii) Causes hydrolysis of neutral lipid through cyclic AMP.

3. **On Circulation :**

Heart :

(i) Heart rate and cardiac output increase.

(ii) Excitability of myocardium is increased.

(iii) Raises the conductivity of Bundle of His in heart.

Blood vessels :

(i) Assists in dialation of vessels of skeletal muscles.

(ii) Helps in constriction of splanchnic vessels.

Blood pressure :

(i) This hormone also causes vasoconstriction and as a result raises the blood pressure.

(ii) Increases the systolic blood pressure but no effect on diastolic pressure.

Blood :

(i) RBC, WBC and platelet count and percentage of haemoglobin are increased.

(ii) Helps in concentration of plasma proteins.

4. **On respiration :**

(i) Helps in relaxation of branchial muscles causing dilation of bronchioles.

(ii) Stimulates the rate and depth of respiration.

(iii) Accelerates the BMR, hence RQ is increased.

5. **On skeletal muscle :**

(i) Adrenalin facilitates the activity of skeletal muscles and delays onset of fatigue in them by increasing the blood supply and metabolism.

(ii) Helps in the conversation of muscle glycogen into lactic acid and discharges into the blood stream.

6. **On kidney** : Epinephrine selectively constricts the efferent glomerular vessels, thus reducing the glomerular flow but increasing the glomerular pressure. Consequently glomerular filtration increases. But in spite of it urine volume is reduced. This is because the rate of reabsorption of water by the renal tubule increases.

7. **On skin :**

(i) Adrenalin produces vasoconstriction and piloerection (erection of hairs) in the skin which help to conserve the body heat by preventing its loss due to radiation through skin.

(ii) Adrenalin acts on sweat gland in the skin of mammals to cause sweating.

8. **On nervous system** : Epinephrine produces a sense of restlessness, anxiety and fatigue.

9. **On digestive system** :

(i) Adrenalin stimulates the salivary gland to secrete more secretion of saliva.

(ii) It inhibits peristaltic movement of the stomach.

(iii) Epinephrine stimulates contraction of gall bladder and helps in the expulsion of bile to release into the small intestine.

> • **Why adrenalin is called emergency hormone?**
>
> The adrenal medullary hormone, adrenalin is known as emergency hormone because it helps the body to fight against (or to adjust with) the emergency conditions by increasing the respiration, circulation along with the activity of skeletal muscles, eyes, etc, i.e., this hormone is responsible for production of physiological reactions such as palpitation, piloerection, pupillary dilation, etc; in conditions of emotion (e.g., fear, anger, pleasure).

(b) **Function of nor-adrenalin (nor epinephrine)**

1. **On carbohydrate metabolism** :

(i) Noradrenalin stimulates glycogenolysis.

(ii) May inhibit the secretion of insulin.

(iii) Blood sugar level is slightly increased owing to the influence of noradrenalin.

2. **On fat metabolism** : Noradrenalin stimulates breakdown of fat into fatty acid and glycerol (i.e., lipolysis) in the blood.

Differences between Epinephrine and Norepinephrine

Subject	Epinephrine	Norepinephrine
1. Cardiac output	1. Increases cardiac output greatly.	1. Has no effect on cardiac output.
2. Heart rate	2. Increases heart rate profoundly.	2. Increases heart rate only slightly.
3. Blood vessels	3. Constriction of the blood vessels of skin, kidney, GI tract, spleen, etc. while relaxation of the blood vessels of liver, skeletal muscle and heart.	3. Constriction of all the blood vessels except the coronary vessels.
4. Peripheral resistance	4. Decreases the overall peripheral resistance.	4. Increases the overall peripheral resistance.
5. Uterine muscle contraction	5. Strong inhibition of uterine muscle contraction is seen.	5. Weak inhibition is noticed.
6. Broncho-dilation	6. Strongly increases.	6. No change is visible.
7. Blood surgar level	7. Moderately increases.	7. No change is noticed.
8. Central nervous system	8. Increase mental anxiety.	8. No effect is seen.
9. Eosinophil count	9. Increased.	9. No effect is seen.
10. Mean blood pressure	10. Slightly increases.	10 Strongly increases.

It is much less potent in producing metabolic effects.

3. **On circulation :**

Heart :

(i) This hormone increases heart rate slightly.

(ii) It has no effect on cardiac output.

Blood vessel : It constricts all blood vessels except the coronary vessels. Thus, noradrenalin is a general vasoconstrictor and it increases the overall peripheral resistance.

Blood pressure : Noradrenalin increases both systolic and diastolic pressures.

Blood : Has no effect on blood cell count.

4. **On respiration :**

(i) Norepinephrine helps to increase the rate and depth of respiration.

(ii) Due to the presence of nor-epinephrine O_2 consumption is slightly increased.

5. **On excretory system :**

(i) Nor-epinephrine helps in constriction of renal vessels.

(ii) It helps to decrease urine volume.

(iii) Helps in dilation of urinary bladder muscle.

6. **On digestive system :**

(i) This hormone may cause contraction of muscles of intestine

(ii) It causes contraction of gall bladder and assists in the expulsion of bile to pass into the small intestine.

7. **On skin :** This hormone acts on sweat gland to cause sweating in mammals.

8. **On CNS :**

(i) Has no effect on CNS.

(ii) Helps in dilation of pupil of eye.

• **Chromaffin cells :** The central portion of the adrenal gland, the medulla is composed of a parenchyma of large, pale-staining epithelioid cells. These cells stain brown with chromic acid. For this property they are known as **chromaffin cells.** They are, in effect, modified neurons. Numerous myelinated, preganglionic sympathetic nerve fibres pass directly to those cells of the medulla. When nerve impulses carried by the sympathetic fibres reach the catecholamine secreting chromaffin cells, they release their secretory products. Therefore, chromaffin cells are considered to be the equivalent of post-ganglionic neurons. These chromaffin cells are housed in the adrenal medulla, paravertebral and prevertebral sympathetic ganglia and various other locations. The scattered groups of those cells located among or near the components of the autonomic nervous system are termed as **paraganglia**.

• **PNMT :** The full of PNMT is phenylethanolamine-O-methyl transferase. It is found in adrenal medullary cytoplasm. It converts norepinephrine to epinephrine by N-methylation.

CHAPTER 5

Histology of Mixed Endocrine Gland

(A) PANCREAS OF MAMMAL

Pancreas is the second biggest gland in the body of mammals which is found in the region of the junction between the stomach and the duodenum. Its broad right extremity is called **head** which lies within the concavity of duodenum. Its main middle portion is termed as body and its narrow left extremity is called tail that lies near the spleen. The human pancreas is a large **retroperitoneal gland** and is both **exocrine** and **endocrine** in its secretory functions. The exocrine cells of the pancreas responsible for the enzyme-rich pancreatic secretion are the **pancreatic acinar cells.** The endocrine cells of the pancreas are found in scattered groups throughout the organ and are commonly designated as the **islets of Langerhans**. This endocrine part was first described by **Langerhans** in 1869 [Fig 5(a).1].

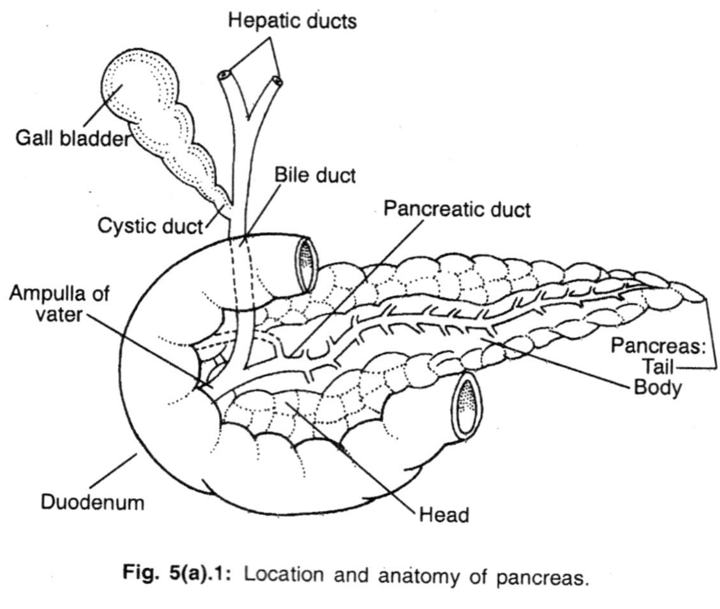

Fig. 5(a).1: Location and anatomy of pancreas.

Development

Pancreas is originated form endodermal lining of the duodenum.

Anatomy

The pancreas is an elongated leafy structure. The gland is creamy white or pale yellow in colour. The gland can be divided into a head, body and tail. However, there is no sharp demarcation between these three parts. The main excretory duct of pancreas is called the **duct of Wirsung** which combines with the common bile duct prior to the opening into the duodenum through the ampulla of vater. The opening of the bile-pancreatic duct is guarded by a ring of smooth muscle fibres called **sphincter of Oddi.**

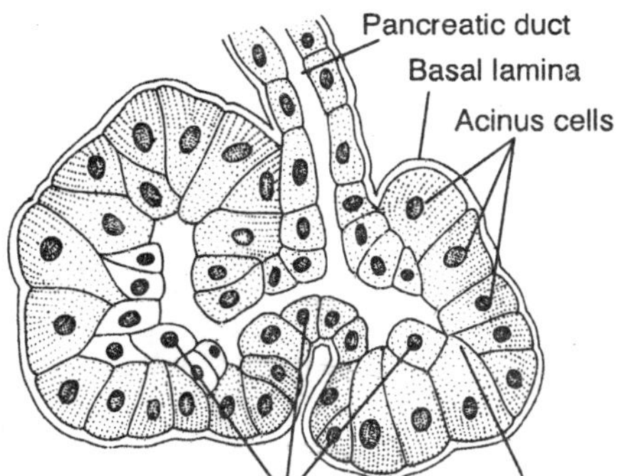

Fig. 5(a).2: T. S. of Pancreas.

Histological structure

The pancreas is a mixed gland, being composed of exocrine as well as endocrine tissues. The gland is diffused in nature and is invested by a thin layer of loose connective tissue. This layer of connective tissue forms a capsule for the gland. From the capsule, septa extend into the the gland, dividing it into ill-defined lobules. Within the lobule, a stroma of loose connective tissue surrounds the parenchymal units. Between the lobules, larger amount of connective tissue surround the larger ducts, blood vessels and nerve fibres.

The main mass of tissue is the **exocrine part** of pancreas within which clusters of **endocrine cells** remain embeded here and there constituting the **pancreatic islets**.

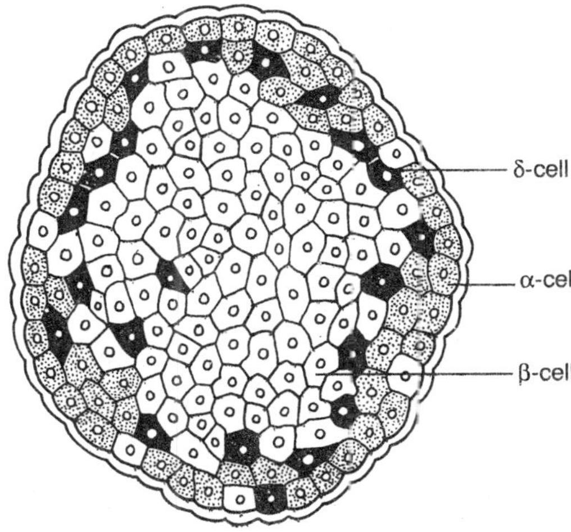

Fig. 5(a).3: Schematic representation of mammallan pancreatic islet.

Exocrine pancreas : Pancreas is practically a complex tubulo-alveolar gland. The exocrine part of this gland is identical to salivary gland and is composed of **acini** and **duct system.** The lobules of acinous gland are bound together by loose connective tissue, through which run blood vessels, nerves, lymphatics, and endocrine ducts. The pancreatic acini are of serous type being composed of secretory **zymogenic cells** which are of pyramidal shape and are arranged around a central lumen. The nucleus is round and situated at the broad part of the cell. Distinct nucleolus is also found inside the cell. The nucleus is acidophilic but the cytoplasm is basophilic. The basophilic nature is due to presence of large quantity of chromatidal material in the mitochondria of the cells. The secretory cells are covered by a basement membrane. Occasionally some **myoepithelial** or **basal cells** may be found in between the secretory cells and the basement membrane.

The acini that produce the exocrine secretory product vary from rounded structures to short tubules. They consist of single row of pyramidal epithelial cells converging toward a central lumen and resting upon a basal lamina supported by delicate reticular fibres. Between the acinar cells are fine secretory capillaries, connected with the central lumen. The acinar cells show rather striking differences in the various stages of secretion. In general, the basal part of the cell is homogeneous or may show a faint striation owing to presence of filamentous mitochondria in it. The apical portion of the cell is filled with highly refractile secretory granules or droplets which vary greatly in number, depending on the degree of secretory activity. The basal region of the acinar cells stains a dark purple whille the secretory granules are bright organe-red. The basophilic materials may have a lamellar or filamentous appearance. The Golgi apparatus is located in the supra-nuclear region. The zymogen granules or droplets arise in the Golgi region, they are particularly numerous in fasting animals and relatively few after a large meal. After discharge of the zymogen droplets, the Golgi apparatus enlarges as new secretory droplets are formed. The Golgi complex consists of stacks of parallel isternae, numerous small vesicles and condensing vacuoles containing secretory material of relatively low densily. The basal-half of acinus cell is occupied by tubular elements of granular endoplasmic reticulum and extensive parallel arrays of cisternae. Free ribosomes are abundant in the cytoplasmic matrix. The long mitochondria have well-developed cristae and numerous granules. The free surfaces of the acinar cells usually bear a few short, irregularly oriented microvilli. The apical cytoplasm is crowded with zymogen granules, some are found in the process of discharging their contents into the lumen of the acinus. The acini cells are covered with vascular network and nervous network.

Centroacinar cells form the begining of the **duct system.** These cells are continuous with the cells of the short **intercalated duct** that lies outside the acinus. The intercalated ducts are short and drain to interlobular collecting ducts. The complex, branching network of these ducts drains to the larger intralobular ducts which are lined with a columnar epithelium having goblet cells in between them. The interlobular and intralobular ducts drain directly into the main **pancreatic duct** [Fig 5(a).2 and 3].

Endocrine pancreas : The endocrine tissues of pancreas are called **islets of Langerhans** that remain scattered here and there in between the acinar tissue. The islets are made up of closely packed mass of cells. These are not connected with duct system of the gland but are richly supplied with blood capillaries. The islets constitute about 2 per cent of the volume of pancreas but are most numerous in the tail portion of this gland.

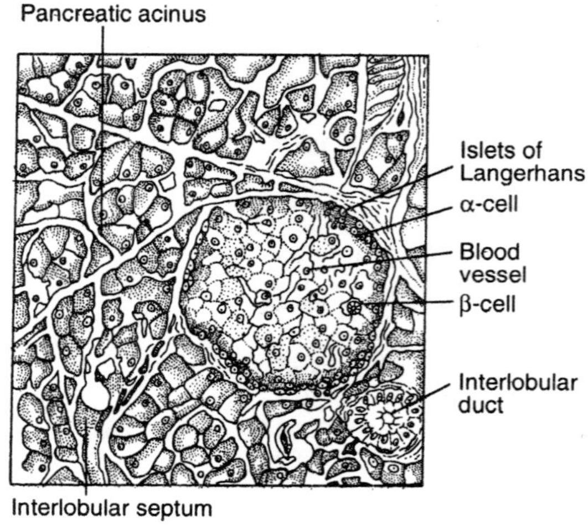

Fig. 5(a).4: A section of the pancreas showing a pancreatic islet cell.

Lacy and Greider (1972) have indentified the presence of three distinct islet cell types after **Mallory Azan Method**—α or A_2-cells (10-15%), β or B-cells (30-40%) and δ or A_1-cells (5-10%) [Fig 5(a).4]. Electron microscopy reveals that islet cells are of two categories—

(a) **Major cell types :** Three kinds of cells can be distinguished in islets on the basis of solubility and staining.

(i) **α-cells or A-cells :** These are fairly numerous (15-20 per cent) in most islets. Cells are tall and cylindrical. The α-cells contain rather course granules which are coloured red with acid fuchsin. These granules are about 250 μm in diameter and the granules are oval in shape and invested by lipoprotein membrane. The granule is oval in shape and bears high electron density. Here the nucleus is lobulated. The cytoplasm contains a well-developed Golgi complex, a moderate amount of granular ER, and occasionally free ribosomes. A few small filamentous mitochondria are encountered in the cytoplasmic matrix. These secrete **glucagon** hormone [Fig 5(a).5].

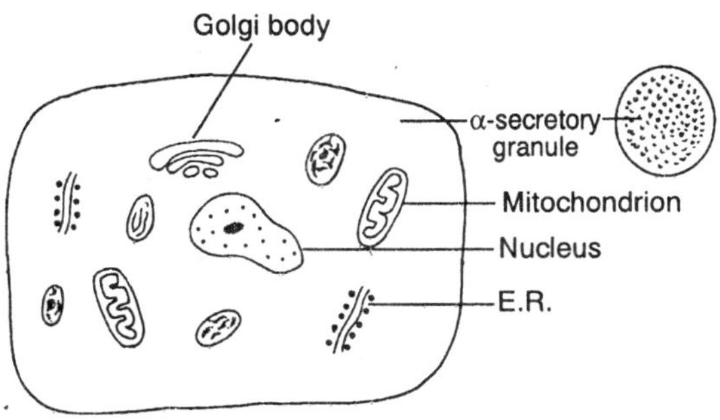

Fig. 5(a).5: E.M. structure of α-cell.

(ii) β-cells or B-cells : These are smaller and usually much more numerous (forming 70 per cent of total islet cells) and are aggregated in the middle part of islet. They possess many granules which are stained brownish orange with Mallory-Azan. The granules are hexagonal and lined by double-layered membrane and are generally similar in size (about 300 μm in diameter) to those of α-cells. Cells are more or less round or irregular in shape with centrally round nucleus. The cytoplasmic inclusions are more ER and free ribosomes than α-cells. Golgi bodies and mitochondria are apparent. They secrete **insulin** hormone [Fig 5(a).6].

(iii) δ-cells or D-cells : These cells constitute about 5-10 per cent of the total pancreatic endocrine tissue and are housed peripherally in the islet. The cells are large spindle shaped and are stained blue with Mallory-Azan stain. These cells contain numerous, small membrane-enclosed granules of moderately low density. The granules are about 325 μm in diameter. Nucleus of this type of cell is elliptical in shape. The cytoplasmic inclusions like ER, ribosomes, mitochondria, Golgi bodies are apparent. Few glycogen molecules and lipid droplets are visible. δ-cells secrete **somatostatin.**

(b) **Minor cell/other cell types :**

(i) X or F-cells : After light microscopy, **Bencosme and Leipa** (1955) first identified the presence of argyrophil cell type other than A_1-(δ)-cells and β-cells in the uncinate process of dog. They called them the X-cells. E.M. studies of **Munger et al.** (1965) suggested the term F-cells.

Functional importance of these cells have not established.

(ii) **E-cells : Thomas** (1937) and **Munger et al.** (1965) suggested the presence of this cell type with very large granules in islets of Opossum.

(iii) **C-cells :** The presence of C-cell in guineapig's pancreas was identified as a

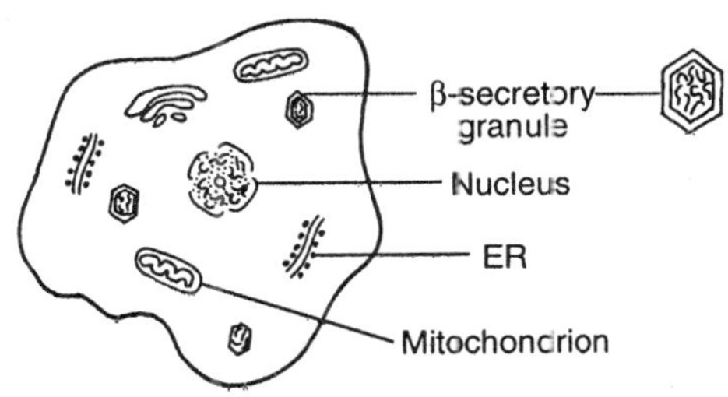

Fig. 5(a).6: E.M. structure of β-cell.

distinct cell type and considered as functional phase of α and β-cells. **Fujita** (1968) opined that this cell type are nothing but δ-cells or A_1-cells. **Watari, Tsukagoshi** and **Honma** (1970) have identified in the yellowtail fish that C_1-cells contain a large number of vacuoles, the diameter of which is almost the same as B_1-cell granules.

- **What is Houssay animal?**

A hypophysectomised and pancreatectomised animal is known as Houssay animal. Houssay observed that the hyperglycemia (increased blood sugar level) caused by pancreatectomy (removal of pancreas) can be corrected by hypophysectomy (removal of pituitary). Such a hypophysectomy and pancreatectomised animal is known as Houssay animal. It serves as an excellent model for studying the relationship between the functions of insulin and pituitary hormones.

Functions of Pancreas

The pancreas is unique among the glands of our body as it performs both **exocrine** as well as **endocrine functions.**

I. Exocrine functions :

The exocrine part or the acini secretes an enzyme-rich digestive juice, the pancreatic juice. It contains hydrolytic enzymes for digestion of carbohydrates, proteins and fats.

(a) **Digestive functions :**

(i) Pancreatic amylase acts on glycogen, starch and dextrin to convert them into maltose.

(ii) Trypsin acts on protein to convert it into amino acids through proteoses, peptones, polypeptides and peptides.

(iii) Chymotrypsin is one of the protein splitting enzymes which coagulates milk.

(iv) Pancreatic lipase almost completes the fat digestion in duodenum. This enzyme in presence of bile salts hydrolyses fat into fatty-acid and glycerol.

(b) **Splitting of nucleic acids :** Pancreatic nucleotidases like DNA-ase and RNA-ase, that act on DNA and RNA respectively into simpler components.

(c) **Neutralizing property :** The bicarbonate content of pancreatic juice tends to neutralise the acid of chyme coming from the stomach. Thus, it helps enzymatic activities.

II. Endocrine functions :

The pancreas secretes three hormones—**glucagon, insulin** and **somatostatin.** Glucagon and insulin regulate various metabolic functions. Somatostatin inhibit the secretion of GI hormones and digestive juices as well as motility of the GI tract.

Functions of glucagon : It is a **catabolic hormone,** i.e., it stimulates the catabolism of carbohydrate, protein and fat, thereby depleting the reserve food stores of the body. It has the following actions :

(1) **Carbohydrate metabolism :** The principal function of glucagon is to increase the blood sugar level. Hence, it is also called **hyperglycaemia** factor of pancreas. Glucagon raises blood sugar level by stimulating the breakdown of glycogen to glucose **(glycogenolysis).**

It increases the **neoglucogenesis** in the liver from proteins by inducing pyruvate carboxylase and FDPase.

(2) **Protein metabolism :** It increases the catabolism of amino acids in liver and urinary excretion of nitrogen thereby causing a negative nitrogen balance, i.e., it reduces protein synthesis by depressing the incorporation of amino acids into peptide chains.

(3) **Fat metabolism :** (i) Glucagon activates the enzyme lipase present in liver and adipose tissue as a result of which lipids are broken down and free fatty acid level of blood is increased.

(ii) Glucagon has ketogenic effects, i.e., it increases fatty acid oxidation and ketosis to supply more fatty acids to the liver.

(4) **BMR :** It increases heat production or BMR in the body because of its catabolic effects.

(5) **Mineral metabolism :** (i) Glucagon promotes cellular release of potassium, inorganic phosphate and calcium.

(ii) It tends to reduce hypercalcaemia and hyperphosphataemia by increasing calcitonin.

(6) **Actions on heart :** Glucagon has no ionotropic effect on cardiac tissue and in-

creases the cardiac output, arterial blood pressure and myocardial contraction.

Functions of insulin : Insulin is essentially an **anabolic hormone** because it assists to increase the storage of food in the body. It has the following actions in the body.

> **What is insulin? Where is it formed? Who discovered insulin?**
>
> Insulin is a protein hormone containing two polypeptide chains joined by disulfide bonds. It is formed in the β-cells of islets of Langerhans. (**Bantin & Best** discovered insulin).

(1) **Carbohydrate metabolism :** The main function of insulin is to reduce the blood sugar level. Insulin is the only hormone that has a blood sugar lowering effect; hence, insulin is also called **hypoglycaemic factor.** The hypoglycaemic effect of insulin is achieved in the following ways :

(i) **Oxidation of sugar :** It increases combustion of sugar in the tissues and assists in the transport of glucose into the cells. So it is effective on the skeletal muscle mass.

(ii) **Glycogen formation and storage :** Insulin increases glycogenesis from sugar and lactate, both in the liver and muscles. Generally in animal tissues glycogenesis occurs via the uridine diphosphate glucose pathway. Insulin increases the activity of synthetase to synthesise amylase, the acceptor being glycogen. Insulin promotes the uptake of glucose inside the cells and intracellular phosphorylation of glucose to glucose-6-phosphate which appears to be a specific activator of glycogen synthetase.

(iii) Insulin regulates hepatic neoglucogenesis by inducing glucose-6-phosphatase and carboxylase.

(iv) It increases the permeability of different tissues to glucose so as to facilitate the transport of glucose from blood to tissues.

(2) **Protein metabolism :**

(i) It increase the permeability of tissues to amino acids like that of glucose and helps in the entry of amino acids from blood to tissues.

(ii) Insulin stimulates synthesis of proteins from amino acids entering into the tissues.

(iii) It depresses protein catabolism and reduces the process of gluconeogenesis from protein.

(3) **Fat metabolism :**

(i) It stimulates lipogenesis, i e., accumulation of depot fat.

(ii) It decreases the cholesteraemia and lipaemia. It also prevents accumulation of excess lipid in liver and breakdown of lipid in adipose tissue.

(iii) Insulin stimulates to increase ketone bodies from fatty acids in liver. The presence of ketone bodies can cause severe acidosis and coma in patients.

(4) **On growth :** It induces the growth of the body by virtue of its protein anabolic effects because growth is not possible without protein synthesis. Insulin is essential for the growth promoting action of STH.

> **• Complimentary interactions of insulin and glucagon in maintaining blood glucose level in the body.**
>
> In response to elevated glucose level, insulin, after release from β-cells, interacts with its receptors at different cell types. Within the liver, insulin activates glycogen synthetase, and produces a direct flow of glucose toward glycogen formation.
>
> Conversion of intracellular glucose to glucose-6-PO_4 prevents glucose release from hepatocytes. In fat cells insulin-stimulated glucose uptake results in enhanced catabolism of the sugar to glycerol.
>
> The biological actions of glucagon are essentially the opposite of those of insulin. Glucagon stimulates hepatic glucose synthesis and release through a glycogenolytic action or through neoglucogenesis.

Distinguish between Insulin and Glucagon

Subject	Insulin	Glucagon
1. Source	1. β-cells of islets of Langerhans.	1. α-cells of islets of Langerhans.
2. Chemistry	2. It is a polypeptide made up of 51 amino acids having two chains joined by disulfide (S-S) linkages.	2. It is a single chain polypeptide having 29 amino acids and is devoid of disulfide (S-S) linkage.
3. Functions	3. It is an anabolic hormone which lowers the blood sugar level. It stimulates glycogenesis, lipogenesis and protein synthesis. It inhibits gluconeogenesis.	3. It is a catabolic hormone which increases blood sugar level. It stimulates glycogenolysis and lipolysis. It stimulates gluconeogenesis.

Functions of somatostatin :

(i) Somatostatin secreted from δ-cells of pancreas inhibits the secretion of insulin and glucagon from the pancreatic islands in a paracrine fashion, i.e., it functions locally on the β-and α-cells without entering the circulating blood.

(ii) Somatostatin is also released into the circulating blood which inhibits secretion of gastrin, secretin, motilin, etc. from the gastrointestinal mucosa and may regulate the peristaltic activity of GI tract.

(iii) It may also directly inhibit the secretion of both bicarbonates and enzymes in pancreatic juice.

- **What is diabetes mellitus? Differentiate between diabetes mellitus and diabetes insidipus?**

Ans. Diabetes mellitus is a pathological condition due to deficiency of insulin secretion and is characterised by hyperglycaemia and glycosuria as a consequence of disordered carbohydrate metabolism.

Distinguish between Diabetes Mellitus and Diabetes Insidipus

Subject	Diabetes Mellitus	Diabetes Insidipus
1. Cause	1. It is caused by deficiency of secretion or action of insulin.	1. It is caused by deficiency of secretion or action of ADH.
2. Symptoms	2. Blood sugar level is high, i.e., hyperglycaemia occurs.	2. Hyperglycaemia does not occur.
	3. Glycosuria occurs, i.e., sugar is eliminated through urine.	3. Glycosuria does not occur.
	4. Large volume of urine is excreted, i.e., polyuria occurs but the specific gravity of urine is high.	4. Large volune of urine is excreted (polyuria) but the urine is dilute having low specific gravity.
	5. Abnormally intense thirst (polydipsia) and excessive hunger (polyphagia) are noticed.	5. Polydipsia occurs but polyphagia is not observed.

• Osteocalcin

Osteocalcin is a noncollagenous protein found in serum dentin. It is secreted by osteoblasts and thought to play a role in mineralization and calcium ion homeostasis. It has been stipulated that osteocalcin may also function as a negative regulator of bone formation, although its role is unknown. .

In August 2007, it was reported that osteocalcin acts as a hormone in the body, causing beta cells in the pancreas to release more insulin, and at the same time directing rat cells to release the hormone adiponectin, which increases sensitivity to insulin.

Use as a biochemical marker for bone formation : As osteocalcin is manufactured by osteoblasts, it is often used as a biochemical marker, or biomarker, for the bone formation process. It has been routinely observed that higher serum-osteocalcin levels are relatively well correlated with increases in bone mineral density (BMD) during treatment with anabolic bone formation drugs for osteoporosis, such as **Forteo.** In many studies, Osteocalcin is used as a preliminary biomarker on the effectiveness of a given drug on bone formation.

(B) THE TESTIS

Reproduction is one of the basic life process by means of which living organisms can produce new individuals of their own kind to maintain continuity of the living races. In an individual, the organs concerned with reproduction together constitute the **reproductive system.** Like other vertebrates, in humans also the sexes are separate, i.e., they are sexually distinguished into male and female individuals having separate reproductive system. The male reproductive system consists of the testes, genital excurrent ducts, accessory sex glands and penis. The accessory sex glands comprise the seminal vesicles, prostate, and bulbourethral glands. The two principal functions of the testis are the production of sperm, male gametes and systhesis of androgens or sex hormones.

Anatomy

The testis consists of paired somewhat flat, oval bodies, one on each side, remaining inside the **scrotum.** In early foetal life, they remain within the abdomen. During the third week of gestation, the testis move caudally from their position high in the abdomen, then gradually migrate and descend in the scrotum.

The primary sex organ of human males is called **testis.** It is a compound tubular gland enclosed in a thick fibrous capsule. The male accessory sex organs are divisible into three groups—(i) the **reproductive tract** consisting of epididymis, vas deferens, ejaculatory duct and urethra; (ii) the accessory sex glands including seminal vesicle, prostate gland and Cowper's gland; and (iii) the male external genitalia or penis.

Among the aforesaid primary and accessory sex organs, prostate gland, urethra and penis are present in singles while the remaining ones are paired. In mammals testes are ovoid or walnut-shaped in appearance. Testes are creamy white in colour and well vascularised with genital arteries, and veins. Each testis is covered by a tough, compact, and fibrous capsule, the **tunica albuginea** from which trabeculae descend and divide the gland into a number of pyramidal lobules. The lobules are filled up with convoluted seminiferous tubules, each about 500 mm long. Several tubules unite to form a straight tubule which again unite forming the rete testis [Fig 5(b).1].

• **Rete testis :** The seminiferous tubules of each testicular lobule unite to form a straight tubule. The straight tubules of the different lobules join in an irregular manner to form a network like structure, called the **rete testis,** which leads into the vasa efferentia emerging from the testis.

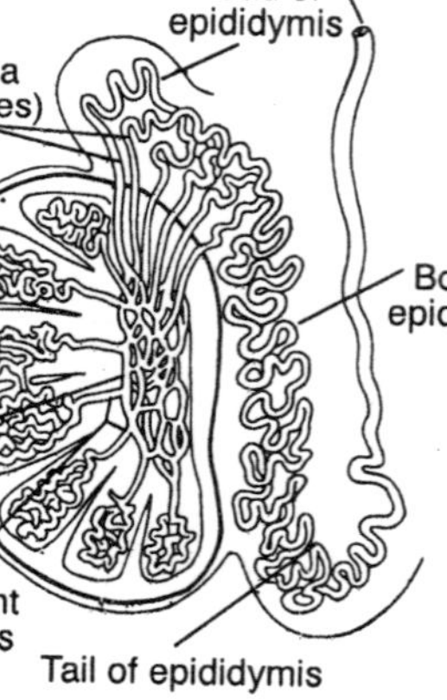

Fig. 5(b).1: Longitudinal section of testis.

Development

The testes originate on the posterior wall of the abdomen and later descend into the scrotum. They develop in close association with the urinary system retroperitoneally, on the posterior wall of the abdominal cavity. Testes are derived from three sources : (i) **intermediate mesoderm** that forms the urogenital ridges on the posterior abdominal wall; (ii) **mesodermal epithelium** that lines the urogenital ridges; (iii) and primordial germ cells that migrate from the yolk sac in to the developing gonads, where they divide and differentiate into spermatogonia.

Location

Testes are paired male gonads. In vertebrates other than mammals testes are housed on either side of the vertebral column in the abdominal region. They are held in position by ligaments and mesenteries. These organs are attached with the peritoneal muscle.

In mammals the testes are located within the **scrotal sac** which is situated on the anterior aspect of the body near the junction of the legs with the abdomen. They are attached with the scrotum wall by ligaments, called **mesorchium.**

• **Cryptorchidism :** In the embryonic life, the testis begins to develop in the abdominal cavity and then descends into the scrotum before birth. It is a condition in which the testis fails to descend into the scrotum, i.e., retention of one or both of the testes in the abdominal cavity of an individual.

Histology

The testis is composed of three elements :

(1) **Tunica albuginea :** The testis has an unusually thick connective tissue capsule, the tunica albuginea. The inner part of this capsule, the **tunica vasculosa,** is a loose connective tissue layer that contains blood vessels. Tunica albuginea is composed of collagenous connective tissue with an admixture of elastic tissue. There is a thin layer of squamous cells on the outer surface of this coat, which is mesothelial lining of the scrotal sac reflected over the testis. Along the posterior surface of the testis, the tunica albuginea thickens and projects inward as the **mediastinum testis.** Blood vessels, lymphatic vessels and the genital excurrent ducts enter or leave the testis through the mediastinum. The tunica albuginea, the fibrous covering, from which trabeculae or septa descend into the mass of the testis, dividing it into a number of pyramidal lobules. Each lobule contains one to four highly convoluted **seminiferous tubules,** which produce spermatozoa and loose connective tissue, called the **interstitial tissue.** In human each testis contains of about 400-600 seminiferous tubules which measure about 150-250 μm in diameter and 30-80 cm in length.

(2) **Seminiferous tubules :** Inside the testis two main structures are noticed—**Leydig cells** and **seminiferous tubules.** Each seminiferous tubule is externally bounded by a basement membrane within which lie the **germ cells** at different stages of maturation. The seminiferous tubule is a complex stratified epithelium, i.e., the wall of the seminiferous comprises an outer capsule or **tunica propria** which is made up of elastic connective tissue and flattened fibroblast cells. The basal lamina separates the epithelium from the tunica propria. Below the basal lamina few flattened smooth muscle cells are found, called **Myoid cells.**

Internally the seminiferous tubule contains living stratified epithelium or **spermatogenic cells** and **Sertoli cells.**

(i) **Spermatogenic cells** are lined by four to eight layers of cells, each layer representing a particular stage in the development of spermatozoa. From outside inwards the following five layers are found; the **spermatogonia, primary spermatocytes, secondary spermatocytes, spermatids** and **spermatozoa.**

The spermatogenic cells contain spherical nucleus with granular chromatin and are about 12 μm in diameter. The spermatogenic cells are organised in poorly defined layers of progressive development between adjacent sertoli cells. The most immature spermatogenic cells, the **spermatogonia** or **stem cells** rest on the **basal lamina.** The most mature cells, the **spermatids,** are attached to apical portions of the sertoli cell. There are two kinds of spermatogenic cells—A-type and B-type cells.

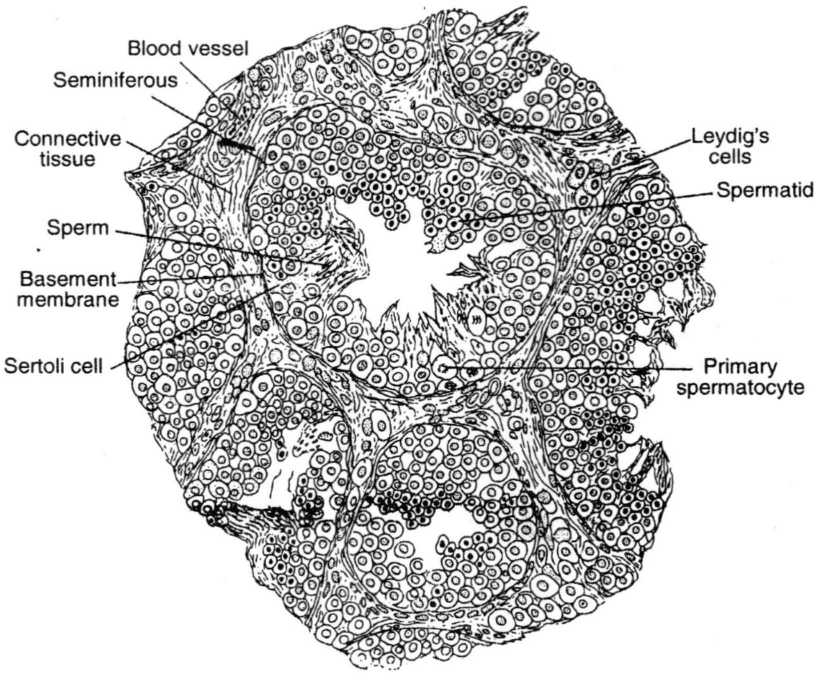

Fig. 5(b).2: T. S. of testis.

A-type cells are with one or two nucleoli at the inner surface of nuclear envelope. These spermatogenic cells are reserve cells, whereas the B-type cells have central nucleolus and mitotic in nature. The nucleus is spherical in shape. They divide into **primary spermatocytes,** which are large cells and have very large vesicular nuclei. The primary spermatocytes measure about 17-19 μm in diameter. These cells divide meiotically into **secondary spermatocytes.** They are larger than primary spermatocytes with distinct chromatin materials. The secondary spermatocytes undergo further division and form the **spermatids.** The spermatids, therefore, contain only half the number of chromosomes (i.e., 23). They are small about 9 μm in diameter. Cells have distinct nucleus, Golgi apparatus and centrosome. The spermatids do not divide any more. They gradually mature into spermatozoa and they contain distinct nucleated head and tail [Fig 5(b).2].

- A-type is distinguished into dark Ad and pale Ap types. Both types are provided with slightly ovoid nuclei. The nucleus measures about 6-7 μm in diameter. Type Ad can be recognised from AP type by the more intense staining of the nucleoplasm and the presence of large pale staining nuclear vacuole [Fig 5(b).3].

(ii) **Sertoli cells** are also known as **supporting** or **sustentacular cells.** They are tall columnar cells with extensive apical and lateral processes that surround the adjacent spermatogenic cells and occupy the spaces between them. The nucleus of this kind of cell is situated towards the base and is ovoid or triangular in shape and may have one or more deep infoldings. The nucleus of it contains a unique tripartite structure which comprises of a RNA containing nucleolus flanked by a pair of DNA bearing bodies, known as **karyosomes**.

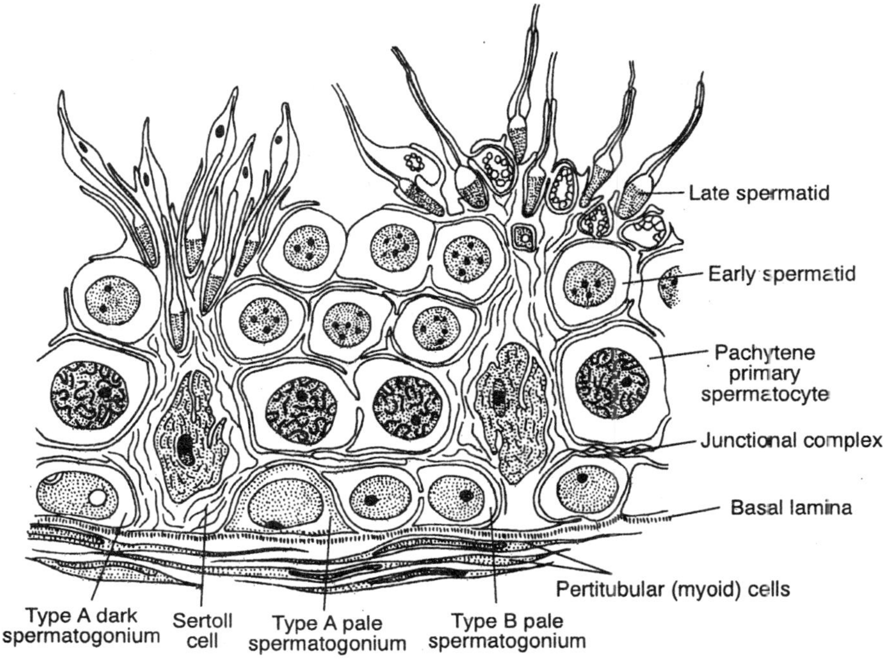

Fig. 5(b).3: Schematic drawing of human seminiferous epithelium. This figure shows the relationship of the Sertoli cells to the spermatogenic cells.

There is a special sheath of 70-90 Å filaments which surrounds the nucleus and separates it from other organelles. The cytoplasm bears selender mitochondria, Golgi bodies, ER, lysosomes, lipid droplets, glycogen granules and fine filaments. The apical end of sertoli cell is provided with invagination which provides the nutrition to the early spermatozoa. Sertoli cells give structural organisation to the tubules as they extend through the full thickness of the seminiferous epithelium.

• **Spermiation** is the process of release of mature sperms into the lumen of the seminiferous tubules from the sertoli cells, under the influence of LH of adenohypophysis.

Seminiferous tubules are avascular. Within the testis special junctional complexes between the adjacent sertoli cells near the base of the seminiferous epithelum are seen. These complexes are provided with many parallel lines of fusion of the apposed cell membranes which effectively prevent the entry of substances into the system of intercellular clefts. So the sertoli junctional complex is referred to as the site of **blood testis barrier** which divides the tubular epithelium into two portions—(i) a basal one bearing spermatogonia and primary spermatocytes and (ii) an adluminal one containing secondary spermatocytes, spermatids and spermatozoa. This kind of barrier helps to conserve certain product of sertoli cells, such as androgen binding protein (ABP) [Fig 5(b).3].

• **Function of sertoli cells :** These cells serve as "nurse" cells for differentiating spermatogenic cells. That's why they assist in the exchange of metabolic substrates and wastes between the developing spermatogenic cells and the circulatory system. Sertoli cells phagocytise any spermatogenic cells that fail to differentiate completely. In addition, these cells secrete fluid that facilitates the passage of maturing sperm into the intertesticular duct and also secrete ABP (androgen binding protein) which is necessary to concentrate testosterone hormone in the lumen of the seminiferous tubule. It is essential for the normal maturation of developing sperm.

(3) **Leydig cells (interstitial cells) :** These cells are referred to as the endocrine part of the testis. Leydig cells are large, polygonal, eosinophilic cells that typically contain lipid droplets. Lipofuscin pigment is also frequently found in these cells. They also contain distinctive, refractile, rod-shaped cytoplasmic crystals, the **crystals** of **Reinke,** of unknown function. Like other steroid-secreting cells, Leydig cells have an elaborate smooth endoplasmic reticulum (SER). The enzymes necessary for the synthesis of testosterone from cholesterol are associated with the SER. Mitochondria of Leydig cells have the characteristic tubulovesicular cristae. The cytoplasm of this cell also contains Golgi apparatus, ribosomes, lipid droplets, protein crystals, etc.

Leydig cells are arranged at the angular position of the seminiferous tubules of the testis. There are two types of cells in the mass—**fusiform cells** having relatively few organelles and **large cells** containing more organelles and vesicles.

• **Cryptorchidism** : Cryptochidism is unilateral or bilateral absence of the testes from the scrotum because of failure of normal testicular descent from the genital ridge through the external inguinal ring.

Functions of Testis

It performs both **exocrine** and **endocrine functions.**

A. Exocrine function :

The exocrine function of the testis is the formation of mature sperm from the seminiferous tubules of testis, i.e., **spermatogenesis.**

Spermatogenesis occurs in two stages. Firstly, **Spermatids** are formed from germ cells or mother cells and secondly, sperms are produced from spermatids which is known as **Spermiogenesis.**

(a) **Formation of spermatid :** The primary germ cell or mother cell is diploid cell produced from the testis and it gives rise to spermatids. The process takes place in three stages :

(i) **Multiplication phase :** The primary germ cell undergoes mitotic division and gives rise to a large number of spermatogonial cells. The spermatogonium is diploid.

(ii) **Growth phase :** In this phase mitotic division ceases and spermatogonia increase in size and they are called primary spermatocytes. During this phase crossing over and splitting of chromosomes are completed.

(iii) **Maturation phase :** In this phase primary spermatocyte undergoes maturation division. At first maturation process by meiotic division gives rise to haploid number of chromosome and reduction in cell size occurs. These cells are referred to as secondary spermatocytes. The secondary spermatocyte then gives rise to two haploid spermatids. Each spermatid then develops into one spermatozoon.

(b) **Spermeogenesis :** The transformation of spermatids into spermatozoon is known as spermeogenesis. So this process causes structural modifications of spermatids to form mature sperms with acrosome, middle piece, tail, etc. that are necessary for motility and penetrating ability of the sperms. Spermatogenesis is controlled by FSH of anterior pituitary and androgen of testis.

The immature sperms remain attached to the sertoli cells which nourish them. After maturation sperms are released into the lumen of the seminiferous tubules from the sertoli cells. The phenomenon of release of sperms from sertoli cells is called **spermiation** which is controlled by LH of anterior pituitary.

B. Endocrine function :

The interstitial cells of Leydig secrete the male sex hormone, called **testosterone**. This hormone is also secreted to some extent from sertoli cells of testis. It performs several functions :

(i) **Effects on growth of seminiferous tubule and spermatogenesis :** Androgen stimulates this spermatogenesis jointly with FSH. Normally hormone stimulates spermatogenesis in a paracrine fashion by diffusing into the seminiferous tubules directly from the Leydig cells. Sertoli cells play an important role in this. Both FSH and androgen stimulate the sertoli cells to release ABP within the seminiferous tubule. This maintains a high and stable supply of androgen in the tubular fluid which enables the androgen to promote spermatogenesis.

(ii) **On accessory sex organs and glands :** Testosterone stimulates the growth and functions of necessary sex organs of males, e.g., epididymis, seminal vesicle, prostate gland, Cowper's gland, vas deferens, urethra, etc. Thus, it helps in the maturation and full growth of the male reproductive system and maintain its proper functioning.

(iii) **Effect on secondary male sex characters :** Testosterone helps to develop and maintain the secondary sex characters like beards, mustache, masculine voice, distribution of hairs over the pubis, chest, back, etc. and distribution of pigments on the skin. It also causes emotional make up (characteristic feature of man) and sexual activities.

(iv) **On bone growth and musculature :** Testosterone increases the synthesis of muscle proteins for well-built musculature. It also increases the formation of bone matrix and deposition of calcium salts in the bones for their growth.

(v) **On blood :** Androgen stimulates the formation of RBC and for this reason, the total count of RBC in males is slightly higher than that in females.

(vi) **Effect on sperms :** Testicular hormone increases the span of life and fertilizing power of the spermatozoa.

• **Capacitation :** Full fertilizing power is achieved only after travelling within the uterine tube. This power is known as **capacitation** and the capacitation is acquired only after staying in the uterine cavity for a few days, because ejected sperm into the vagina has got a little fertilising power.

(vii) **Effect on BMR :** Androgens are protein anabolic in nature and they stimulate protein synthesis. Androgens, for protein anabolic activity, increase BMR. For this reason, the BMR of males is higher than females.

(viii) **On sexual behaviour :** Androgens maintain the sexual behaviour of males, e.g., attraction for opposite sex, sexual desire, etc. Deficiency of androgen may lead to impotence.

Structure of the mature sperm

A mature spermatozoon is a highly specialised type of cell. The greater part of its total volume is represented by nuclear material. The sperm is characterised by the presence of a propulsive system in the form of an axial filament powered by energy obtained from the mitochondria. The mature human sperm is about 60 μm long.

A typical mammalian sperm comprises the following main parts : head, neck, middle piece or body and tail.

Head : The sperm head is flattened and pointed, i.e., spoon-shaped and measures 4.5 μm long and 3 μm wide. The head is composed of an elongated nucleus which is covered by a chromosomal membrane. This nucleus occupies the major part of the head. The anterior tip of the head is differentiated as the **acrosome** which plays an important role in the penetration of the spermatozoon through the egg membrane and the activation of the egg during fertilization. The acrosomal cap that covers the anterior two-third of the nucleus contains hyaluronidase, neuraminidase, acid phosphatase and a trypsin-like protease, called acrosin.

Neck : The neck is very short connecting the head with the middle piece or body and contains a centeriole known as proximal centriole. There is another centriole lying at the junction of body and tail; this is known as distal centriole or ring centriole. The distal centriole gives rise to the axial filament of the flagellum of the spermatozoon for which it serves as a basal granule or a starting point. The cytoplasm forms a condensed layer, known as **manchette**, around the posterior part of the nucleus [Fig 5(b).4].

Middle piece or body : E. M. reveals a highly complex architecture in the middle piece. The most important internal structure is the **axial filament** which comprises two **central fibres** surrounded by ring of nine double **inner fibres.** In mammals the nine pairs of longitudinal fibres are surrounded by nine thick outer fibres. Still more external are **mitochondria,** arranged spirally around the rings of filaments.

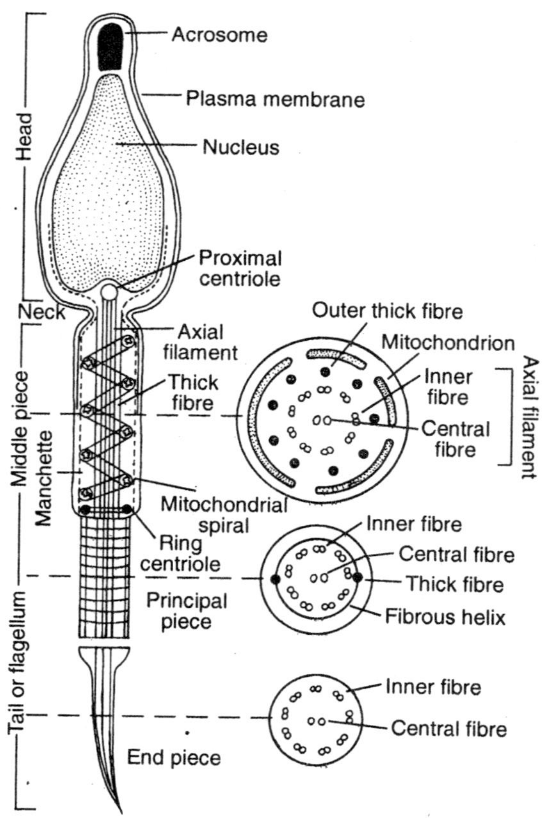

Fig. 5(b).4: Semi-diagrammatic view of a mammalian spermatozoon.

Tail : The main piece of tail is in continuation of axial filament. The mitochondrial sheath is anclosed by semicircular group of fibrils. This portionn is responsible for the movement of the sperm.

The end or terminal piece of tail consists of axial filament enclosed by a plasma membrane and a thin layer of cytoplasm. It has no covering sheath [Fig 5(b).5].

• **Roles of Leydig cell and sertoli cell in spermatogenesis :** During hormonal regulation of spermatogenesis, FSH interaction with sertoli cell plasmalemmal receptors results in the synthesis of ABP. The ABP is then secreted into the lumen of the seminiferous tubules. In response to LH, testosterone is synthesised in the Leydig cells, because sertoli cells are connected by tight junctions, thus providing a blood testis barrier. Testosterone may be taken up by the sertoli cells by an active transport or facilitated diffusion. Within the sertoli cells testosterone is bound to ABP. This binding protein may provide a mechanism for testosterone sequestration close to the spermatocytes whose maturation is androgen dependent. Because germ cells lacking androgen receptors develop into fertile spermatozoa in the presence of normal sertoli cells. It is presumed that the hormonal effects of testosterone on spermatogenesis are mediated via the sertoli cells. ABP may also provide a mechanism for the accumulation of androgen within sertoli cells, which then can be released (via vesicular exocytosis) into the lumen of the seminiferous tubules. Within the lumen ABP may function to transport testosterone to epididymis where they

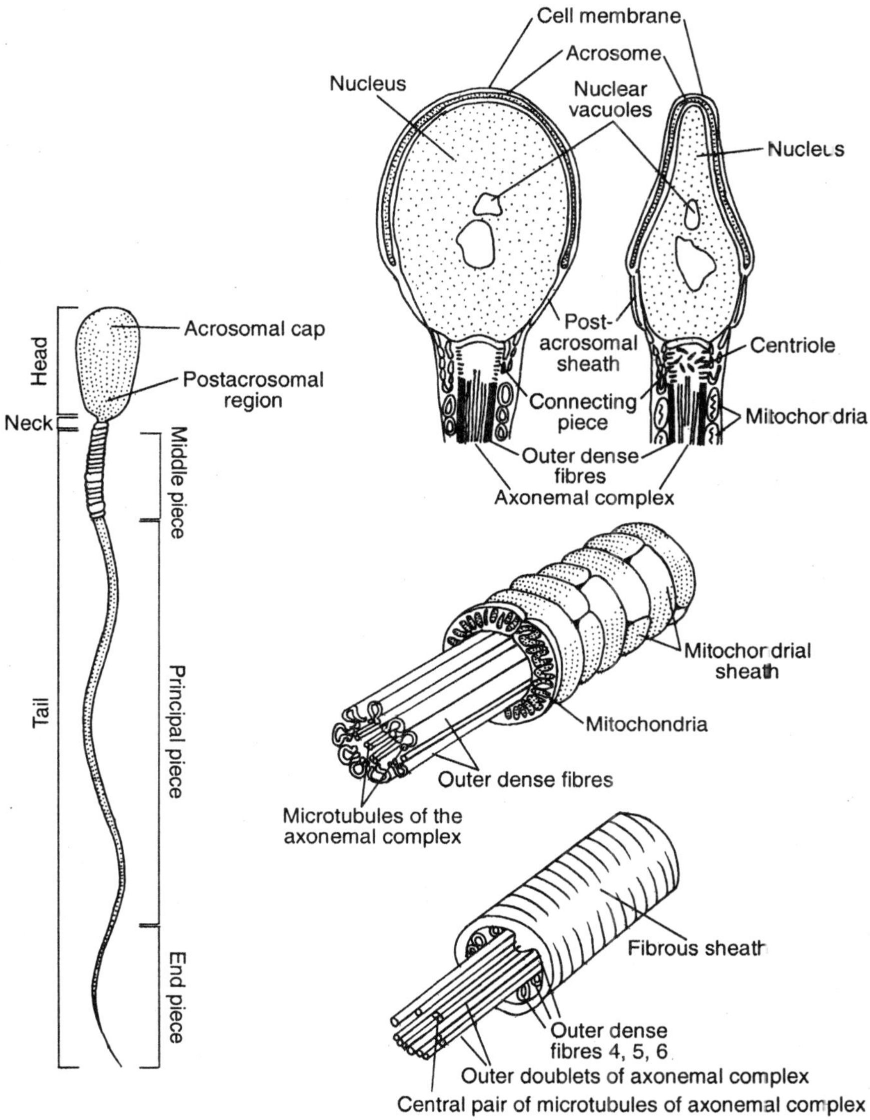

Fig. 5(b).5: Diagram of a human spermatozoon.

develop the potentiality for fertilization and motility. Meiosis II is hormonally independent. FSH participates in spermiogene-sis. Estradiol and DHT are also involved in the spermatogenic process. The Leydig cells synthesise and secrete testosterone.

Blood testis barrier : The seminiferous tubules of testis are avascular. Within the testis, there are specialised junctional complexes between adjacent sertoli cells just near the base of the seminiferous epithelium. These complexes comprise many parallel lines of fusion of the apposed cell membranes, which prevent effectively the entry of substances into the system of intercellular clefts. This is termed as **blood testis barrier**, which divide the tubular epithelium into two compartments—a **basal one** bearing the spermatogonia and primary spermatocytes and **adluminal one** bearing secondary spermatocytes, spermatids and spermatozoa.

It conserves certain products such as androgen binding protein (ABP) of sertoli cells within the seminiferous tubules.

(C) THE OVARY

The female reproductive gonads are ovaries. Production of female gametes and steroid hormones like estrogens and progesterones are the two major functions of the ovary.

Anatomy

There are two somewhat bean-shaped bodies, one on each side, near the free end of the fallopian tube, hanging from the broad ligament by a fold of peritoneum, called the **mesovarium.** In the region of attachment, known as the **hilus,** are found smooth muscle fibres, numerous large blood vessels and lymphatics. The tissue of the broad ligament is continued into the ovary, where it spreads out as the **stroma.** The free surface of the ovary is covered with surface epithelium, the modified mesothelium of the visceral peritoneum.

Location

Each ovary is situated on either side of the pelvic cavity near the free end of the fallopian tube and remains suspended by three ligaments namely the broad ligament, the ovarian ligament and suspensory ligament of the corresponding side. The ovary is attached to the broad ligament by a fold of peritoneum, the mesovarium. The ovarian ligament connects the ovary with the uterus and through this ligament large blood vessels, lymphatics and nerves enter into the ovary. The suspensory ligament attaches the ovary with the posterior wall of the pelvic cavity.

Ovarian histological structure

There is no organ in the female body which shows so much histological variations at different phases of life. The following is a brief description of a normal mature ovary. A section through the ovary reveals two distinct regions cortical region or cortex and medullary region or medulla.

(1) **Cortex :** It is located in the peripheral portion of the ovary surrounding the medulla. The cortex contains the **ovarian follicles** embedded in a richly cellular connective tissue. Scattered smooth muscle fibres are found in the stroma around the follicles.

(2) **Medulla :** It is located in the central portion of the ovary and contains loose connective tissue, a mass of relatively large contorted blood vessels, lymphatic vessels and nerves.

(i) **Germinal epithelium :** The surface of the ovary (i.e., the cortex) is covered by a single layer of cuboidal epithelium. This cellular layer is known as **germinal epithelium** and it is continuous with the mesothelium that covers the mesovarium. Cells of germinal epithelium are joined by a cementing substance, called **hyaluronic acid.**

(ii) **Tunica albuginea :** Below the germinal epithelium, dense fibrous connective tissue layer is found, called tunica albuginea.

(iii) **Stroma :** It is a connective tissue network continuous with the tunica albuginea and containing spindle-shaped cells with a few involuntary muscle fibres. It supports the essential ovarian structures and carries blood vessels, lymphatics and nerves [Fig 5(c).1].

(iv) **Vesicular follicles or ovarian follicles :** Scattered throughout the cortex are vesicles of different sizes. Histologically three different kinds of ovarian follicles can be identified on the basis of developmental state—primordial follicles, growing follicles, and mature or graafian follicles.

(a) **Primordial follicle :** It is the earliest stage of follicular development. In the mature ovary they are present in the stroma of the cortex just beneath the tunica albuginea. A single layer of squamous follicle cells surrounds the oocyte. The outer surface of the follicle cells is bounded by a basal lamina. Here the oocyte and the surrounding follicle cells are closely apposed to one another. The oocyte of the follicle has a large, eccentric nucleus that contains finely dispersed chromatin and one or more large nucleoli. The ooplasm of the oocyte contains

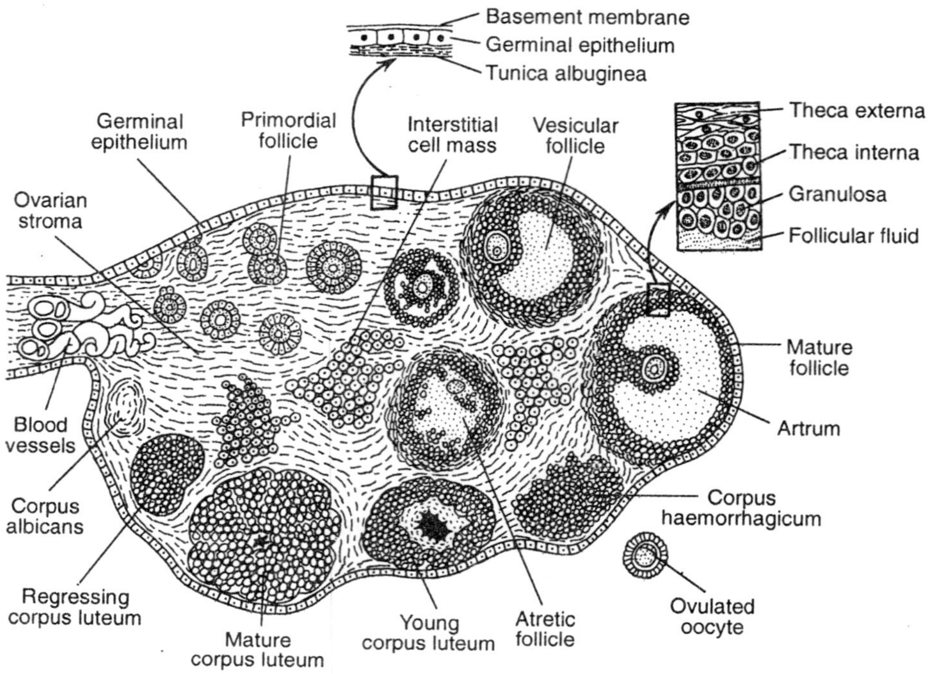

Fig. 5(c).1: Section of mammalian ovary.

a **Balbiani body.** E. M. study reveals that Balbiani body is a localised accumulation of Golgi membranes and vesicles, E.R., numerous mitochondria and lysosomes. Human oocytes also contain annulate lamellae, and numerous small vesicles are scattered throughout the ooplasm along with small spherical mitochondria [Fig 5(c).2].

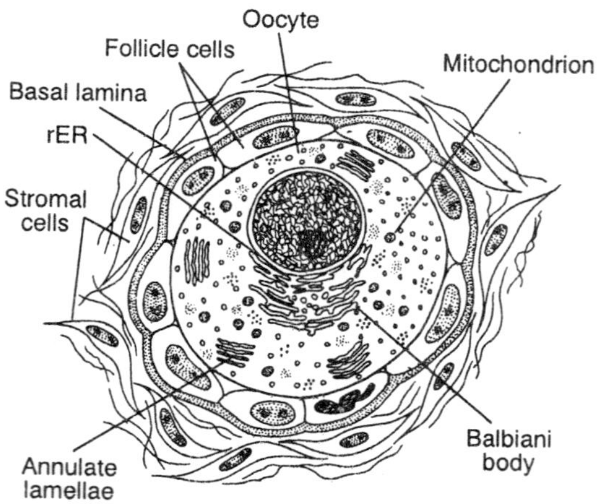

Fig. 5(c).2: Primordial follicle.

(b) **Growing follicles :** These are of two kinds—primary and secondary follicles.

Primary follicle : It is the first stage in the development of the growing follicle. The oocyte is enlarged than that of primordial follicle and the surrounding flattened follicle cells proliferate and become cuboidal in shape. A homogeneous deeply staining acidophilic, refractile layer, called the **Zona pellucida,** exists between the oocyte and adjacent follicle cells.

In the late primary follicle, instead of a single layer of follicular cells, a stratified **stratum granulosa** is found around the oocyte. A sheath of connective tissue cells forms the **theca folliculi layer** around the primary follicle. Theca folliculi consists of two layers—**theca interna** (a highly vascularised inner layer of cuboidal secretory cells) and **theca externa** (an outer layer of connective tissue cells containing smooth muscle cells and bundles of collagen fibres) [Fig 5(c).3].

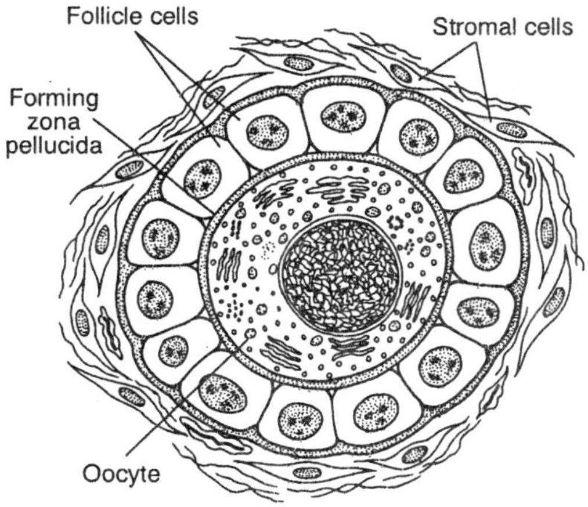

Fig. 5(c).3: Primary follicle.

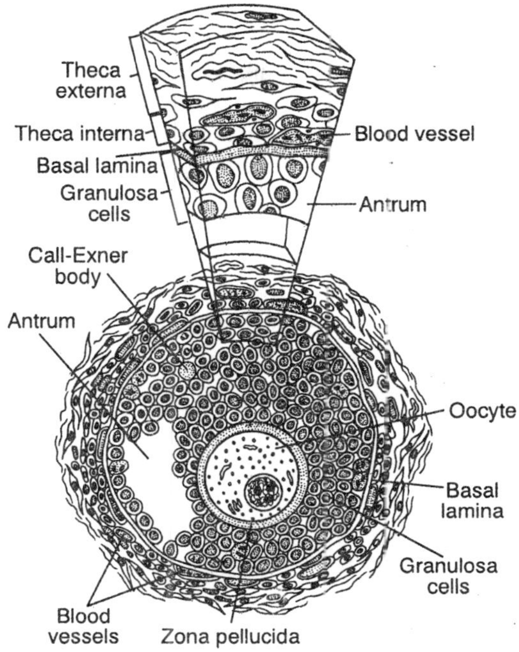

Fig. 5(c).4: Secondary follicle.

Secondary vesicle : The secondary follicle is characterised by a **fluid-containing antrum.** Now the vesicle is enclosed by 6-12 layers of granulosa cells. As the **hyaluronic acid-rich fluid,** called **liquor folliculi,** continues to accumulate among the granulosa cells, the cavities of the follicle begin to coalesce, finally forming a single crescent-shaped cavity, called the **antrum.** The follicle is now identified as a **secondary vesicle.** In this condition the oocyte is eccentrically positioned and no further growth occurs. The inhibition of oocyte growth is achieved by the presence of a small peptide called **oocyte maturation inhibitor** or **OMI.** OMI is secreted by the follicular granulosa cells in the antral fluid.

As the secondary follicle increase in size, some granulosa cells form a thickened mound around oocyte which is called **cumulus oophorus** that projects into the antrum. The cells of **cumulus oophorus,** that immediately surround the oocyte, form a layer called **corona radiata.** The corona radiata is composed of cumulus cells that send penetrating microvilli throughout the zona pellucida to communicate via gap junctions with microvilli of the oocyte [Fig 5(c).4].

(c) **Graafian follicle :** The mature follicle is known as Graafian follicle. Because of its large size (about 10 mm in diameter), it extends through the full thickness of the ovarian cortex and causes a bulge on the surface of ovary. When fully mature, the Graafian follicle ruptures to release the ovum. This is called **ovulation.**

While the growing follicle gradually enlarges by cell proliferation, the oogonium is converted to oocyte and the granulosa cells become many layered. These layers then split and lead to the formation of a cavity inside the Graafian follicle, called **antrum.** This antrum divides the granulosa cells into two layers—outer **membrana granulosa** and an inner or central **cumulus oophorus** (or discus proligerus). With the maturation of the Graafian follicle, the stroma cells surrounding the follicle are also differentiated into two layers—an outer fibrous layer, called **tunica fibrosa** or **theca externa** and an inner vascular layer, called **tunica vasculosa** or **theca interna.** The theca externa is made up of fibrous tissue and few spindle-shaped cells with distinct nucleus. The theca interna is made up of loose connective tissue, epithelial cells and blood vessels. Epithelial cells are ovoid and spindle-shaped and the nuclei of those cells are with distinct nucleoli. Granulosa layer is separated from theca interna by a prominent membranous structure, called **basal lamina.**

In Graafian follicle the cells of cumulus oophorus that immediately surround the oocyte and remain with it at ovulation are referred to as the **corona radiata** cells. Corona radiata possess **microvilli.** It is to be noted that lipid droplets appear in the cy-

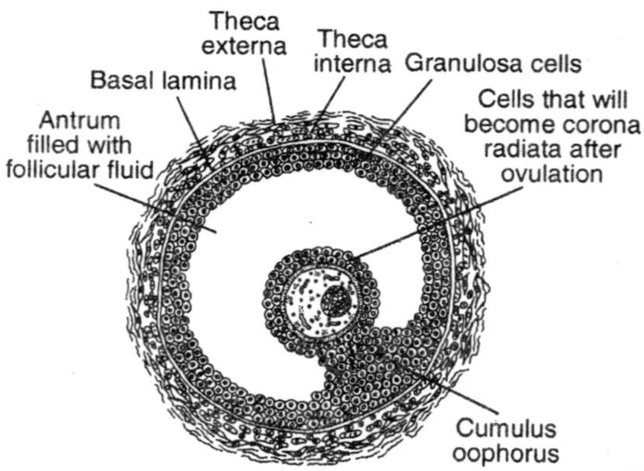

Fig. 5(c).5: Structure of a Graafian follicle.

toplasm of theca interna cells during maturation [Fig 5(c).5].

(v) **Corpus luteum :** Just after discharge of the ovum from the mature Graafian follicle, the collapsed follicle undergoes reorganisation and looks like blood filled cavity and is called **corpus haemorrhagicum.** Soon after this clotted blood is reabsorbed and the cells in the remnant of the ruptured follicle multiply rapidly to fill up the cavity and forms a solid mass of cells, the **corpus luteum.** It consists of granulosa lutein cells and theca lutein cells. The corpus luteum is so named because the cells present in it contain a pinkish-yellow pigment granules, called **lutein.** This pink coloured corpus luteum secretes estrogen and progesterone.

• **Corpus albicans :** The corpus luteum degenerates and undergoes a slow involution after pregnancy or menstruation. The cells of this gland become loaded with lipid droplets, decrease in size, and undergo autolysis. Then it looks like a **white scar** due to fatty infiltration. This is called **corpus albicans.** A white scar is formed and the intercellular hyaline material accumulates among the degenerating cells of the corpus luteum. Corpus albicans sinks deeper into the ovarian cortex region as it slowly disappears over a period of several months.

(vi) **Interstitial cells :** The central part of ovary is known as **medulla.** The main connective tissue mass is stroma and it consists of reticular fibres, spindle shaped fibroblast cells, blood vessels and mass of polyhedral interstitial cells.

The groups of polyhedral interstitial cells containing lipid granules develop from the stroma cells or from the cells of the unruptured follicles. These cells probably secrete estrogen.

Structural changes in the ovary with age : In **childhood** the ovaries are made up of spindle-shaped stroma cells, a cubical, called germinal epithelium and a large number of primordial follicles. The maturing follicles and corpora lutea are absent. There is no ovulation. At **puberty,** the germinal epithelium contains flattened cells, a large number of maturing follicles at different stages of development and corpora lutea. During pregnancy the ovary additionally contains a large corpus luteum. At menopause, the ovaries atrophy, become smaller in size, the follicles disappear and are replaced by fibrous tissue scars. The interstitial cells degenerate and very little estrogen is formed.

Functions of ovary

The ovaries have two major functions (a) **Exocrine function** (formation of ovum, the female gamete) and (b) **Endocrine function.** The secretion of three ovarian hormones (estrogen, progesterone and relaxin) which are essential for the development of female reproductive system.

(a) **Exocrine function** : The formation of female gamete or ovum is called oogenesis. During this process the Graafian follicle of the ovary develops into ovum. The primary germ cells in the germinal epithelium give rise to ovum. There are three phases in the development of ovum.

(i) **Multiplication phase** : The diploid primary germ cells divide mitotically and give rise to large number of cells. These cells are known as **oogonium.**

(ii) **Growth phase** : In this phase the growth of the oogonium takes place. The nucleus enlarges and the cell size also increases. These cells are called primary oocyte.

(iii) **Maturation phase** : The primary oocyte now enters into the maturation phase. Here maturation and reduction in size of primary oocyte occur by the first meiotic division. An unequal two haploid daughter cells consisting of a large **secondary oocyte** and a **first polar body** occur. In the second meiotic division **secondary oocyte** divides to give rise to a **mature ovum** and **second polar body.** The first polar body also divides and gives rise to **secondary polar** bodies. The polar bodies are non-functional. The primary oocyte thus gives rise to a **single ovum** and **three polar bodies.** This ovum is the actural female gamete which takes part in female reproduction.

(b) **Endocrine functions** : The secretions of hormones are the endocrine functions. The hormones are estrogen, progesterone and relaxin.

(1) Functions of estrogens : The chief source of estrogen secretion is Graafian follicle. The ovarian interstitial cells also seem to secrete estrogen.

(i) **On ovary** : Estrogen helps in the maturation of Graafian follicle in the ovary. It also assists in release of ovum from the mature Graafian follicle (i.e., ovulation) by causing a surge of LH secretion from the adenohypophysis.

(ii) **On female sex characters** : Estrogen stimulates the growth and development of brest, fallopian tube, uterus, vagina etc. at puberty. The external genitalia become enlarged by the effect of estrogen with the deposition of fat.

(iii) **On secondary sex characters** : Estrogen is responsible for development of secondary sex characters and pubertal changes in females, for example—development of mammary glands, appearance of hair in axilla and pubes, fat deposition on thigh and hip and formation of a feminine body. In mammany gland, it causes proliferation of the duct system.

(iv) **On reproductive cycle** : Estrogen takes important part in the regulation of menstrual cycle. The chief function is the onset of menstruation and the first half of this cycle, i.e., follicular phase is dependent on estrogen. Estrogen promotes the pituitary release of LH for ovulation.

(v) **On bone growth** : Estrogen conserves calcium and phosphorus and encourages bone formation. After menopause lack of estrogen may cause ostroporosis.

(vi) **On metabolism** : Estrogen is a protein and fat anabolic hormone, thus helps in the syntheis of protein. This hormone stimulates in deposition of fat in the subcutaneous tissue.

(vii) **On sexual desire** : Oestrogen induces sexual heat or **oestrus** in lower animals. In woman it plays a minor role in determining sex desire. Progesterone is one of the female sex hormones which is secreted from corpus luteum.

(2) Functions of progesterone :

(i) **On uterus** : Progesterone acts jointly with estrogen to maintain the growth of uterus and prevents the disintegration of uterine endometrium.

(ii) **On menstrual cycle** : It controls the second half of the cycle, i.e., the luteal phase of the menstrual cycle. It helps in the regulation of menstrual cycle.

(iii) **On implantation and pregnancy** : It stimulates to prepare the endometrial bed for implantation of the ovum and maintenance of pregnancy. The earlier and later parts of pregnancy are maintained by the progesterone levels secreted from the ovary and placenta respectively. Progesterone inhibits the uterine movements to prevent expulsion of foetus from the uterus.

(iv) **On mammary gland development** : Progesterone acts synergistically with estrogen to facilitate the proliferation and development of mammary glands. This hormone stimulates the growth of alveolar system of the mammary glands.

(v) **On ovary** : Surge of progesterone inhibits the maturation of ovarian follicle and ovulation probably by suppressing the release of gonadotrophic hormones like FSH and LH from the anterior pituitary. This is why maturation of follicle and ovulation does not occur during pregnancy when the placenta secretes large quantities of progesterone.

(3) Function of relaxin : Relaxin is secreted at the terminal stage of pregnancy. It stimulates to cause enlargement of birth canal by relaxing the pelvic ligament and cervix and thus helps in parturition, i.e., expulsion of the foetus.

STRUCTURE OF OVUM

In the female sex the first stage of the development of gametes is similar to that found in spermatogenesis. The oogonia—the cells eventually giving rise to the eggs—undergo proliferation by mitotic divisions. They then become oocytes and enter a period of growth.

The oocytes are surrounded during the whole time of their growth and maturation by special cells of the ovary, the follicle cells.

Follicle cells : In mammals, the follicle cells are derived from the germinal epithelium of the ovaries, and initially the young oocyte is surrounded by one layer of follicle cells, forming a simple cuboidal epithelium around the oocyte. later the number of follicle cells increases greatly, the cells are arranged in several rows. As the egg approaches maturity, an eccentric cavity appears in the mass of the follicle cells and the cavity is filled with fluid secreted by the cells of the follicle. The follicle at this stage is known as **Graafian follicle.**

The oocyte is surrounded by follicle cells not only in mammals but in other vertebrates as well. It might be that the follicle cells actively assist the growth of the oocyte by secreting substances which are taken up by the oocytes.

The structural relationship between the follicle cells and the oocytes, revealed by E.M. studies in recent years, is very peculiar. Originally there is a simple opposition of the follicle cells and the oocyte, similar to the one existing between oridinary epithelial cells. The cytoplasmic membranes of the adjoining cells are separated only by a narrow gap of about 80 Å.

EGG MEMBRANE

Eggs are covered by cell membrane or plasmalemma. E.M. reveals that the plasma lemma is surrounded by accessory envelopes called **egg membranes.** This cell membrane is formed of two layers of electron dense material, about 50 Å thick separated by a less dense interval of about 60 Å. Sometimes the plasmalemma is surrounded by special membrane depending on their origin. They are further classified into three groups.

(a) Primary membrane : The primary egg membranes are formed by the ovum itself. These develop around the plasma membrane of the egg in the space occupied by the interdigitating microvilli of the oocyte and follicle cells. The primary egg membrane of insects, molluscs, amphibians and birds is called **vitelline membrane.** It is usually thin and transparent and is closely applied to the surface of the underlying plasma membrane.

The primary egg membrane is so called, **zona radiata** because of its striated appearence and represents the zone of interdigiting microvilli around the oocyte. Zona radiata has a wide distribution among verebrate eggs, notably those of the sharks, certain bony fishes, amphibians and reptiles. In birds it is not evident, but in mammals it is usually conspicuous around an early oocyte.

The primary egg membranes usually closely adhered to the surface of the oocyte, but at a later stage a space filled with fluid may appear between the cytoplasm and the membrane, this space is called the **perivitelline space.**

Zona pellucida is unstriated and takes the place of zona radiata of young mammalian oocyte. Towards the time when the oocyte reaches its full size a dense material of fibriller structure appears in between the interdigitating processes of the oocyte and the follicle cells. The materials become consolidated, eventually fills most of the space between the follicle cells and the oocyte, and becomes the zona pellucida [Fig 5(c).6 and 7].

(b) Secondary membrane : Thicker membrane secreted by the follicle cells on top of the vitelline membrane is called chorion—in insects.

In mammals an egg escaping from the ovary carries with it on the surface of the zona pellucida a layer of follicle cells, known as the **corona radiata.** The cells of the corona radiata are peeled off later, as the egg descends the oviduct.

At certain points, the two cytoplasmic membranes show a close connection in the form of **desmosome**. Here the plasma membranes of the adjoining cells are thickened and the space in between, appears to be filled by a denser substance which presumably holds the two-cell membrane together (**Andarson** and **Beams**, 1960; **Wartenberg,** 1962). At a later stage a wide space appears between the follicle cells and the oocyte. The follicle cells, however, retain contact with the oocytes at the points where the desmosomes could be noticed in the previous stage.

The cytoplasm of the follicle cells becomes drawn out into elongated processes or microvilli reaching across the space separating the follicle cells and the oocyte.

At the same time the surface of the oocyte is drawn out into numerous finger-like microvilli projecting into the space between

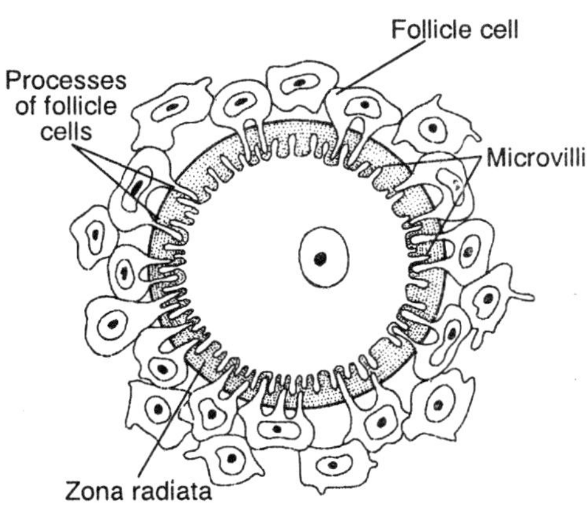

Fig. 5(c).6: Young oocyte of a mammal surrounded by follicle cells.

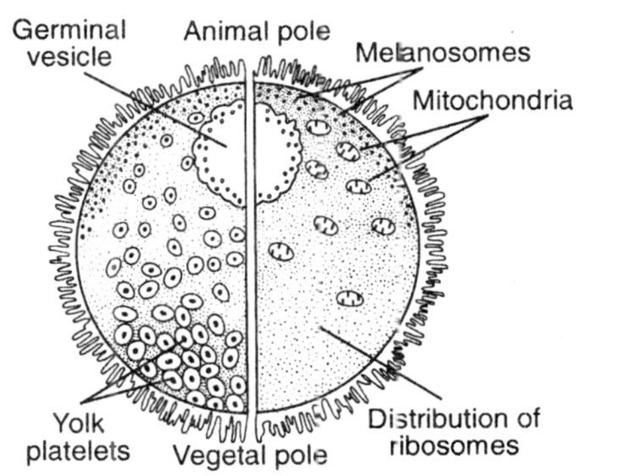

Fig. 5(c).7: Representation of gradients of cytoplasmic organelles in the amphibian oocyte.

the oocyte and the follicle cells. The microvilli of the oocyte integrate with those of the follicle cells (**Sotelo** and **Porter**, 1969). These (microvillus) greatly increase the surface area of the oocyst, and it seems to facilitate metabolic turnover between the oocyte and its environment. Small inpocketing of the oocyte cytoplasm may often be observed at the base of the microvilli, and these are interpreted as an indication that the oocyte is taking in fluids and the dissolved substances from the space between itself and the follicle cells by means of pinocytosis or "cell drinking" (**Anderson** & **Beams**, 1960).

When the oocyte reaches its full size a denser material, often of fibriller structure appears in between the processes of the oocyte and the follicle cells. The material becomes consolidated and eventually fills most of the space between the follicle cells and the oocytes, becoming the egg membrane.

In the last stage of oocyte maturation, the cytoplasmic process of the oocyte and of the follicle cells may be withdrawn, and the space between the two is taken up by the egg membrane. This is the case in all vertebrates and in mammals in particular (**Oder**, 1969).

(c) Tertiary egg membranes are formed by the oviducts, or the uterus or other accessory glands of the female genital system while the egg is passing from the ovary of the exterior. These membranes have different form and consistency. Thus, for example, in reptiles, birds and egg-laying mammals (Monotremes), their eggs are provided with three envelopes: the egg albumen, the shell membranes and the hard porous calcareous shell.

CYTOPLASM

The **cytoplasm** in young oocyte is rather poor in complex inclusions possessing practically none of the specialised structures found in the adult oocyte and mature egg.

A large amount of nucleic acids, mainly in the form of DNA but possibly with some amount of RNA are present in the cytoplasm of the young oocyte. The cytoplasm is finely granular as seen under EM.

Mitochondria are fairly scarce in the young oocytes but may increase in number very considerably during the growth of oocytes and may, in some animals (amphibia, birds), be arranged in the form of large "mitochondrial clouds". (**Balinsky, Devis,** 1963).

Golgi bodies are found in younger oocytes around the controsome. In the oocytes of some mammals Golgi-type membranes form a large spherical mass while later disperses in Guineapig etc., **Odor**, 1969.

In the advanced oocytes small Golgi bodies become scattered throughout the whole cytoplasm or they may be located in the sub-cortical cytoplasm, sometimes distributed at fairly regular intervals. In mature oocytes Golgi bodies sometimes disappear completely (**Odor**, 1969) possibly indicating that these organoids have been used up or transformed into some other structures.

Endoplasmic reticulum, in the form of double lamellae with ribosomes attached to their outer surfaces, is very rarely found in the young oocytes. Instead of that numerous vesicles surrounded by a simple membrane attached with ribosomes on its surface are found, believed to be equivalent to or to be a modification of the endoplasmic reticulum. Different kind of membranous structures often found in oocytes which are of double membranes, sometimes in parallel, and sometimes in spiral arrangements without any attachment of ribosomes but instead are perforated by pores which closely resemble with pores of the nuclear membrane (**Rebhun**, 1961) might have derived from the nuclear membrane (**Kessel**, 1963).

Yolk appears in the oocytes at the second period of their growth; Perivitellogenesis period and Vitellogenesis period (**Raven**, 1961). Growth is very rapid at the second period. Yolk is the main source of food storage and consisting of proteins, phospholipids and very few neural fats. The yolk, might be 'protein yolk', contains variable amounts of lipids as well as protein and fatty yolk which in addition to phospholipid may contain some admixture of proteins.

Glycogen is present in the egg cytoplasm in the form of small granules. Fat may be stored in the egg particularly in the vertebrates for nourishment of the developing embryo.

Yolk nuclei in different animals are not similar in nature as revealed by E.M. It might be that the E.R., Golgi bodies, and mitochondria are responsible for the formation of yolk but it is contradictory. The yolk platelets are formed inside modified mitochondria in the amphibians and fishes.

• **Discharge of ovum from mature ovarian follicle :** Through a signal transduction cascade initiated by LH, proteolytic enzymes are secreted by the follicle that degrade the follicular tissue at the site of the blister, forming a hole, called the **stigma.** The cumulus-oocyte complex (COC) leaves the ruptured follicle and moves out into the peritoneal cavity through the stigma, where it is caught by the fimbriae at the end of the fallopian tube.

• **Formation and degeneration of corpus luteum :**

Formation : After rupture of the mature follicle and liberation of the ovum during ovulation, the follicle promptly fills up with blood forming what is called a corpus haemorrhigicum. The granulosa and thecal cells rapidly increase in number and the clotted blood is absorbed. Vascular elements from the theca peretrate the granulosa cells. The granulosa cells begin to accumulate large amount of cholesterol; this lutinization process leads to formation of corpus luteum. The mature corpus luteum of some species appears to contain a number of distinct cell types. Cells derived from the theca interna migrate into granulosa–derived areas of the luteal tissue soon after ovulation to give rise to small luteal cells, thecal lutein cells and fibroblasts. The large luteal appears to be derived from granulosa cells.

Degeneration : CL usually regresses about 12 days after ovulation during an infertile cycle in primates. CL is maintained by LH that induces the production of progesterone by the luteal cells that maintains the CL. If there is fertilization, the HCG from placenta maintains the CL because HCG receptors are identical to LH receptors at the CL. Thus, no fertilization leads to the decline of progesterone production and eventual degeneration of CL.

CHAPTER 6

Biosynthesis of Hormones

Chemically, hormones may be grouped into three categories : Polypeptides, Steriods and Amino-acid derivatives. The synthesis of hormone is an important event of hormone action. Secretion of endocrine gland can be released directly into the extracellular fluid and circulation. Like enzymes, hormones cannot be stored and are not continuously synthesised. Thus, hormones are released in the blood and can reach all cells and tissues, but function only on genetically differentiated cells of the body, the **target cells.**

BIOSYNTHESIS OF T_3 AND T_4 (THYROID HORMONES)

Thyroid follicular cells secrete two iodinated amino-acids as hormones, viz; thyroxine or T_4 (3, 5, 3′, 5′-tetraiodothyronine) and triiodothyronine or T_3 (3, 5, 3′-triiodothyronine). These hormones are synthesised by the iodination and further modification of some of the 115 tyrosine residues of a 19S dimeric glycoprotein, thyroglobulin. TSH stimulates all the following reactions for the synthesis of the thyroid hormones. [Fig. 6.1]

(a) **Synthesis of thyroglobulin** : Thyroglobulin (TG) is only found in the plasma. It is an iodinated glycopeptide of molecular weight 680,000. TG is translated by polysomes on the granular ER in the basal part of the thyroid cells and glycosylated in the smooth ER and Golgi-cisternae. Small membrane bound vesicles containing TG are then pinched off from the Golgi-cisternae, migrate towards the apical plasma membrane and fuse with the latter, releasing their contents into the colloidal substances of the thyroid follicles.

(b) **Trapping of iodide** : Trapping of iodide from circulation is an important phenomenon in the synthesis of thyroid hormones. Thyroid follicular cells have the unique abilities to trap iodide from the circulating blood. These follicular cells actively collect inorganic iodides (I^-) from the blood against steep electro-chemical gradients with the help of an **iodide pump** located in the basal plasma membrane in association with $Na^+ - K^+$ – ATP-ase which provides an energy for its running. The transport mechanism is often called **iodide trapping mechanism** on iodide pump. For this active transport energy is required. The iodide pump obeys hyperbolic saturation kinetics which collects about 33% of the body I^- in the thyroid and concentrates I^- in the thyroid cells by 25-50 times the serum I^- concentration. This iodide pump is dependent upon ATP-ase system. Uptake of iodide can be inhibited by some anions, notably perchlorate and thiocynate. TSH stimulates iodide uptakes by the gland. The normal daily intake

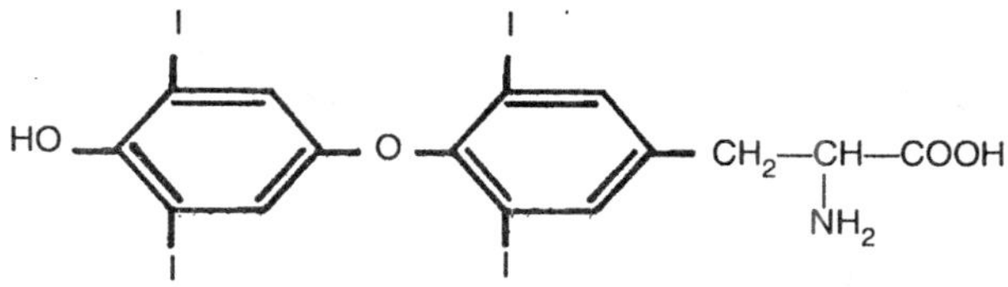

L–Thyroxine (T_4)

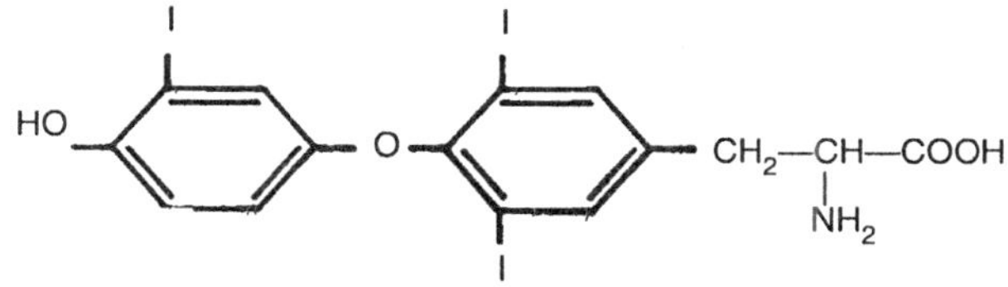

L–3, 5, 3' Triiodothyronine (T_3)

Fig. 6.1: Thyroid hormones

of iodide is 100-150 µg and mainly absorbed from the small intestine and subsequently transported in the plasma in loose attachment to protein. [Fig. 6.2]

(c) **Oxidation of iodide :** Within the thyroid, the iodide that is taken up the follicular cells is quickly oxidised to an active form of iodine, catalysed probably by a tetrameric heme enzyme, thyroperoxidase in presence of H_2O as a source of oxygen.

Oxidation of iodide to nascent form of iodine is : $2I^- \rightleftharpoons I_2$ or $I^o + 2e$

Peroxidase system :

$H_2O_2 + 2I + 2H^+ \xrightarrow{\text{Peroxidase}} 2$ 'oxidised active I' + $2H_2O$

TSH is active in stimulating this reaction. The enzyme thyroperoxidase uses H_2O_2 as a co-substrate and the reaction is chiefly occurred in the microvilli of the follicular

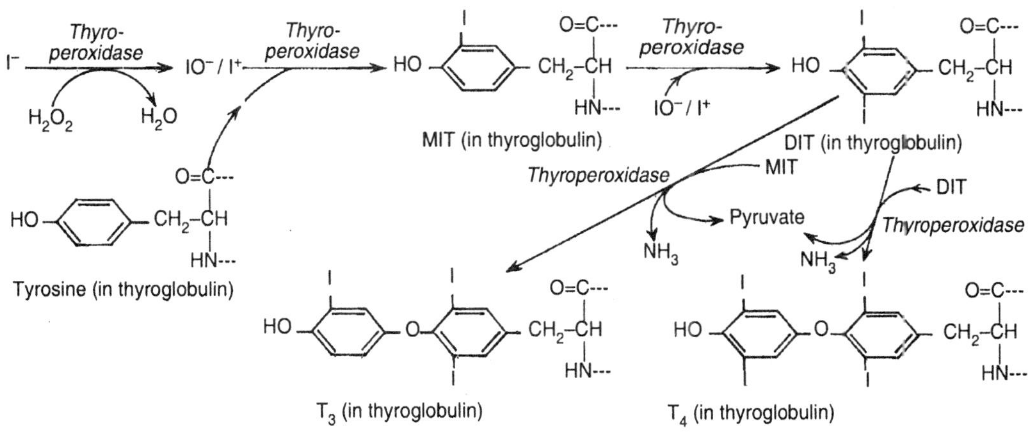

Fig. 6.2: Biosynthesis of thyroid hormones

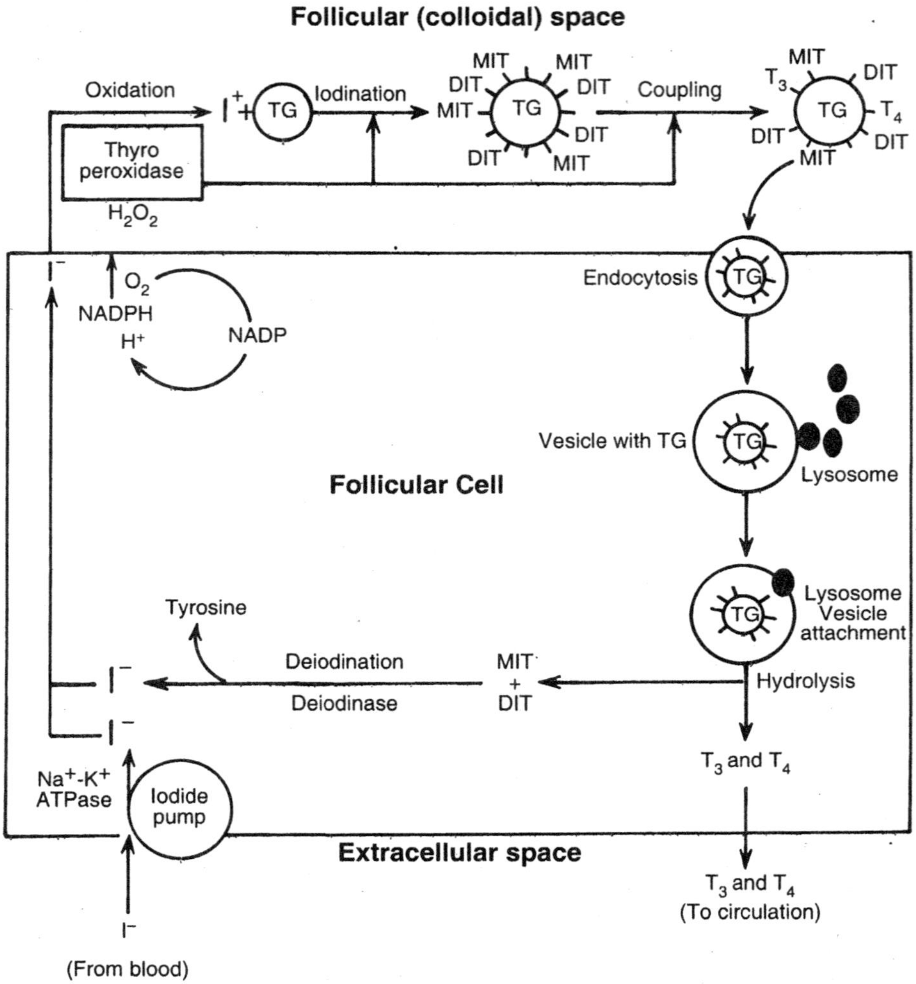

Fig. 6.3: Schematic representation shows T_3 and T_4 biosynthesis in thyroid follicle (TG-Thyroglobulin)

cells. The active iodine may be **iodinium ion (I^+)**, hypoiodate (IO^-) or free iodine radical (I).

(d) **Iodination of tyrosine** : The Thyroperoxidase enzyme probably catalyses the step, **'organification of iodine'.** The iodination of tyrosine in thyroglobulin takes place first at 3 position and then at 5 position of aromatic nucleus, forming respectively the monoiodotyrosine (MIT) and di-iodotyrosine (DIT). In these reactions, thyroperoxidase probably uses H_2O_2 again to oxidise the tyrosine and MIT residues respectively to free tyrosine radical and free MIT radical before they may interact with **'active iodine'.** Thyroperoxidase may also iodinate a few histidine residues of thyroglobulin to N^3–monoiodohistidines (MIH). Normally MIT and DIT molecules are present in equal concentration. [Fig. 6.3]

(e) **Coupling of iodotyrosines in thyroglobulin :** Two di-iodotyrosine molecules thus undergo oxidative condensation with the liberation of alanine residue and the formation of thyroxine (T_4), still in peptide linkage to thyroglobulin. It is claimed that tri-iodothyronine (T_3) is formed by condensation of MIT with DIT. This process is called

coupling. Under normal conditions, coupling takes place readily between adjacent iodo-tyrosine residues on the surface of thyroxine binding globulin (TBG) molecules. Loss of iodine atom from thyroxine molecule may possibly produce T_3.

It is known that thyroperoxidase first oxidises iodotyrosine residues with H_2O_2 to form iodotyrosine-free radicals. Probably the C–C bond between the phenylring of an iodotyrosine radical and its alanine side-chain is next cleaved and this phenyl ring is transferred to the phenolic OH of another diiodotyrosyl radical of the thyroglobulin molecule to produce an iodothyronine residue. During this coupling, an alanine is cleaved off, which is later catabolised to pyruvate and ammonia (NH_3).

Storage and release : Thyroglobulin with thyroid hormones (T_3 and T_4) that are formed in the follicular epithelium are discharged within the follicular lumen and stored there until these are required.

Transport : The hormones which are released in the bloods are transported as such but in binding with plasma proteins thyroxine (T_4) is bound much more firmly than tri-iodothyronine (T_3) and for this reason T_3 is quick acting and short lasting but the T_4 is slow acting but long lasting. Thyroxine (T_4) is transported entirely with the plasma proteins—thyroxine-binding globulin (TBG), thyroxine-binding prealbumin (TBPA) and serum albumin. T_3 is carried through TBG only. Both thyroxine and tri-iodothyronine are transported through blood to the tissues.

Catabolism : The liver and kidneys are the principal organs concerned in the catabolism of thyroid hormones. The free T_4 and T_3 enter within the liver and other tissues where 80% is deiodinated by the enzyme deiodinase. T_4 on deiodination yields T_3. The iodide is recirculated to thyroid and excreted through urine. Near about 35% T_4 is excreted through bile either in free form or in conjugated form with glucuronates or sulfates. In case of tri-iodothyronine (T_3), 75-80% is deiodinated and 20-25% is excreted through faeces.

Control of thyroid hormone secretion : Regulation of thyroid hormone secretion is very essential because of delayed and prolonged action of the thyroid hormones. The synthesis and secretion of T_4 and T_3 are chiefly controlled by co-ordination of hypothalamus and adenohypophysis. The release of thyroid hormones is regulated by TSH and the secretion of TSH is stimulated by TSH-RH. The secretion of thyrotropin releasing hormone (TRH) by hypothalamus is influenced by feedback actions of TSH and T_4 and T_3.

The secretion of TSH-RH is inhibited by hypersecretion of TSH by negative feedback mechanism. The excess secretion of thyroxine (T_4) and triiodothyronine (T_3) regulate the secretion of TSH by negative feedback mechanism. Again, the drugs like thiourea, thiouracil, and their substituted derivatives and propylthiouracil inhibit the thyroxine formation. [Fig. 6.4]

BIOSYNTHESIS OF PARATHORMONE (PTH)

Parathormone is the principal hormone of parathyroid gland. This hormone is secreted from the chief cells of parathyroid gland. Parathormone is not stored in the parathyroid gland but it is synthesised and secreted continuously. It is a polypeptide having a linear chain of 84 amino acids and its molecular weight is about 9.5 kd.

Synthesis : PTH, a polypeptide of 84 amino acids long, is derived from a precursor molecule of 115 amino acid residues. As the polysomes on the RER membrane translate a 115 amino-acid precursor known as pre-pro PTH, the N-terminal end of the latter protrudes into the ER lumen and the so-called pre-pro PTH then undergoes proteolytic cleavages to yield a pro-PTH of 90 amino acid in the ER, from which 6 (six)

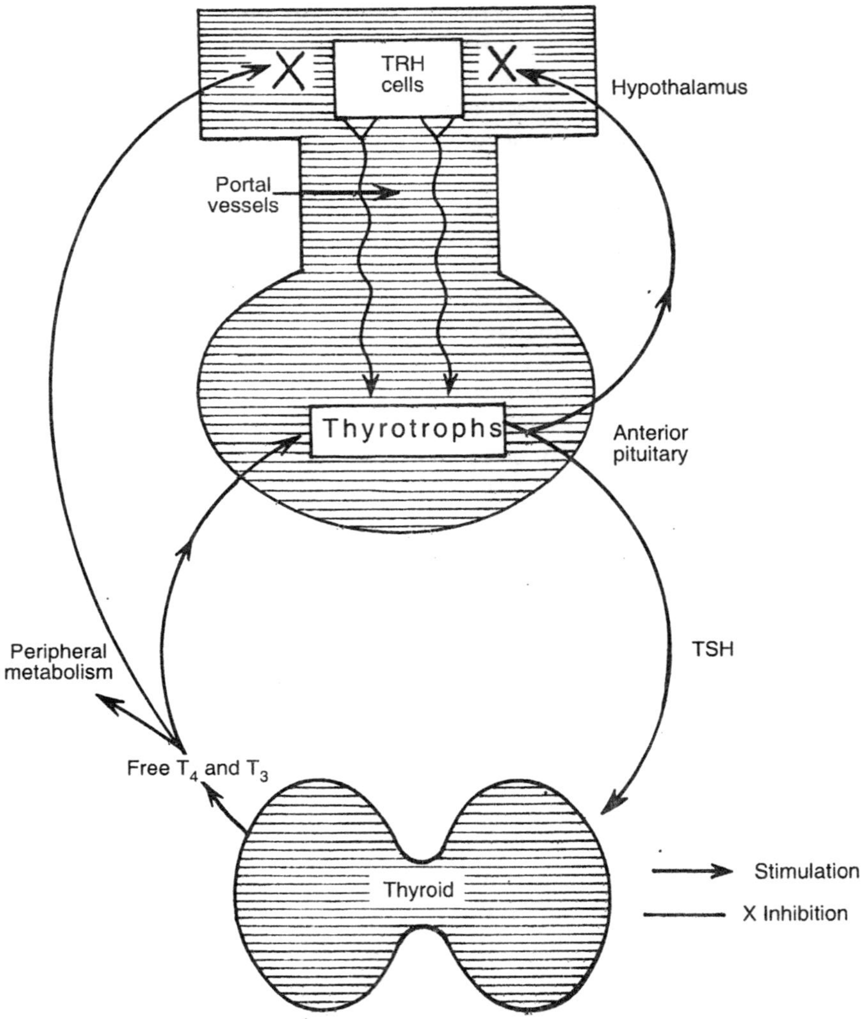

Fig. 6.4: An overall view of the factors regulating thyroid secretion T_4 = thyroxine; TSH = thyroid stimulating hormone; TRH = thyrotrophin releasing hormone

amino acid residues are then removed to yield the definitive hormonal product. [Fig. 6.5]

The pro-PTH, an intermediate form, is then transferred to Golgi-cisternae. After its transfer from ER to the Golgi-cisterane, the N-terminal basic hexapeptide segment of pro-PTH is hydrolytically cleaved off by the enzyme, clipase B (a trypsin-like protease) and leads to 84 amino acids containing PTH. The hormone is then packaged into secretory vesicles that migrate to the periphery of the

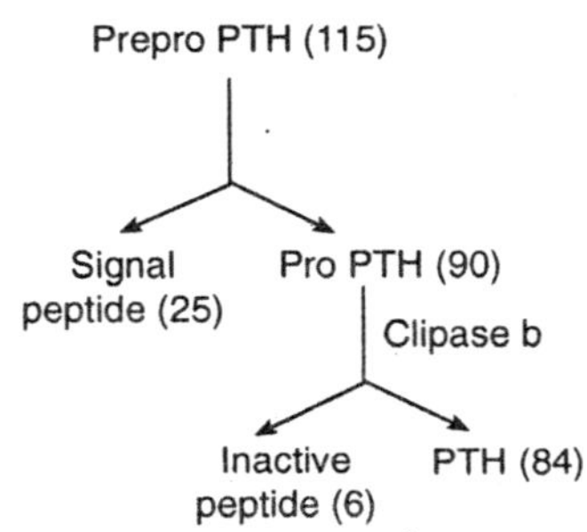

Fig. 6.5: Biosynthesis of PTH

cell where the hormone is secreted by a mechanism of vesicular exocytosis.

The intact hormone of the peripheral circulation is cleaved into two major fragments, one of which, PTH (1-34), retains some biological functions. Studies using radiolabeled bovine PTH in calves exhibited an initial rapid disappearance of most of the hormones with a half-life of 3 to 4 minutes. In humans, PTH has approximately the same half-life as measured after parathyroidectomy.

Catabolism : Parathormone (PTH) in most cases is degraded in the parathyroid gland itself by the enzymes, cathepsins and other peptidases into a C-terminal 48-amino acid 7~KD fragment, released in the blood, and several small N-terminal fragments like di- and tri-peptides.

When PTH released in the blood is mostly degraded by cell-surface cathepsins of hepatic kupffer cells into similar small N-terminal and C-terminal fragments, the latter being subsequently eliminated in the urine.

Control of PTH secretion : The secretion of PTH is controlled by a negative feedback mechanism, relating to the level of calcium in the plasma of blood. Abrupt decrease of PTH concentration takes place after administration of Ca^{++} and rises after administration of EDTA (ethylenediaminetetra acetate) when circulating ionised calcium is lowered. The decrease in PTH secretion owing to high serum Ca^{2+} results from a Ca^{2+}-dependent activation of a G protein of parathyroid plasma membrane, leading to enhanced proteolytic degradation of PTH stored in parathyroid cells.

EDTA lowers the blood calcium by chelation. The relation is reciprocal. Parathyroids regulate Ca metabolism while blood calcium controls parathyroid secretion. Sometimes, thyroid may also influence the parathyroid secretion as in hyperthyroidism mobilisation of Ca level from bones occurs.

BIOSYNTHESIS OF INSULIN

Insulin is 5.7 KD heterodimeric protein hormone consisting of 51 amino-acids contained within two polypeptide chains, secreted by β-cells of Islets of Langerhans of pancreas.

Chemical structure : It has been isolated from pancreas and prepared in crystalline form. For crystallization, it requires Zn^{++}. Zinc is also a constituent of stored insulin and normal pancreatic tissue is relatively rich in Zn. Insulin molecule is composed of two polypeptide chains, called 'A' chain and 'B' chain, containing total of 51 amino acids. 'A' chain comprises of 21 amino acids and 'B' chain with 30 amino acids. In A-chain, N-terminal amino acid is glycine and C-terminal is asparagine. In B-chain, N-terminal amino acid is phenyl alanine and C-terminal is threonine.

Disulfide bridges : Both the chains are held together by two s-s linkages. Cys 7 and Cys 20 of A-chain are joined to Cys 7 and Cys 19 of B-chain respectively. In addition, the A-chain carries an "intra-chain" s-s linkage between Cys 6 and Cys 11. [Fig. 6.6(a)]

Importance of s-s bridges : Breaking of the disulfide bonds with alkali or reducing agents inactivate insulin. Digestion of insulin protein with proteolytic enzymes also inactivates the hormone. [Fig. 6.6(b)]

Synthesis : Biosynthesis of insulin takes place in β-cells of the islets of Langerhans. It is presumably similar to protein synthesis in other cells and it occurs through the following steps :

1. **Transcription of code :** The human insulin gene is located on the short arm of chromosome 11 coding and the insulin is synthesised by the ribosomes of the granular endoplasmic reticulum (GER) under the control of triplet nucleotide sequences of mRNA.
2. **Translation of the code :** In the cytoplasm of the pancreatic β-cells, a long precursor molecule, **pre-pro insulin** is first translated. This pre-pro insulin is translated by polysomes on the GER membrane. It is constituted by a long chain of 10 g amino-acid residues and molecular weight is 11.5 KD. The pre-pro insulin is produced by DNA/RNA

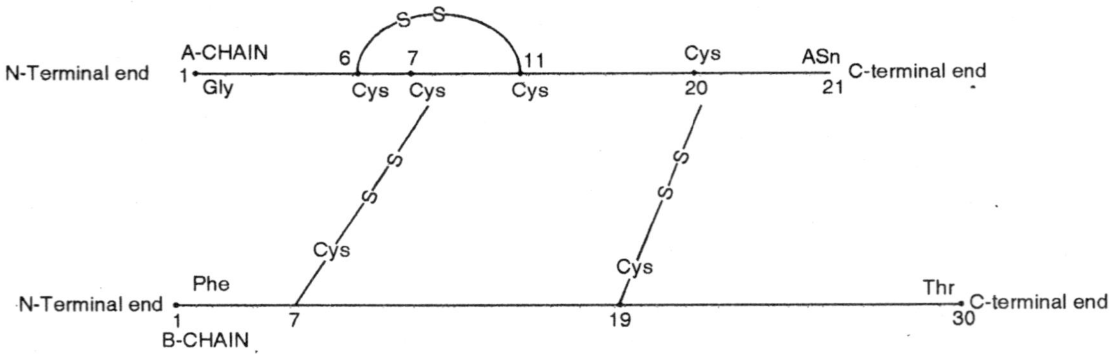

Fig. 6.6(a): Shows structure of insulin schematically

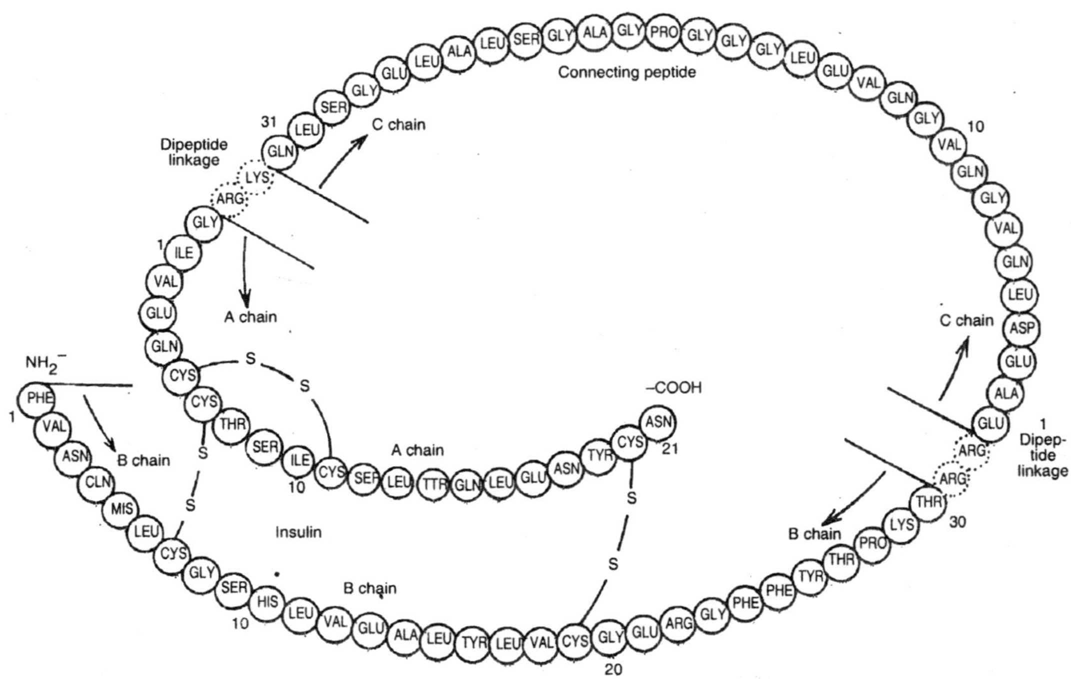

Fig. 6.6(b): Structure of human proinsulin C-peptide and insulin molecules connected of two sites by dipeptide bonds

directed synthesis in the GER of pancreatic β-cells.

3. **Separation of signal sequence :** Immediately after translation this molecule (pre-pro insulin) enters into the lumen of GER and from its hydrophobic N terminal signal peptide, 23 amino acid sequence is hydrolysed away by a signal peptidase of the GER membrane to produce 86-amino acid **pro-insulin** (~ 9 KD). It has three intra-chain disulfide bonds.

4. **Transfer of pro-insulin :** Pro-insulin is transported from GER to the Golgi complex.

5. **Splitting of pro-insulin :** In the Golgi complex, the pro-insulin is hydrolysed by a trypsin like endopeptidase to yield a 33-amino acid pro-C peptide and a 53 amino acid long **insulin precursor.**

Under conditions of excessive stimulation, pro-insulin is also released by vesicular exocytosis along with the insulin from the β-cells of pancreas. [Fig. 6.7(a) & (b)]

6. **Formation of insulin :** The insulin precursor thereby comes to consist of A and B peptide chains, interlinked by two of the S-S bonds of pro-insulin. The third S-S bond of pro-insulin continues as an intrachain S-S bond of the A chain. An endopeptidase eventually hydrolyses the C-terminal peptide bonds in the pro-C peptide and the insulin precursor. This yields two C-terminal basic amino-acids from each. Two molecules of Arg. are driven out from the insulin precursor and lead to the formation of **active insulin** (containing 51 amino acids) with a molecular weight of 5.7 KD. From pro-C-peptide two amino

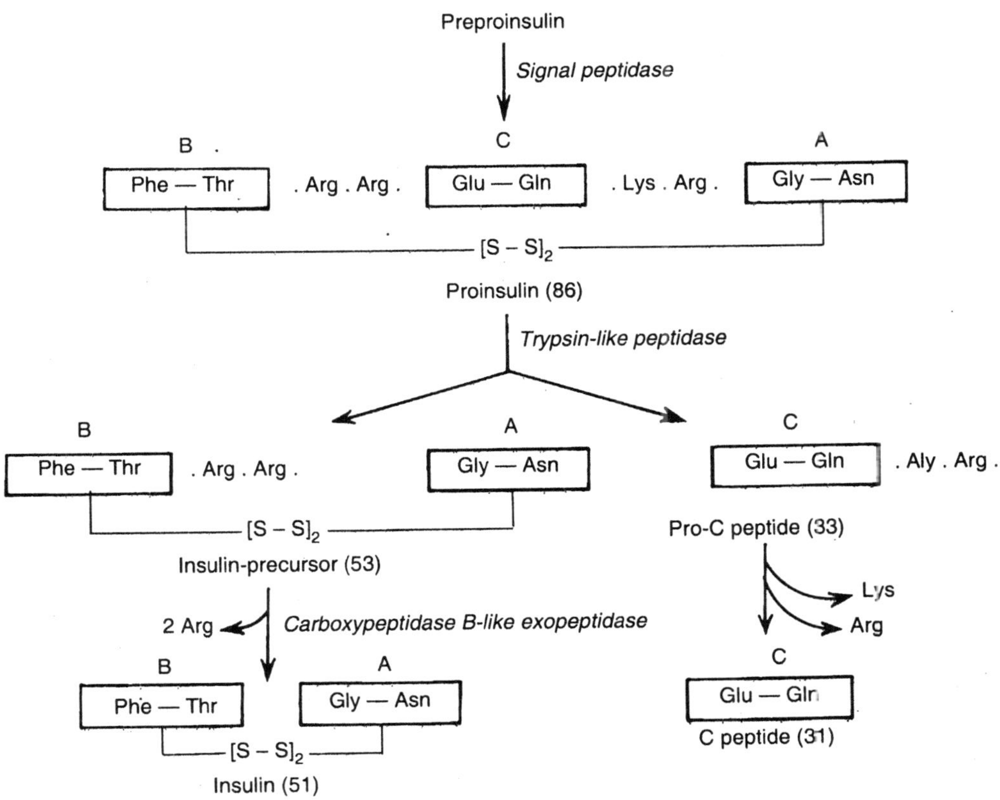

Fig. 6.7(a): Biosynthesis of insulin

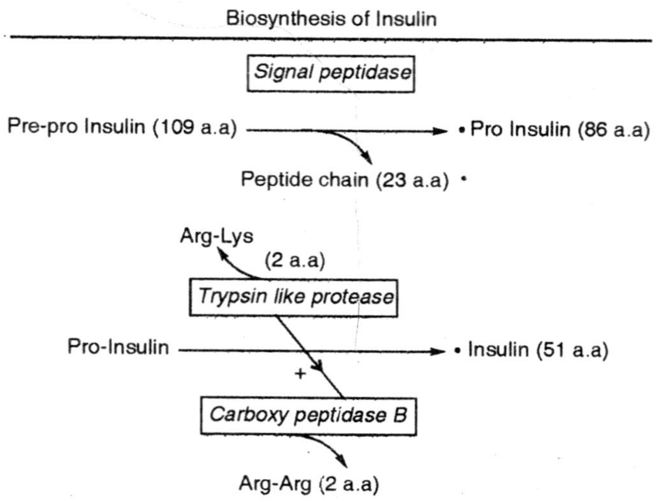

Fig. 6.7(a): Biosynthesis of insulin

acids, Lysine (Lys) and Arginine (Arg) are separated and leads to the formation of connecting peptide or C-peptide containg 31 amino acids.

Insulin and C-peptide are found to be present in the secretory granules of Golgi complex. In some species, insulin is complexed with zinc within the β-cells of pancreas. After stimulation insulin is released by exocytosis. There is some evidence that the C-peptide may subserve some functions along with insulin, in glucose homeostasis (**D. F. Steiner** and **H. Rubenstein**, 1997).

Note :

- Pro-insulin is comparatively inactive biologically, but it can cross-react with antisera prepared against insulin.
- Plasma pro-insulin is not elevated in human diabetes or in normals after glucose stimulation, but it may be the predominant circulating form in some subjects with islet-cell tumours.

Catabolism : Insulin has a short half-life of 3-10 minutes in the plasma. It is destroyed in blood and tissues by degradation process. Mostly all the tissues can degrade insulin. Liver, kidneys, pancreas, testes and also the placenta can degrade the insulin greatly. After it binds to insulin receptors on its target cell membrane, the receptor-insulin complex is internalised into the cell by absorptive pinocytosis. Insulin is then rapidly hydrolysed by an enzyme, **lysosomal insulin-specific protease. Glutathione-insulin transhydrogenase** activity is of great importance in insulin degradation by liver. This enzyme is specially essential for reductive cleavage of disulfide bonds of insulin to release reduced **A-chain** and reduced **B-chain.** This is the first step of degradation.

There are certain compounds which inhibit degradation of insulin such as α-corticotrophin, growth hormone, glucagon, vasopressin, oxytocin, prolactin, etc.

Regulation of secretion : For insulin secretion there is no pituitary trophic hormone control. Its regulation is regulated by several factors :

(a) **Nervous control :** It has been shown that stimulation of vagus increase the release of insulin. Normally blood sugar adjusts the vagal tone and modifies insulin release. High blood sugar stimulates and low blood sugar depresses the vagus. But this is least effective and is only a means for fine adjustment.

(b) **Hormonal control of blood glucose level :**

(i) The blood sugar concentration of arterial blood entering the pancreas is the best controller for the secretion of insulin by β-cells of islets of Langerhans. There is some evidence that intake of carbohydrate rich food leads to raise the blood glucose which is the signal for increased insulin secretion.

(ii) In response to dietary glucose and amino acids, the intestinal mucosa secretes gastric inhibitory polypeptide (GIP) which in turn stimulates insulin secretion from the β-cells.

(iii) High levels of GH, ovarian steroids, gluco-corticoids, vasoactive intestinal polypeptide (VIP), β-adrenergic effect of catecholamine stimulate insulin secretion.

(iv) Pancreatic somatostatin (secreted from D-cells of islets of Langerhans) regulates the secretion of α-cells and β-cells of pancreas.

(v) Low blood sugar level stimulates the secretion of glucagon for glycogenolysis, which in turn inhibits the synthesis of insulin.

(vi) The release of insulin is degraded by negative feedback mechanism of epinephrine in stress condition.

(c) **cAMP as modulator :** cAMP is another important modulator of insulin secretion. Glucose is shown to induce cAMP formation directly. Elevations of cAMP, however, will not stimulate insulin secretion in absence of glucose.

BIOSYNTHESIS OF MELATONIN

The hormone melatonin, an indoleamine, is secreted from the pineal gland. It is chemically N-acetyl-5-methoxytryptamine and has been named melatonin because it lightens the skin of tadpoles by an action on the melanophores. It is generally believed that the pineal gland secretes a hormone that has antigonadotropic properties. [Fig. 6.8(a)]

Pineal Melatonin Biosynthesis : Pineal gland contains high concentration of melatonin. The aminoacid tryptophan is the precursor of melatonin. Indole amine biosynthesis involves use of the amino acid, tryptophan, which is converted to 5-hydroxytryptophan by the enzyme tryptophan hydroxylase. The enzyme 5-hydroxytryptophan decarboxylase acts on 5-hydroxytryptophan to form 5-hydroxytryptamine (5-HT, serotonin), which is converted to N-acetylserotonin by the action of N-acetyltransferase. The N-acetylserotonin formed is methoxylated by the enzyme, hydroxyindole-O-methyltransferase (HIOMT) to yield N-acetyl-5-methoxytryptamine (*melatonin*). [Fig. 6.8(b)]

It is believed that the increase in N-acetylserotonin concentration acts by a mass action effect to enhance the production of melatonin. Pineal melatonin is chiefly regulated by N-acetyl transferase activity, which may be the rate-limiting event in the production of indoleamine.

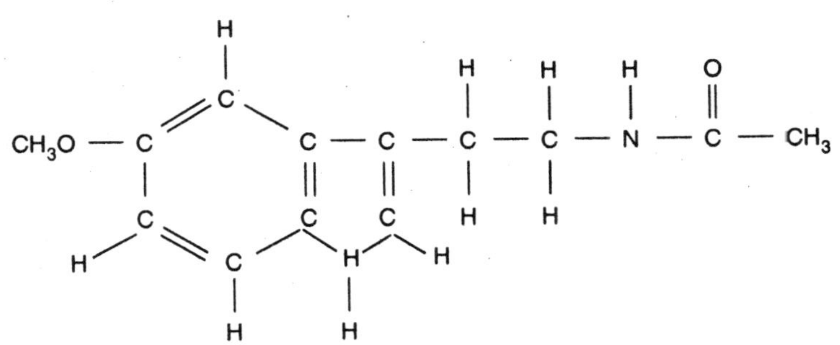

Fig. 6.8(a): Structure of melatonin

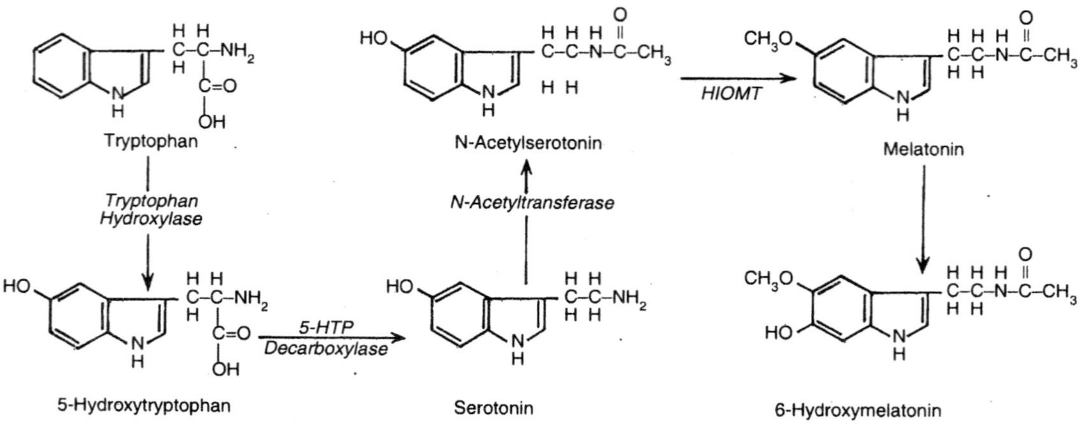

Fig. 6.8(b): Biosynthesis of melatonin

Regulation of secretion : Melatonin synthesis of pineal gland is dramatically affected by photic stimulus received by the lateral eyes. It has been shown that decreased day length increases the melatonin release from pineal gland whereas increased day length decreases the melatonin secretion.

At night there is an increase in the activity of N-acetyl transferase, which is 10 to nearly 100-fold greater than values in the light.

The concentration of N-acetylserotonin is increased to values 10 to 30 times greater than those day conditions. HIOMT is also increased which results in elevated levels of pineal melatonin. Pineal serotonin levels reveal marked diurnal changes with highest levels during the day length hours and those levels are depressed after darkness.

Catabolism : Circulating melatonin is metabolised to 6-hydroxy-melatonin in the liver and other metabolites in the brain by the enzyme melatonin hydroxylase and converted to a sulfate or glucuronide for urinary excretion.

BIOSYNTHESIS OF ADRENO-CORTICAL HORMONES

The adrenal gland is composed of steroidogenic as well as chromaffin tissue. In many mammals, the steroidogenic tissue forms a cortical mass surrounding an inner medullary component of chromaffin tissue. In humans and many other mammals these tissue components may appropriately be referred to as the adrenal cortex and adrenal medulla.

The adrenal cortical tissue can be divided into three morphologically and functionally different layers : the **zona glomerulosa** secretes the mineralocorticoid, aldosterone while the second layer **zona fasciculata** produces the glucocorticoids, cortisol and corticosterone. The inner layer, **zona reticularis** synthesizes sex steroids, like androstenedione, DHEA and progesterone.

Biosynthesis of steroid hormones : The synthesis of adrenocortico steroid hormones are complicated phenomena and can be discussed through the following steps :

(a) **Zones and steroidogenesis :** Because of enzymatic differences between the zona glomerulosa and the inner two zones, the adrenal cortex functions as two separate units, with differing regulation and secretory products. Thus, the zona glomerulosa, which produces aldosterone, lacks 17 α-hydroxylase activity and cannot synthesise 17 α-hydroxypregnenolone and 17 α-hydroxyprogesterone which are the precursors of cortisol and the adrenal androgens. The synthesis of aldosterone by this zone is primarily regulated by the renin-angiotensin system and by potassium.

The zona fasciculata and zona reticularis produce cortisol, androgens and small amounts of estrogens. These zones primarily regulated by ACTH, do not contain the enzyme aldosterone synthetase and therefore cannot convert 11-deoxycorticosterone to aldosterone. [Fig. 6.8(c)]

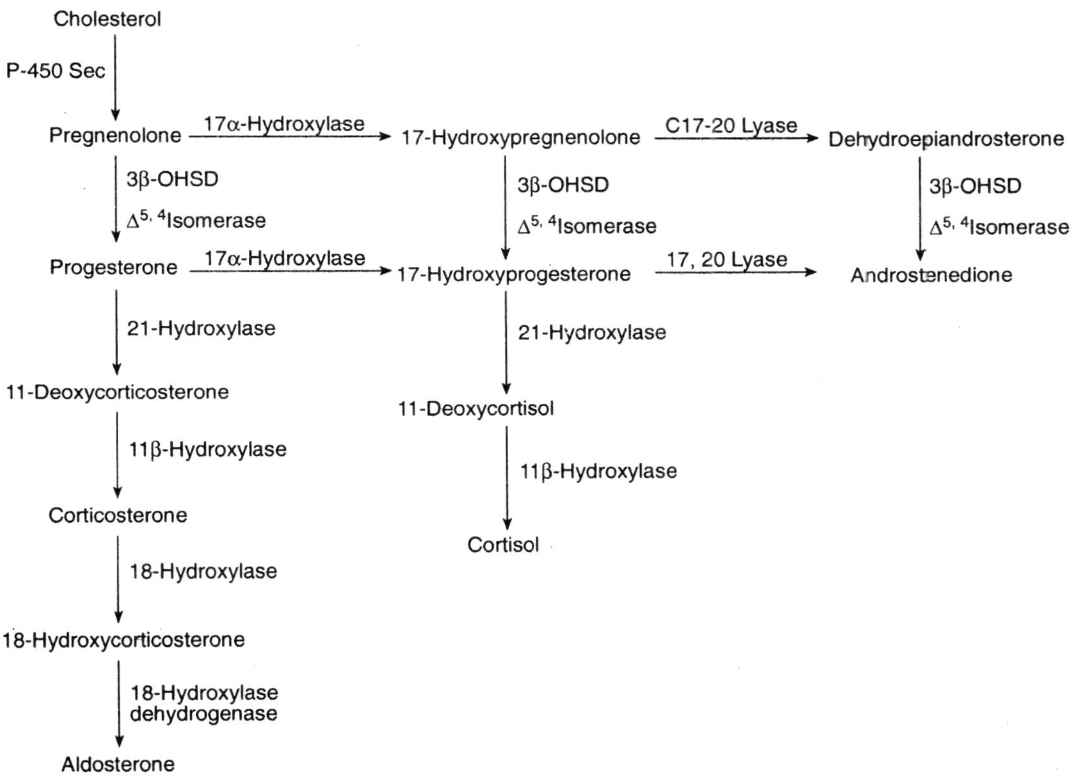

Fig. 6.8(c): Biosynthesis of adrenocorticosteroids

Conversion of cholesterol to pregnenolone : Cholesterol is the source of all steroid hormones. It is formed in the liver and endocrine glands via a number of intermediate steps (squalene, lanosterol etc) from the acetyl CoA. Plasma lipoproteins are the major source of adrenal cholesterol, though synthesis within the gland from acetate also occurs. A small pool of free cholesterol within the adrenal is available for rapid synthesis of steroids when the adrenal is stimulated. When stimulation occurs, there is also increased hydrolysis of stored cholesterol esters to free cholesterol, and increased cholesterol synthesis within the gland [Fig. 6.9(a)].

The conversion of cholesterol to pregnenolone is the rate limiting step in adrenal steroidogenesis and the major site of ACTH action on the adrenal gland. This step occurs in the mitochondria and involves two hydroxylations. Upon stimulation of the adrenal by ACTH or cAMP, an esterase is activated and the free cholesterol (formed) is passed into the mitochondrion, where P-450 side chain cleavage enzyme mediates this process; each step requires molecular oxygen and a pair of electrons. The latter are donated by NADPH to adrenodoxin reductase, a flavoprotein, and then to adrenodoxin, an iron-sulfur protein, and finally to P-450 sec. Within the mitochondrion cytochrome P-450 side chain cleavage enzyme (P-450 sec) converts cholesterol to pregnenolone. It acts as a pivot for synthesis of all adrenocorticosteroids. Pregnenolone is then transported outside the mitochondria before further steroid synthesis occurs and enter into smooth ER [Fig. 6.9(b)].

Conversion of pregnenolone to different adrenocorticosteroids : Pregnenolone is changed successively into three different kinds of hormones by the following reactions :

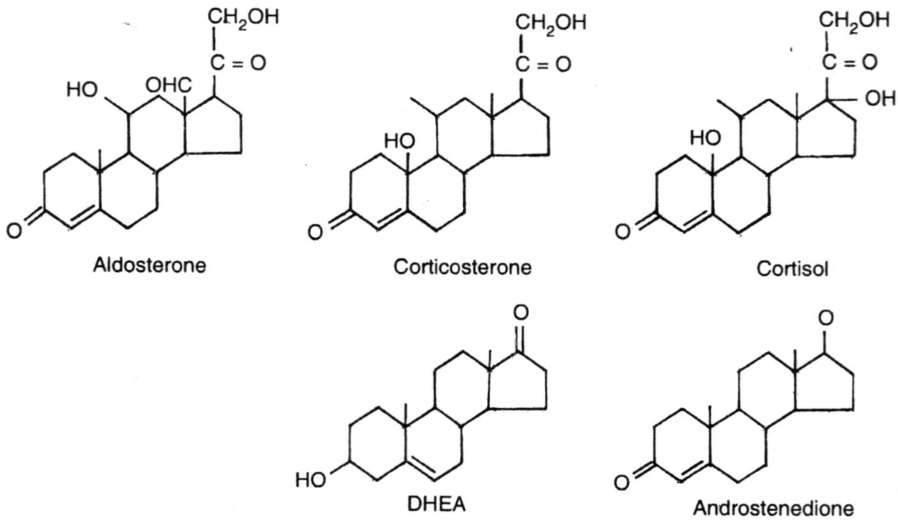

Fig. 6.9(a): Structural configuration of glucocorticoids and mineralocorticoids

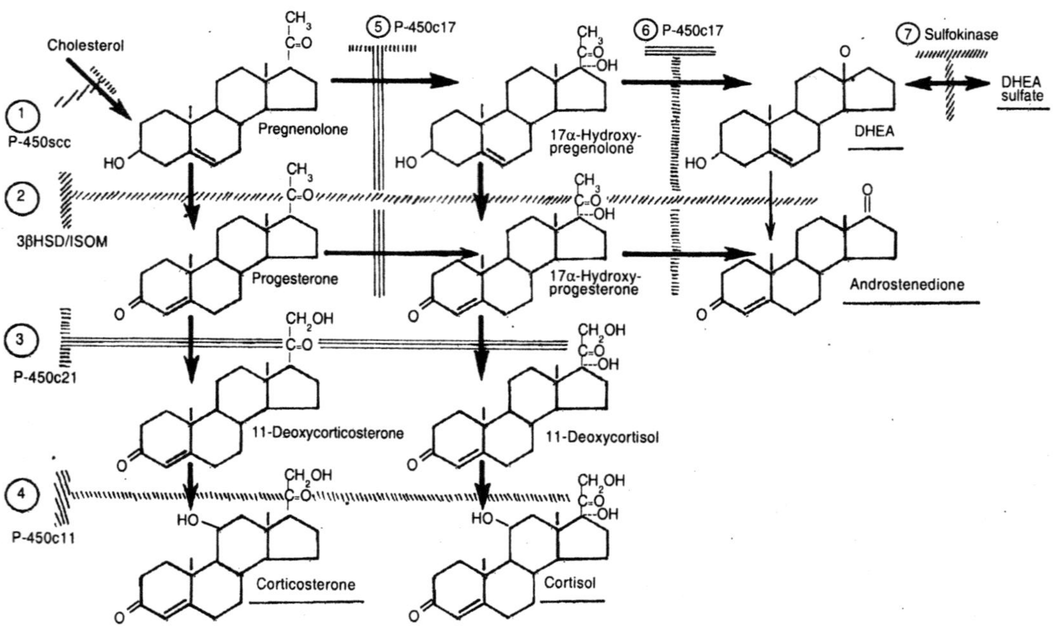

Fig. 6.9(b): Biosynthesis of adrenocorticosteroids

1. **Synthesis of glucocorticoids or cortisol :** In the cells of zona fasciculata, within smooth ER, pregnenolone is changed to 17 α-hydroxypregnenolone by 17 α-hydroxylase. (The adrenal contains 17-, 21-, and 11-hydroxylases, enzymes which introduce a hydroxyl group into the steroid molecule at the carbon atom indicated by the number). This steroid molecule is then converted to 17 α-hydroxyprogesterone after conversion of its 5, 6 double bond to a 4, 5 double bond by the 3β-hydroxysteroid dehydrogenase. Pregnenolone is converted successively through 17-hydroxypregnenolone and 17-hydroxyprogesterone to 11-deoxycortisol by the actions of microsomal enzymes, 17 α-hydroxylase, 3β-OHSD, $\Delta^{5,4}$-isomerase (located within smooth ER) and 21-hydroxylase respectively. An alternative but apparently less important pathway in zonae fasciculata and reticularis is from pregnenolone → progesterone → 17 α-hydroxyprogesterone.

In the next step 11-deoxycortisol is then translocated to mitochondria, where it is hydroxylated by mitochondrial enzyme, 11 β-hydroxylase to form cortisol. The zonae fasciculata and reticularis also produce 11-deoxycorticosterone (DOC), 18-hydroxycorticosterone and Aldosterone.

2. **Mineralocorticoid synthesis or Aldosterone synthesis :** In the zona glomerulosa, pregnenolone is changed successively to progesterone and 11-deoxycorticosterone on their smooth ER by the actions of microsomal 3βHSD (3 β-hydroxysteroid dehydrogenase) : 5, 4-isomerase pair and 21-hydroxylase, respectively. 11-deoxycorticosterone is then transferred into mitochondria where the successive actions of 11 β-hydroxylase and 18-hydroxylase convert it through corticosterone to 18-hydroxycorticosterone. The latter is then oxidised to **aldosterone** by 18 HSD.

18-hydroxylase and 18-hydroxysteroid dehydrogenase occur only within the mitochondria of glomerulosa cells. However, as noted above, the absence of the mitochondrial enzyme P-450 aldo (aldosterone synthetase, P-450 cmo) prevents production of aldosterone by these zones of the adrenal cortex (zonae fasciculata and reticularis).

3. **Sex corticoid synthesis :** The production of adrenal androgens from pregnenolone and progesterone requires prior 17 α-hydroxylation (P-450c 17) and thus, does not occur in the zona glomerulosa. The major production of androgens is by conversion of 17 α-hydroxypregnenolone to the 19 carbon compounds (C_{19} steroids), dehydroepiandrosterone (DHEA) and its sulfate (conjugate DHEA sulfate). Thus, 17 α-hydroxypregnenolone undergoes removal of its two-carbon side chain at C_{17} position by microsomal 17, 20-desmolase, yielding DHEA with a keto group at C_{17}. DHEA is then converted to DHEA sulfate by a reversible adrenal sulfokinase. The other major adrenal androgen, androstenedione, is produced from 17 α-hydroxyprogesterone by 17, 20 desmolase and to a lesser extent from DHEA. Androstenedione can be converted to testosterone, though adrenal secretion of this hormone is minimal. The adrenal androgens, DHEA, DHEA sulfate and androstenedione, have minimal intrinsic androgenic activity, and they contribute to androgenecity by their peripheral conversion to the more potent androgens, testosterone and dihydrotestosterone [Fig. 6.9(c)].

Transport : Adrenocorticosteroid hormones are transported mostly in bound form and only a small quantity is free. Glucocorticoids are circulated through plasma α-globlulin, called corticosteroid binding globulin (CBG) or transcortin. Mineralocorticoid does not have a specific plasma transport protein but it makes a very weak association with albumin. The sex steroids (i.e., oestradiol and testosterone) are carried via the plasma proteins; β-globulin—a sex hormone binding globulin (SHBG) or gonadal steroid binding globulin (GSBG). CBG binds steroid with Δ^4–3 ketone and 20-ketone groups, while SHBG or testosterone oestra-

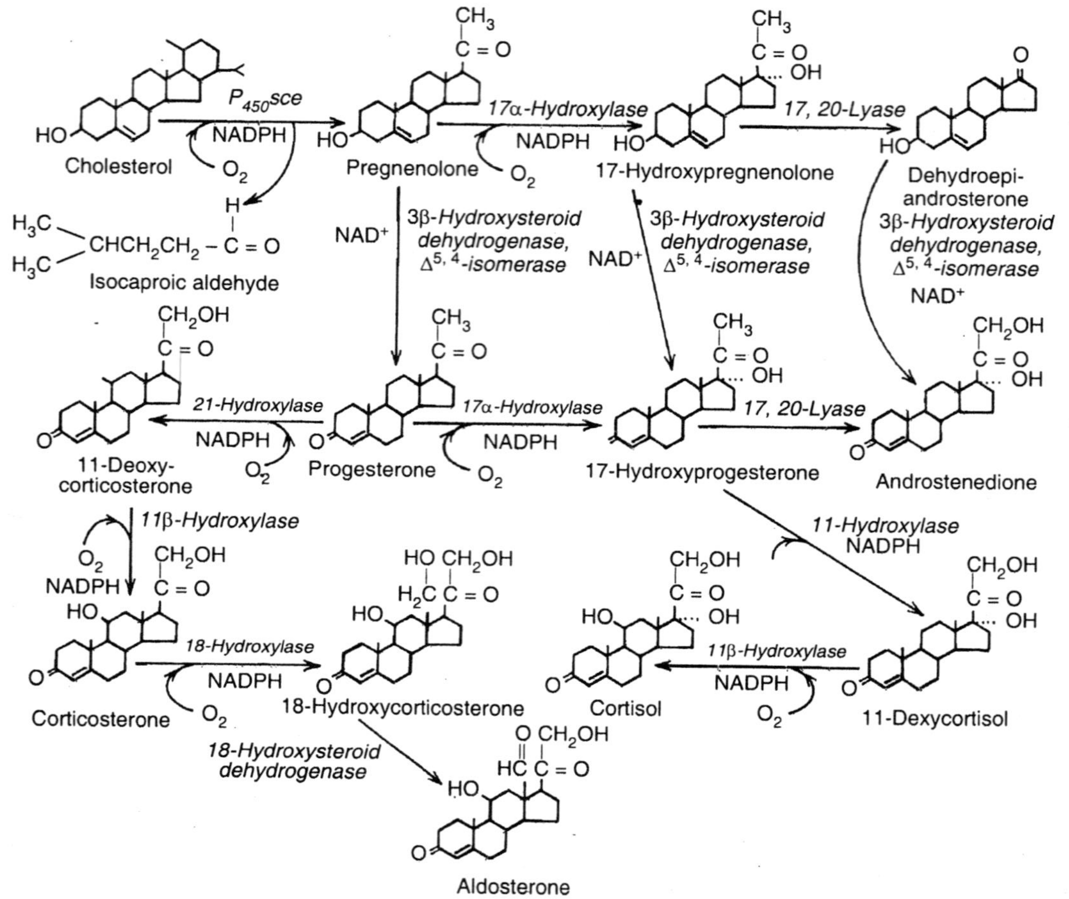

Fig. 6.9(c): Pathways of adrenal steroid hormone biosynthesis

diol binding globulin binds oestrogens and androgens with a 17 β-OH group. A minor degree of binding to albumin also takes place.

Catabolism : Adrenal cortical hormones are metabolised in the liver, kidney and gut. The cortisol is converted in the liver to cortisone. Both are reduced in the liver to dihydrocortisol and dihydrocorticosterone respectively and loose the double bond between C_4 and C_5. These compounds are hydroxylated at C_3 to tetrahydrocortisone and tetrahydrocortisol which are transformed to glucuronide in the liver by conjugation at the C_3 hydroxyl group. This is finally excreted through urine.

Aldosterone weakly bound to plasma protein which is separated in liver and is converted into tetrahydro-aldosterone glucuronide. It is excreted through urine. Androstenedione and DHEA are oxidised to 17-ketosteroids and they are excreted through urine in conjugated form as sulfates.

Control of secretion : The synthesis and release of adrenocortico steroids are regulated by ACTH of adenohypophysis. Increase in the concentration of glucocorticoids in blood inhibits the secretion of ACTH by negative feedback mechanism. In the hypothalamus corticotrophin releasing factor secretion is influenced by negative feedback control from the cortisol level of blood.

A direct feedback regulation of corticotrophin producing cells in the hypophysis by cortisol is also found [Fig. 6.9(d)].

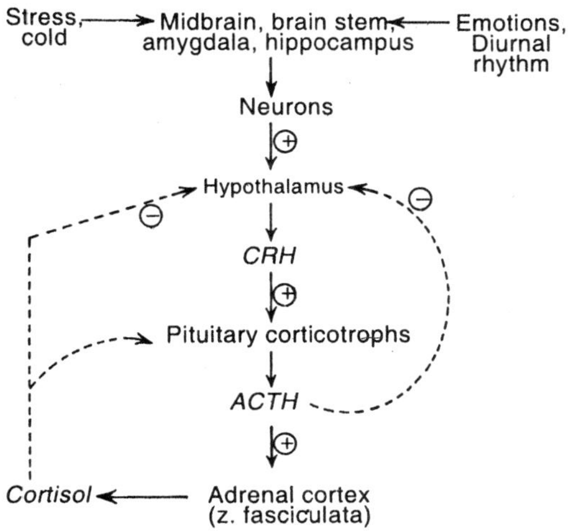

Fig. 6.9(d): Control adrenocorticosteroids

ACTH-RH of hypothalamus regulates the secretion of pituitary ACTH. The different factors like cold, excitement, stress, diurnal rhythm, etc. regulate the secretion of hypothalamus.

The synthesis and secretion of mineralo corticoids are controlled by plasma concentrations of Na^+ and K^+, renin-angiotensin system and to some extent, corticotrophin also.

BIOSYNTHESIS OF ADRENAL MEDULLARY HORMONES

Adrenal madulla is histologically made up of chromaffin cells. These cells synthesize two catecholamines, **adrenaline** or **epinephrine** (E) and **noradrenaline** or **norepinephrine** (NE). In mammals, epinephrine is synthesised mainly in the adrenal medulla but also in the central nervous system and in the peripheral sympathetic nerves. **Dopamine,** the precursor of norepinephrine, is found in the adrenal medulla and in noradrenergic neurons.

Synthesis : Two catecholamines, adrenaline (epinephrine) and noradrenaline (norepinephrine), are secreted by adrenal medullary chromaffin cells and also released at adrenergic axon terminals. The proportions of epinephrine and norepinephrine found in the adrenal medulla vary with the species. In humans, the adrenal cortex contains 15-20% norepinephrine. Catecholamines are amine derivatives of catechol nucleus (dehydroxylated phenyl ring). Catecholamine synthesis takes place in the following steps :

1. **Conversion of Tyrosine to DOPA :** The catecholamines are derived from the amino acid, phenyl alanine in the liver which is hydroxylated by phenylalanine hydroxylase (enzyme) to **tyrosine**. This tyrosine is either derived from ingested food or synthesised from phenylalanine in the liver. It enters neurons and chromaffin cells by an active transport mechanism and is converted to **dihydroxyphenylalanine (DOPA).** The reaction is catalysed by tyrosine hydroxylase which is transported via axonal flow to the nerve terminal. Activity of tyrosine hydroxylase is a reliable marker of intact sympathetic nerve tissue and neurotransmitter synthesis.

2. **Conversion of DOPA to Dopamine :** Dopa is then decarboxylated to dopamine by the enzyme aromatic L-amino acid decarboxylase. This enzyme is observed in all tissues with the highest concentration in liver, brain, kidney and vas-deferens.

3. **Conversion of Dopamine to Norepinephrine :** The conversion of dopamine to norepinephrine is catalysed by dopamine β-hydroxylase, a copper oxidase having mixed functions—requiring oxygen and an external electron donor. This enzyme does not occur in tissues outside the neuron. The conversion takes place within the granule of chromaffin cell.

Part of the biologic specificity of dopamine β-hydroxylase may result from its compartmentalization. Newly synthesised dopamine β-hydroxylase is incorporated directly into storage vesicles that take up, synthesise, and store the catecholamines. Dopamine β-hydroxylase is also present within the granule and is released with norepinephrine during secretion. [Fig. 6.10(a)]

catecholamines and ATP in 4 : 1 molar ratio, several neuropeptides, Calcium, Magnesium

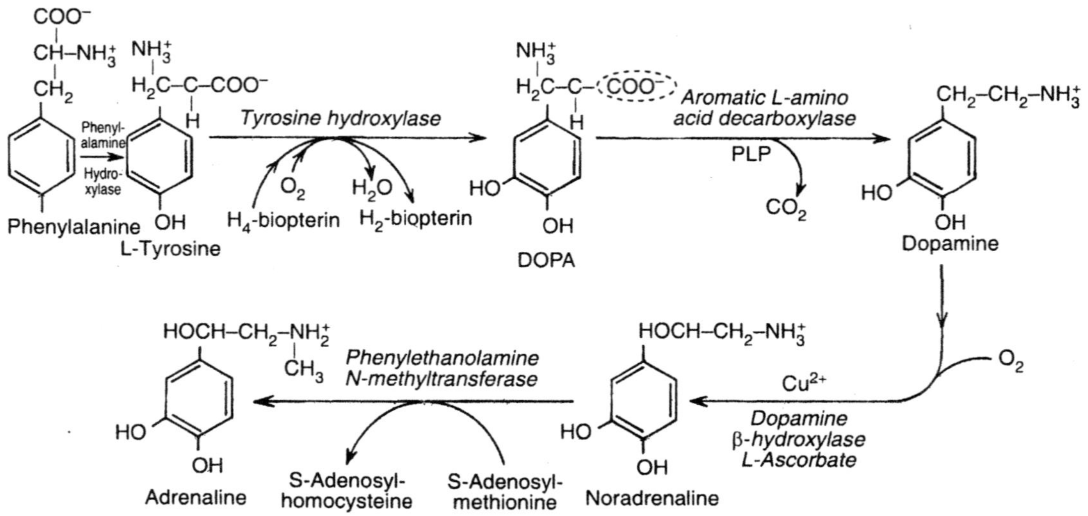

Fig. 6.10(a): Biosynthesis of catecholamines

4. **Conversion of norepinephrine to epinephrine** : Norepinephrine (NE) passes out into cytosol and undergoes methylation by the enzyme, phenylethanolamine-N-methyl transferase (PNMT), using s-adenosyl-methionine as a methyl donor. It is found only in the adrenal medulla and in a few neurons in the CNS. NE after being synthesised from dopamine leaves the granules and after methylation re-enters different granules. This enzyme (PNMT) is induced by the high levels of glucocorticoids found in the adrenal medulla. As the adrenal medulla is cradled by the cortex, it is bathed with very high concentration of glucocorticoids, so that PNMT is available.

The major product of the adrenal medulla is epinephrine and this compound constitutes about 80% of the catecholamines.

Storage and release : The catecholamines are present in the adrenal medulla and various sympathetically innervated organs. They are stored in electron dense granules approximately 1 μm in diameter that contain and water soluble proteins called **chromograins.** The ratio of catecholamines to ATP is much higher in granules. The interior surface of the membrane vesicle comprises dopamine β-hydroxylase and ATPase. The Mg^{++} dependent ATPase facilitates the uptake and inhibits the release of catecholamines by the granules.

Catecholamines are released from the adrenal medulla by a process known as exocytosis. After chemical stimulation, followed by membrane depolarisation, the chromaffin granules discharge catecholamines including ATP and specific proteins, called **chromograins.** The process of exocytosis takes place via the plasma membrane rather than by diffusion through the cell cytoplasm. The vesicle membrane is not discharged with the catecholamines. Ca^{++} is not intimately related to the exocytosis process.

The hydrolysis of ATP in the granules by an enzyme, ATPase might play a role in catecholamines release. It is presumed that ATP assists in keeping the granules intact.

Thus, hydrolysis of ATP causes breaking of the string that holds the package granules together. Acetylcholine does alone cause the release of the catecholamines, but component of intact cell is required.

Catabolism : Catecholamines are metabolised by two enzymes, catecholamine-o-methyl transferase (COMT) and monoamine oxidase (MAO). Norepinephrine and epinephrine are metabolised extracellularly by COMT to normetanephrine and metanephrine respectively. Both metanephrine and normetanephrine are ultimately converted into 3-methoxy-4-hydroxymandelic aldehyde by MAO. This aldehyde is excreted as vanil mandelic acid (VMA). Principal metabolic product either of epinephrine or of norepinephrine that is excreted through urine is the VMA. Normetanephrine and metanephrine are also excreted [Fig. 6.10(b)].

BIOSYNTHESIS OF TESTOSTERONE

Testosterone is the most important male reproductive hormone which is secreted by the testicular Leydig cells. Testosterone is popularly known as androgen. In addition to testosterone, the testis also secretes small amounts of other androgen like dihydrotestosterone and DHEA (dehydroepiandrosterone) and small quantities estradiol, estrone, pregnenolone, etc.

Testosterone is C_{19} steroid and its chemical formula is $C_{19}H_{28}O_2$. It is converted to some extent to a more potent derivative, 5 α-dihydrotestosterone, in extratesticular tissues as well as testes.

Source : Testosterone is secreted by interstitial cells of Leydig in testis. Trace amount is also released by adrenal cortex.

Synthesis : Interstitial cells of Leydig are the target cells that are stimulated by gonadotrophins for an increased synthesis of androgens. The chief products which are secreted into the spermatic venous blood of adult testes are testosterone and smaller quantities of Δ^4–androstenedione and dehydroepiandrosterone (DHEA). Like adrenal steroidogenic tissues, cholesterol serves as the precursor of testosterone biosynthesis in Leydig cells. Within Leydig cells, cholesterol is delivered to inner mitochondrial membrane by steriodogenic acute regulatory protein and then converted to pregnenolone by P_{450} sce (i.e., sce–side chain cleavage. enzyme) of mitochondria. Pregnenolone is then translocated to smooth ER for conversion to testosterone in two pathways :

Progesterone or Δ^4 pathway : Most of the pregnenolone is converted to progesterone in presence of the enzymes 3 β-hydroxysteroid dehydrogenase (3β HSD) and $\Delta^{5,4}$–isomerase in human. Progesterone is then transformed into androstenedione via 17α-hydroxyprogesterone with the help of the enzymes 17α-hydroxylase and 17,20–lyase of smooth ER membrane. In the next step, androstenedione is reduced by the microsomal 17β-hydroxysteroid dehydrogenase into testosterone. [Fig. 6.11]

Dehydroepiandrosterone pathyway or Δ^5 pathway : In another pathway pregnenolone is changed into dehydro-

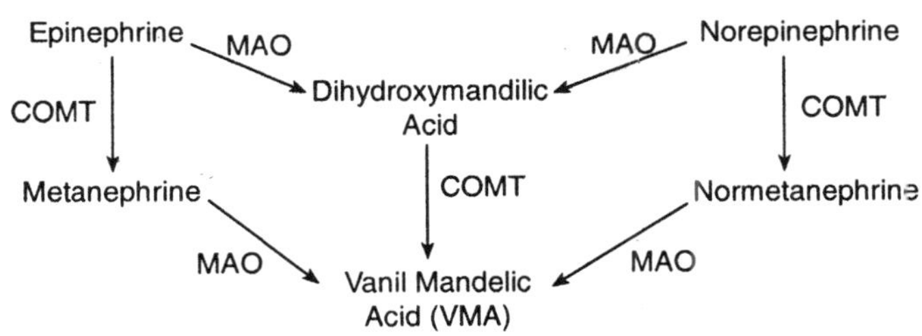

Fig. 6.10(b): Catabolism of epinephrine and norepinephrine

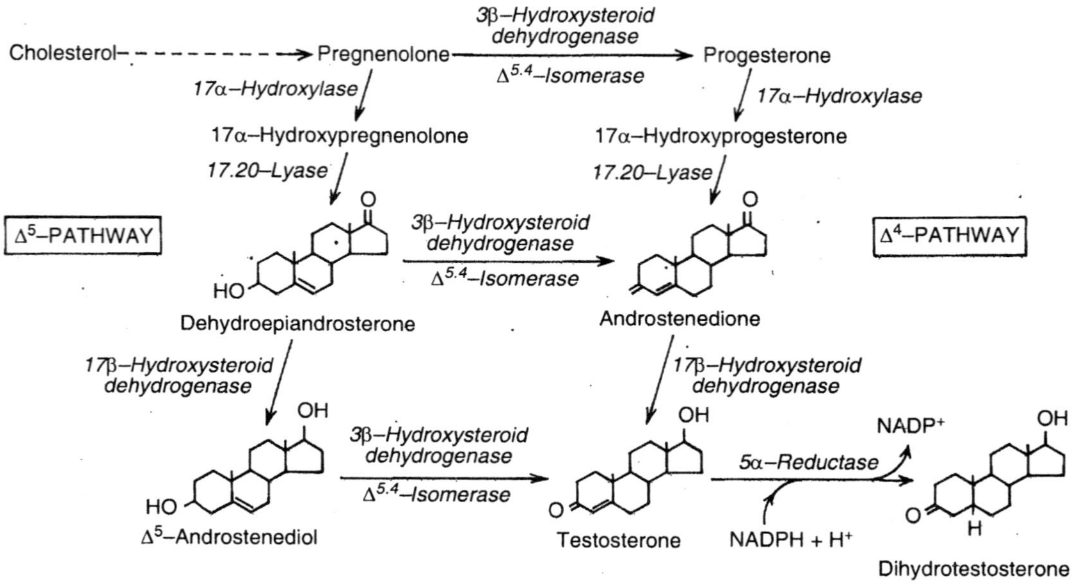

Fig. 6.11: Biosynthesis of testosterone

epiandrosterone (DHEA) through 17α-hydroxypregnenolone by the actions of respectively 17α-hydroxylase and 17,20 lyase of smooth ER membrane. DHEA is then converted to testosterone either through Δ^5–androstenediol in presence of the enzymes 17β–HSD, 3β–HSD and $\Delta^{5,4}$–isomerase or through androstenedione with the help of the enzymes, 3β–HSD, $\Delta^{5,4}$–isomerase and 17β–HSD.

Transport : Testosterone circulates in the plasma bound to plasma proteins. About 4-10 mg of testosterone are secreted in every 24 hours. In men, of the total production about 45% is bound to β-globulin, called sex hormone binding globulin (SHBG) and 40% is bound to albumin and 12-15% to other proteins. Only about 2-3% of testosterone is unbound in peripheral blood and is in the active free form.

Before entering the target tissues the protein bound testosterone get dissociated from the protein and binds to specific receptor.

Catabolism : Testicular androgens or testosterones are mainly catabolised in the liver to 17 ketosteroids such as androsterone and etiocholanolone which are eliminated through urine as glucuronides and sulfates.

Control of secretion : The hypothalamus secretes gonadotrophin releasing hormone (Gn RH) and releases it in pulses every 90-120 minutes into the hypothalamo-hypophysial portal blood. After reaching adenohypophysis, GnRH binds to gonadotrophs and stimulates the release of both LH and, to a lesser extent, FSH into the general circulation. LH is taken up by the Leydig cells where it binds to specific membrane receptors. This leads to activation of adenyl cyclase and generation of cAMP and other messengers that finally result in the secretion of androgens. In turn, the elevation of androgens inhibits the secretion of LH from adenohypophysis through a direct action on the pituitary and an inhibitory effect at the hypothalamic level.

Sertoli cells also release several other substances like inhibin A and B, Gn RH-like peptide, transferrin plasminogen activator, H-Y antigen. Of these, the inhibins can inhibit FSH secretion from the adenohypophysis without affecting LH release.

The major inhibitory effect of androgen on the hypothalamus appears to be mediated principally by estradiol, which may be derived locally through the aromatization of testosterone. Again, stress, emotion, high fever, etc. may reduce the androgen secretion.

BIOSYNTHESIS OF ESTROGEN

Estrogen is a kind of female sex-steroid hormone which plays a great role of female reproductive physiology. Estrogens are compounds which can produce estrus in ovariectomised animals, and are of two varieties, the synthetic and natural. Natural estrogen is secreted by the interstitial cells of the ovary and is called **estradiol.** Other estrogens like **estrone** and **estriol** are found in adult female and are believed to be the derivatives of estradiol. Chemically, estrogens are sterol derivatives, i.e., C_{18} steroids. Three compounds of this group with hormonal activity are—(i) β-estradiol (E_2)—$C_{18}H_{24}O_2$, (ii) estriol—$C_{18}H_{24}O_3$ and (iii) Estrone (E_1)—$C_{18}H_{22}O_2$. Of the estrogens, 17β–estradiol (E_2), estrone (E_1) and estriol have biological potencies in a descending order. [Fig. 6.12(a)]

Source : Estrogen is secreted mainly from the theca interna and granulosa cells of Graafian follicle of the ovary. Estrogens have been extracted from the suprarenal cortex. Small amounts of estrogen have been extracted from testes. In cow and many other mammalian species placenta is the source of estrogen during pregnancy.

Synthesis : The ovarian steroids are synthesised from cholesterol which is the precursor of estrogen biosynthesis. Ovarian steroidogenic cells synthesise pregnenolone and progesterone from cholesterol through steps identical with initial steps in corticosteroid synthesis.

In the biosynthesis of estrogen, cholesterol is metabolised to pregnenolone by P_{450} cleaved enzyme. Pregnenolone formed by this reaction is then either transformed to progesterrone through the action of 3β-HSD and $\Delta^{5,4}$–isomerase or to 17α-hydroxy pregnenolone by 17α-hydroxylase and then to androstenedione by 17, 20 lyase action. The androstenedione is then converted to testosterone by the action of 17β–HSD.

The 17α-hydroxypregnenolone formed by another pathway may also be converted to dehydroepiandrosterone by the action of the enzyme 17, 20 lyase. The latter may produce testosterone via androstenedione [Fig. 6.12(b)].

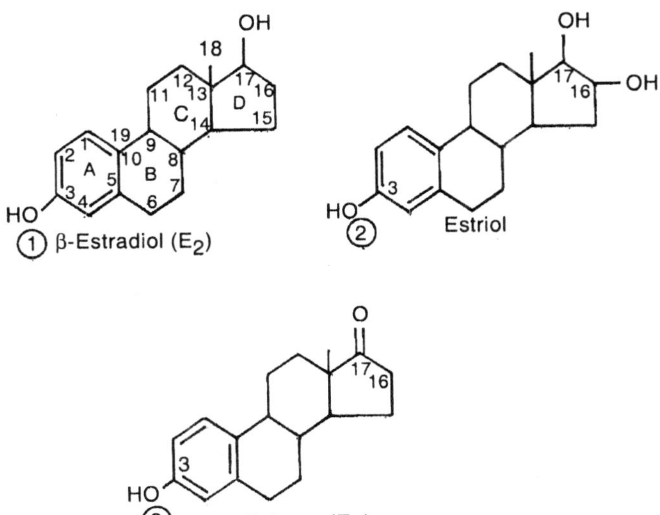

(1) β-Estradiol (E_2)

(2) Estriol

(3) Estrone (E_1)

Fig. 6.12(a): Principal estrogens

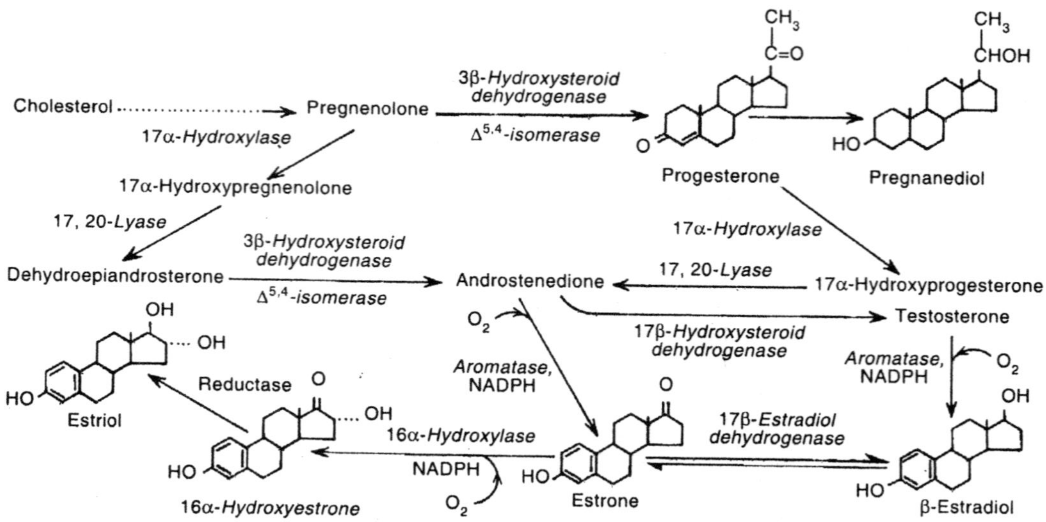

Fig. 6.12(b): Biosynthesis of estrogens

There are different ideas of estrogen synthesis :

1. **Two-cell theory :** This theory states that the production of testosterone (C_{19} androgen) by the stimulation of LH occurs in thecal cells. This C_{19} androgen is then delivered to the granulosa cells wherein this is aromatised to estrogen by NADPH dependent aromatase. It is also observed that granulosa cells of several species release estrogens after stimulation of FSH and the granulosa cells have little or no capacity for producing C_{19} androgens from C_{21} progesterone but do have an active aromatase system. As the follicles become mature the ability of granulosa cells to aromatise androgens increases. The synthesis of estrogens increases during preovulatory phase and becomes highest at the time of LH/FSH surge.

2. **Modified two-cell theory :** This theory states that the androgen production within thecal cells is stimulated by LH. This androgen is then aromatised within the thecal cells but are also made available to the granulosa cells for aromatisation to estrogens. Estrogens of thecal cells are the major source of circulating levels of steroids where as the estrogens, synthesized by granulosa cells, serve locally and possibly assist in the maturation of ova.

Transport : Estradiol is released directly by the ovary in blood stream. Estrone is produced by peripheral conversion of estradiol or androstenedione. Estrone is further metabolised to estriol in liver. About 1-3% of the plasma estradiol and estrone circulate in free active forms. Most circulating estrogens are bound to **sex hormone binding globulin** (SHBG) and transported through plasma.

Catabolism : Estrone and estriol are the principal metabolites of estradiol. These are excreted in bile and urine as glucuronides and sulfates. The excretion of these estrogens is variable at different phases of life. It becomes maximum at the time of ovulation and just before the onset of parturition.

Control : Two main gonadotrophins, LH and FSH from anterior pituitary, regulate ovarian steroidogenesis. FSH promotes the growth of follicles and aromatase activity required for conversion of androgen to estrogen. The LH stimulates production of androgens that are utilised in estrogen production.

BIOSYNTHESIS OF PROGESTERONE

Progesterone is another important hormone which plays an important role in life of female reproductive physiology. Progesterone jointly with estrogen help in the growth and development (maturation) of the reproductive system, regulation of its function and appearance of pubertal changes in females. It helps in the regulation of the menstrual cycle and maintains the persistence of corpus lutenum during pregnancy and serves for implantation. Progesterone acts synergistically with estrogen to facilitate the proliferation and development of mammary glands and it also inhibits ovulation.

Chemically, progesterone is a pregnane derivative and is devoid of keto group. It is a C_{21} steroid and its molecular formula is $C_{21}H_{30}O_2$ [Fig. 6.13(a)].

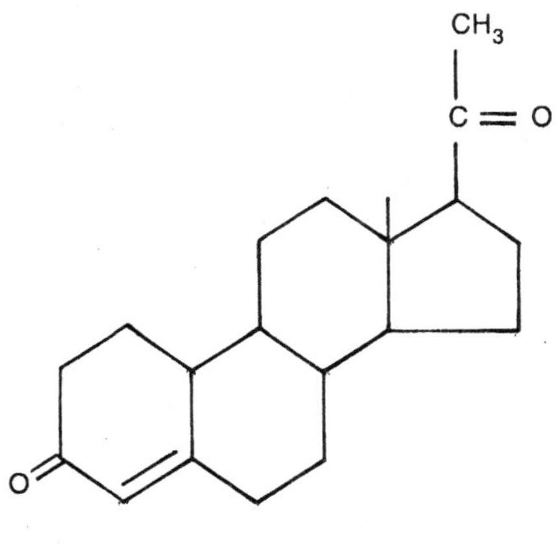

Fig. 6.13(a): Structure of progesterone

Source : The site of formation of progesterone is the corpus luteum, the graafian follicle, the placenta and in males as well, the adrenal cortex.

Synthesis : The biosynthesis of progesterone is an early step in the production of androgen and estrogen within the thecal cells. The corpus luteum formed following ovulation is the major source of circulating progesterone. It is known that the cholesterol is the precursor of this hormone.

Just prior to LH/FSH surge in many species progesterone biosynthesis is initiated within the granulosa cells. During the preovulatory surge, LH acts directly on those cells to initiate luteinisation and it also enhances progesterone synthesis as the luteinised granulosa cells are transformed to corpus luteum following ovulation.

The steroid hormones are synthesised from cholesterol, which is present in the ovary both free and esterified to fatty acids (cholesteryl esters). Cholesterol derived either from circulating lipoproteins or from cholesteryl esters in the gland is converted to pregnenolone by removal of a 6-carbon fragment, isocaproic acid. This reaction or group of reactions is the rate-limiting step and is controlled by LH from the anterior pituitary.

Pregnenolone formed by this reaction may be converted either to progesterone or to 17α-hydroxypregnenolone. The conversion to progesterone requires the action of 3β-HSD and $\Delta^{5,4}$–isomerase, which shifts the double bond from the Δ^5 to Δ^4 position. Progesterone is secreted by the corpus luteum in large amounts following ovulation. However, it is a substrate for 450c 17 (17α-hydroxylase) which converts it to 17α-hydroxyprogesterone in the endoplasmic reticulum then to progesterone. Following 17α-hydroxylation, the two carbon (20-21) side-chain may be cleaved by the $P_{450}C_{17}$ (17, 20 lyase) enzyme to form androgen. [Fig. 6.13(b)]

Transport : Progesterone circulates as bound form with a plasma protein, corticosteroid binding globulin, protein (transcortin).

Control : Two main gonadotrophins, LH and FSH from anterior pituitary, control ovarian steroidogenesis. The secretion of progesterone can be stimulated by those hormones. The granulosa cells acquire LH receptors when the follicles become antral. These cells following stimulation produce

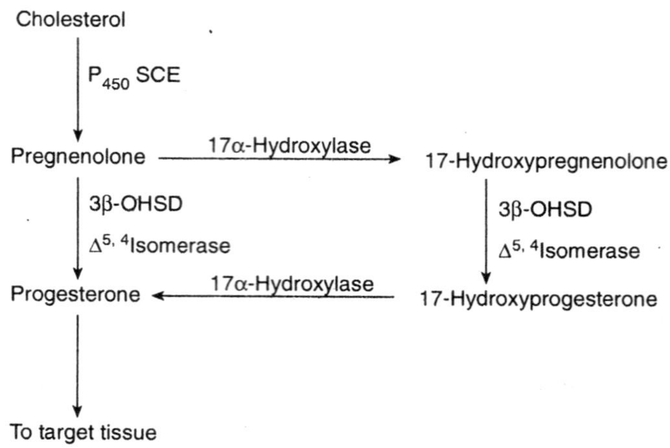

Fig. 6.13(b): Biosynthesis of progesterone

progesterone. During reproductive cycle, just before ovulation, LH surge initiates the synthesis of progesterone.

Catabolism : Small quantities of progesterone are found in blood and urine. During the metabolic processes progesterone gets reduced into an inactive derivative known as pregnandiol. It is conjugated with glucuronic acid and sodium in the liver and appears in the urine as sodium-pregna-ndiol-20-glucuronate.

SYNTHESIS OF STEROIDS

The steroid hormones are derived from cholesterol produced either by de novo synthesis or by uptake of LDL through LDL receptors. When the steroid producing glands are stimulated, the cholesterol is liberated through stimulation of cholesterol esterase and some additional cholesterol is produced through stimulation of cholesterol synthesis by the gland. These glands have particularly high concentrations of LDL receptors that are increased further by steroidogenic stimuli such as tropic hormones.

The rate-limiting step in steroid hormone production is the cleavage of cholesterol to form pregnenolone through the actions of a cytochrome P_{450}-cholesterol side cleavage enzyme (P_{450} sec) located on the inner mitochondrial membrane.

In the adrenocortical zona fasciculata and zona reticularis, pregnenolone is sequentially converted to 17α-OH-pregnenolone, 17α-OH-progesterone and 11-deoxycortisol. The production of 17α-OH-prenenolone from pregnenolone is referred to as the Δ_5 pathway because the –5, 6 double bond is preserved. 11-Deoxycortisol then flows back into the mitochondria where cortisol is formed by 11-β hydroxylation through the actions of cytochrome P_{450} c 11. This enzyme is not found in the gonad.

The adrenal glomerulosa produces progesterone from pregnenolone through the actions of 3β-hydroxy steroid dehydrogenase, and $-\Delta^{4,5}$-isomerase. This is called the Δ^4 pathway. The glomerulosa lacks cytochrome P_{450} c 17 and uniquely contains a mitochondrial corticosterone methyl oxidase I [Fig. 6.14(a)].

For androgen and estrogen production, the side chains at position 17 of 17α-OH pregnenolone or 17α-OH progesterone are removed by C 17, 20-lyase activity to yield DHEA (dehydro-epiandrosterone) and androstenedione respectively. The production of DHEA is a major pathway in both the adrenals

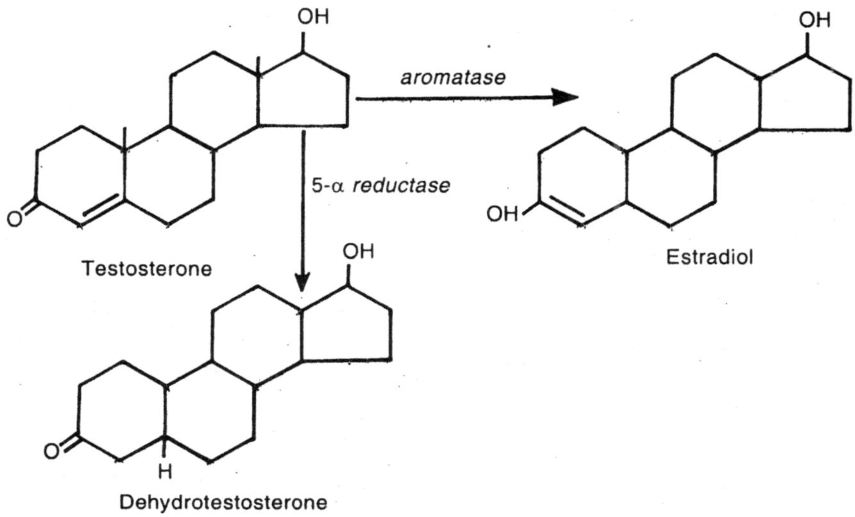

Fig. 6.14(a): Synthesis of estradiol and dihydrotestosterone from testoesterone

and the gonads. Subsequent steps, which lead to the production of the major estrogen, estradiol and the androgen, testosterone, occur in the gonads but to only a minute extent in the adrenal glands [Fig. 6.14(b)].

The major pathway for testosterone synthesis in the male gonad (i.e., testis) is in the Leydig cells via Δ^5 pathway from pregnenolone to DHEA and androstenediol, before the steroids are converted to the Δ^4 derivatives, androstenedione to testosterone and DHEA to androstenediol and then testosterone through the actions of 17β-hydroxysteroid dehydrogenase. It is to be noted that the steroid dihydrotestosterone is produced mostly in the target tissues through the activity of 5α-reductase, and very little is made in the testis.

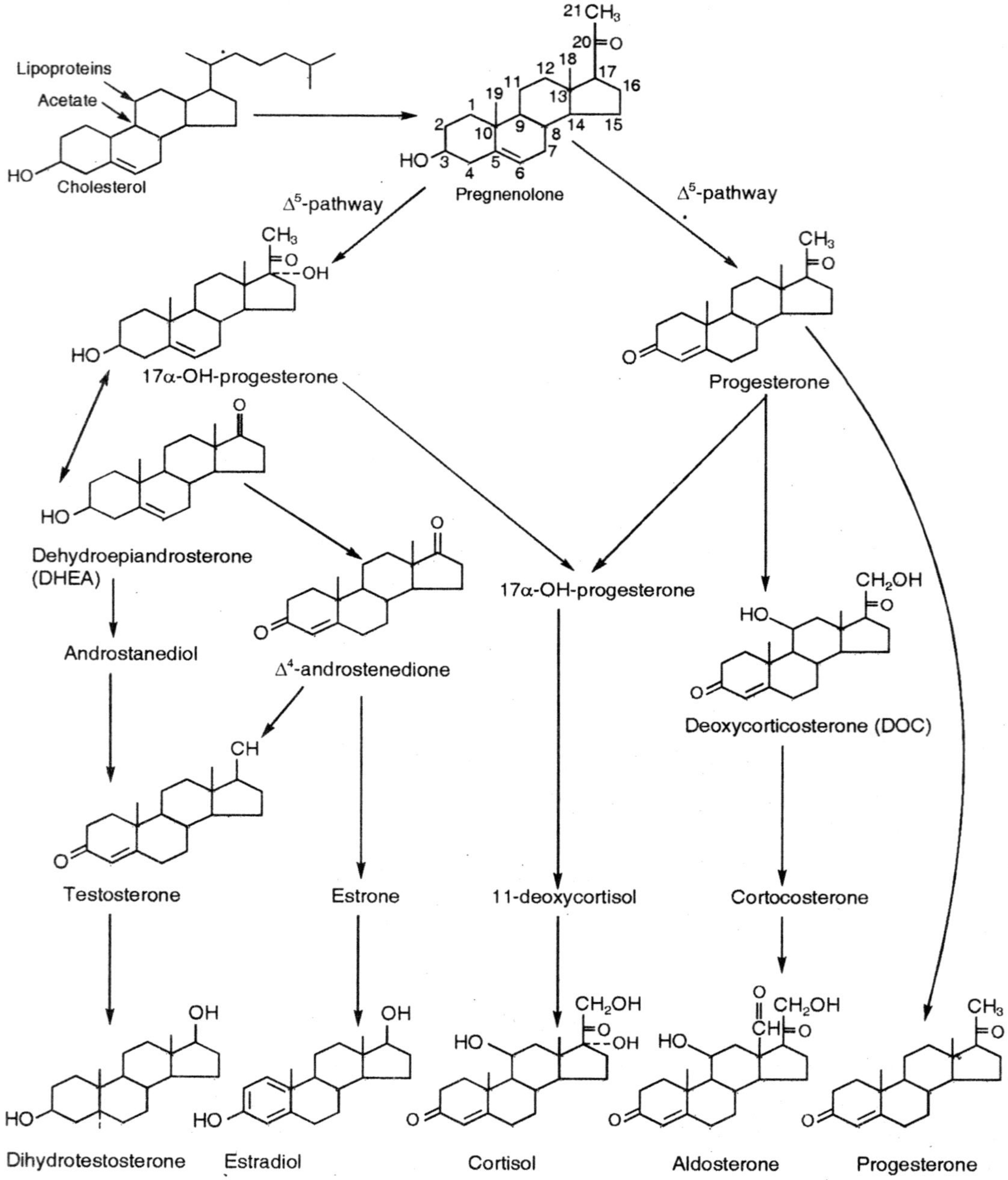

Fig. 6.14(b): Pathways of synthesis of the major classes of steroid hormones. Cholesterol is derived from acetate by synthesis or from lipoprotein particles. The numbering of the steroid molecule is shown for pregnenolone. The major pathways thought to be used are shown

CHAPTER 7

Mechanisms of Hormone Actions

Hormones are organic substances produced naturally within the organism, controlling growth or other physiological functions at a site remote from its place of production and active in minute amounts. **Starling and Bayliss** have considered hormone as a chemical agent which is released from one group of cells and travels via the blood stream to affect one or more different groups of cells. The mode of action of hormones on cells is not yet completely understood. Hormones act through their binding to specific receptors. The **endocrine system** is specialised for the slow, chronic transmission of signals, employing the circulatory system for covering the larger distances within the body. The **messengers** of the endocrine system are the **hormones,** they are synthesised in hormone-producing cells and act either on a subordinate hormone gland or on non-endocrine cells (the **target organ** or **target cells**, respectively). Since all hormones circulate more or less together in the blood there has to be some way of ensuring that the hormone and its specific target cell recognise one another. For this purpose the target cell is equipped with **specific binding sites (receptors)** for its specific hormone.

The molecular mechanism by which the hormones produce their effects at their target cells is very complicated. The hormones are first bound to their receptors for producing their effects. A hormone can produce its effects in the following ways :

(A) HORMONE ACTION ON PERMEABILITY

Some hormones often referred to as first messengers, act by changing the permeability of their target cells to particular substances. For example—insulin increases the permeability of various tissues to glucose, amino acids, etc. so as to facilitate the entry of these food stuffs into the tissues for their proper utilization; ADH accelerates the permeability of renal tubules to water for stimulating the reabsorption of water.

(B) CELLULAR RECEPTORS AND HORMONE ACTION

Hormones regulate specific target tissues, not all cells in the body. During hormone action, hormone first interact with a specific constituent of the target tissues, known as **receptors.** The receptors provide the specificity for hormone cell interaction. These may be components of the plasma membrane or they may be cystolic or nuclear elements. Receptors provide the means by which hormones initially interact with cells. Hormones act through their binding to specific receptors. The binding of hormones to these receptors in general triggers a conformational change in the receptor such that it conveys information to other specific elements of the cell. These receptors are situated either on the cell surface or intracellularly. The surface receptor-hormone interactions generally signal the formation of 'second messengers' that set off cascade of events which lead to the hormone responses.

The distribution of hormone receptors exhibits enormous variability. Receptors for a few hormones, such as insulin and gluco corticoids are widely distributed, whereas those for most hormones have a more limited distribution. The presence of the receptors is the first determinant of whether the tissue will respond to the hormone. However, molecules that participate in postreceptor events are also critical; these determine not only whether the tissue will respond to the hormone but also the specifics of the response. The latter allow the same hormone to have different responses in different tissues. In addition, different hormones can utilize similar downstream mechanisms such that two

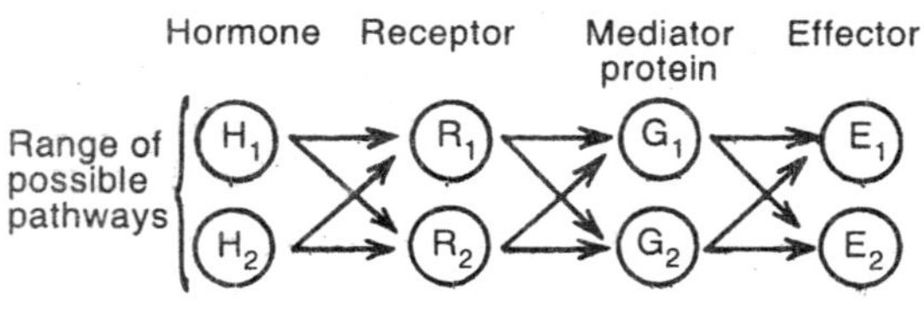

Fig. 7.1: Showing the action of different receptors

different hormones can have the same effect on the same tissue [Fig. 7.1].

Properties of hormone receptor

(i) **Hormone-Receptor Interactions :** Hormones find the surface of the cell through their solubility and their dissociation from plasma binding proteins when present. Hormones that bind to cell surface receptors are then available for binding to the receptors. The steroid hormones appear to penetrate the cell's plasma membrane freely and bind to cytoplasmic receptors. In cases, the hormone also needs to invade the cell nucleus to bind to the nuclear-localised receptors.

In general the hormones bind reversibly and non-covalently to their receptors. This binding is due to three kinds of forces. First, there are hydrophobic influences whereby hydrophobic surfaces on the hormone and receptor interact with each other in preference to water. Second, complementary charged groups on the hormone and the receptors facilitate the interactions. And third, vander Waals forces, which are extremely distance-dependent can contribute to attractive effects on the binding. These influences or forces are important for fitting the hormone into the receptor.

This binding most commonly conforms to a biomolecular reaction as follows : Hormone (H) + Receptor (R) = Hormone-Receptor complex (HRC). The rate of HR formation is proportionate to the concentration of H and R and can be defined by an association rate constant, K_1. Thus,

Rate of association = K_1 [H] [R],

where the brackets indicate concentrations. Similarly, the rate of dissociation of the hormone from the receptor is proportionate to the concentration of HR and can also be defined by a dissociation rate constant, K_2, such that the—

Rate of dissociation = K_2 [HR].

At equilibrium, the rates of association and dissociation are equal, that is

$$K_1\,[H]\,[R] = K_2\,[HR].$$

On rearrangement,

$$\frac{[H][R]}{[HR]} = \frac{K_2}{K_1} = Kd.$$

Kd is also a constant that is known as the **equilibrium dissociation constant.**

From analysis of the binding reaction, other information can be obtained. At low concentrations of hormone, the binding reaction is nearly linear with respect to increasing hormone and when the receptors become more than half saturated, the additional binding decreases progressively until a plateau is reached as the receptor becomes saturated with the hormone.

It is also apparent that for most hormone-responsive systems, the influence of increasing hormones is greatest when the receptors are relatively undersaturated. In some cases, the hormone-receptor interactions are more complex. These mostly occur when the hormone is interacting with a receptor complex with multiple subunits and where binding of the hormone to the first subunit alters the affinity of other subunits for the hormone [Fig. 7.2].

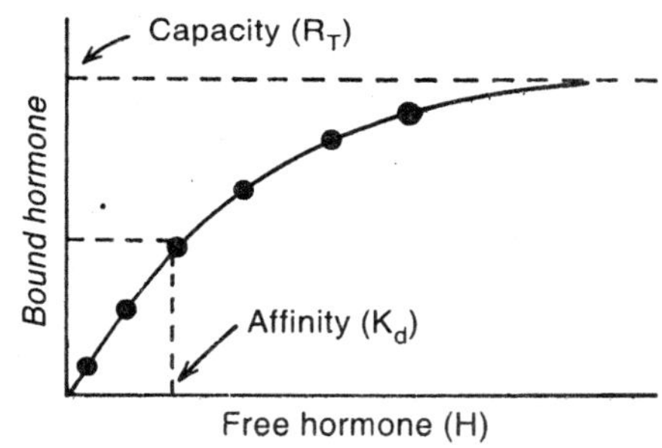

Fig. 7.2: Hormone receptor interaction

(ii) **Receptor specificity** : The essential feature of hormone receptor interaction is the specificity of binding. At the first level of hormone receptor interaction, specific receptor binds to specific hormone within the tissue. For example, insulin binds only to insulin-receptors, glucagon to glucagon- receptors of target cell. At a more subtle level, specificity implies that a hormone and its derivatives bind to their receptors with an affinity that is directly related to its bioactivity.

(iii) **Receptor affinity** : The most characteristic features are that the hormones bind to their receptors with high affinity and specificity and the receptors must have approximately high affinities to achieve significant binding at physiological levels. The affinity of a hormone for its receptor results from noncovalent binding, primarily in the form of hydrophobic interactions that provide the driving force for the binding reaction.

(iv) **Hormone Agonists, Antagonists and Partial Agonists** : Hormones or analogues that bind to receptors and elicit the same biological response as the naturally occurring hormone are called **agonists.** Similarly **antagonists** of a receptor inhibit the actions of its agonists. Molecules that bind to receptors but fail to elicit the normal biological response are known as competitive antagonists as they occupy the receptors and prevent the binding of the biologically active molecules. A partial agonist can produce only a partial biological response on binding to the relevant receptor, i.e., molecules that bind to receptors but are biologically less active than the native hormones are called **partial agonists.**

Substances that interact with the hormone binding site of the receptor can have agonist, antagonist or partial agonist activities. Substances that do not interact with the receptor or interact with it but do not affect the binding of hormones are termed **inactive.** An agonist fully induces the receptors to trigger post-receptor events. An antagonist is able to bind to the receptor and to block the binding of an agonist, but it does not trigger post-receptor responses. In this way it does not elicit a response but it does block the response to the agonist, providing that it is found in a concentration sufficient to block agonist binding. In general, antagonist bind to the same site on the receptor as agonists and prevent agonist binding through direct physical occupancy; however, in some circumtances, antagonist can bind to the receptor at a different site and block agonist binding through allosteric changes in the receptor. A partial agonist (partial antagonist) is intermediate; it binds to the receptors but elicits only a partial change in them such that even when the receptors are fully occupied by the partial agonist, the hormone response will be intermediate. Generally the activities of agonists, antagonists and partial agonists are explained by the fact that agonists induce allosteric changes in the receptors that are not elicited by antagonists.

(v) **Saturation** : The binding of hormone to receptor is a saturable process and this binding must either precede or accompany the biological response and the magnitude of the response must be associated with receptor occupancy.

Relations between hormone receptor binding and responses : The relations between hormone receptor binding and the subsequent response elicited by the hormone is helpful in considering hormone therapy and clinical states.

The nuclear receptors are found in small quantities several thousand per cell and are ordinarily limiting for the magnitude of the hormone response. This indicates that if there were more receptors, the hormone response at concentrations of the hormone that saturate the receptors would be greater. In these cases the relative saturation of the receptors parallels the hormone response. By contrast, the cell surface receptors frequently are not limiting, so that saturation of only a fraction of the receptors results in a maximal hormone response [Fig. 7.3].

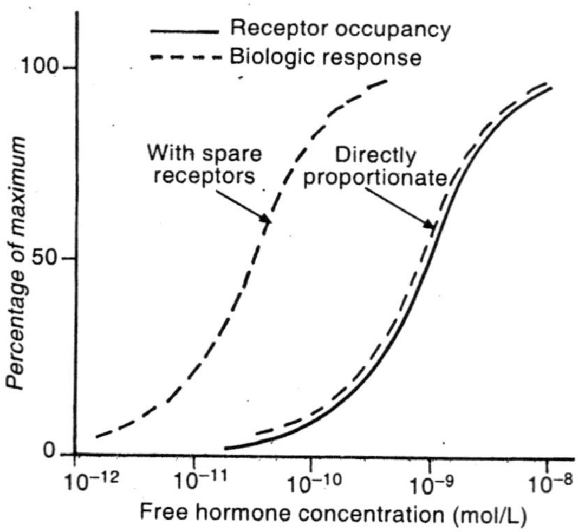

Fig. 7.3: Hormone receptor binding and responses

This situation has been referred to an spare receptor, and the dose response curve is shifted to the left of the hormone-receptor occupancy curve. However, the receptors are not really spare, at hormone concentrations below those which are maximally effective, the hormone response is proportionate to [H] [R]. Thus, in this situation, the response to a given hormone concentration will be greater with more receptors. With cell surface receptors, the generation of second messengers and the ability of each receptor to interact with more than one effector molecule provides an amplification of the response.

Types of hormone receptors : Hormone receptors can broadly be classified on the basis of occurrence into two groups—

I. Membrane receptors or extracellular receptors : These hormone receptors are present on the surface membrane of target cell. These are high in mol. weight (30 KD or more). The protein hormones or catecholamines are hydrophilic or lipophobic in nature and cannot go through the membrane owing to their large molecular weight.

There are four major membrane receptor families, such as—

(a) **Receptor kinase or Tyrosine kinase :** This kind of receptor contains the effector activity, such as tyrosine or serine kinase activity as an intrinsic part of the structure. The best characterised receptors are the protein kinase, as identified by the receptors for insulin, **IGF-1, EGF (epidermal growth factor),** and **PDGF (platelet derived growth factor).**

Each of these receptors is provided with extracellular ligand-binding domain, a **single transmembrane spanning domain** and an **intracellular kinase domain.** Insulin and IGF-1 receptors are linked by disulfide bonds to form dimers. The receptors for many cytokines, interferons and human growth factor are of this kind [Fig. 7.4].

(b) **Receptor-linked kinases :** The membrane receptors for growth hormone prolactin, cytokines (IL-2, IL-4, IL-6 and IL-7), GM-CSF (granulocyte-macrophage colony strimulating factor) are similar in structure to the receptor kinases and contain a single

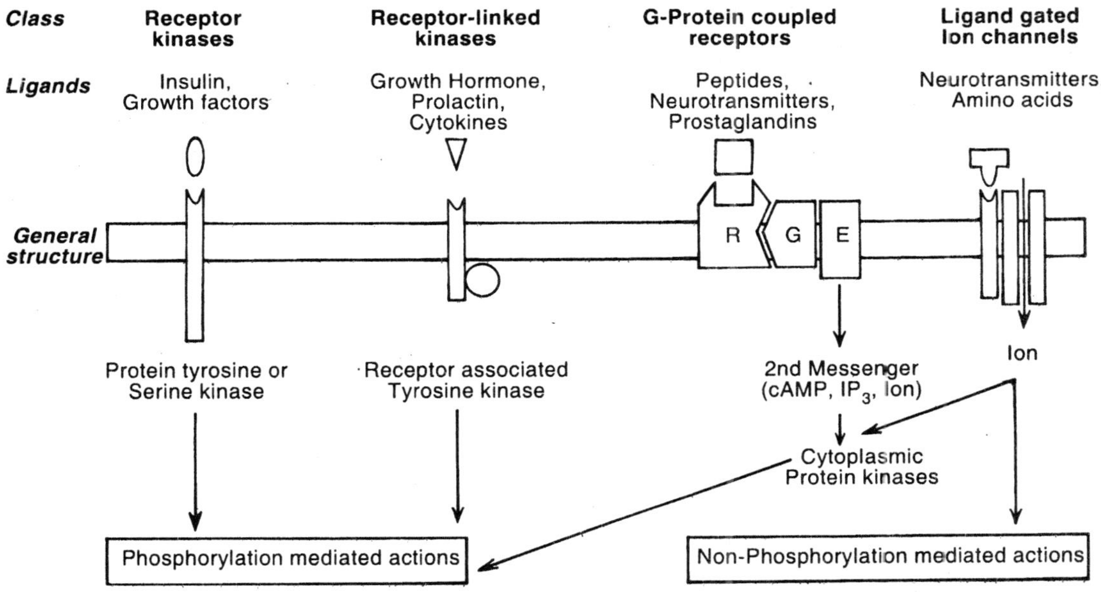

Fig. 7.4: Receptors with intrinsic enzymatic activity

transmembrane spanning domain. These receptors are devoid of intrinsic enzymatic activity but they interact with other membrane or cytoplasmic proteins that possess tyrosine kinase activity.

(c) **G-protein coupled receptors :** GTP dependent membrane protein is known as G-protein (guanine nucleotide-binding protein). Ligand binding activates G-protein, which in turn activates or inhibits an enzyme that generates a specific second messenger or modulates an ion-channel, causing a change in membrane potential. These receptors characteristically comprise of **seven transmembrane domains** and like most membrane receptors, have one or more sites of glycosylation. Seven transmembrane receptors for peptide hormones usually have a large NH_2 terminal extension that participates in ligand binding. The receptors for epinephrine, serotonin and glucagon are examples [Fig. 7.5].

(d) **Ligand-gated ion channels :** Another class of receptor represents the ligand-gated ion channels, of which there are two subtypes : **one subtype** consists of nicotinic acetylcholine, GABA (γ-aminobutyric acid), glycine and kinate receptors. All of which possess four transmembrane spanning domains. The **second subtype** includes ligand-gated ion channels that encode specific conducts for Na, Ca, K-cations and are composed of multiple subunits, each possessing six transmembrane spanning domains that form homomultimers or heteromultimers.

Ligand binding changes the conformation of the receptor so that only specific ions flow through it. The resultant ion movements alter the electric potential across the plasma membrane. The acetyl-choline receptor at the neuromuscular junction is an example [Fig. 7.6].

II. Intracellular receptors : The receptors located on the cell surface or in the cytoplasm are called **intracellular receptors.** The steroid hormones, thyroxine and retinoids are lipophilic or hydrophobic in nature and are transported by carrier proteins in the blood. These hormone receptors are soluble proteins and they are also known as **mobile receptors.** After dissociation from these carriers, such hormones diffuse across the

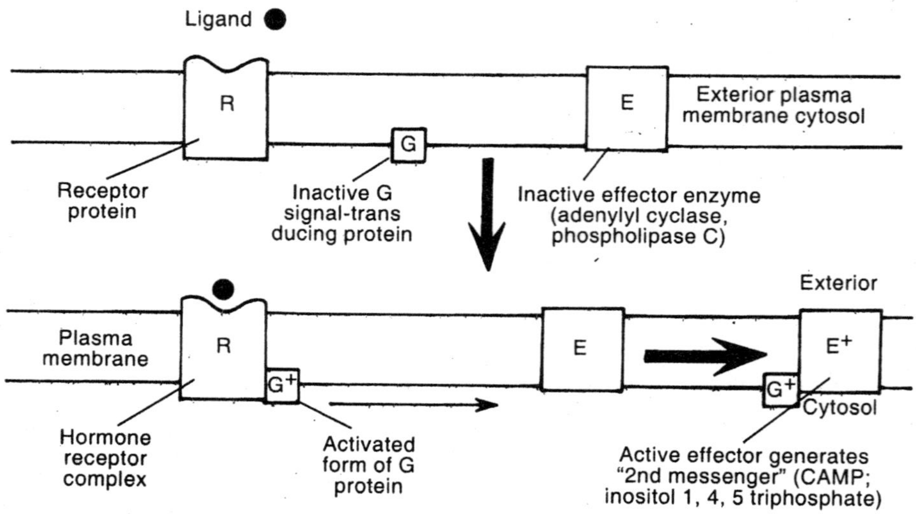

Fig. 7.5: G-Protein coupled receptors

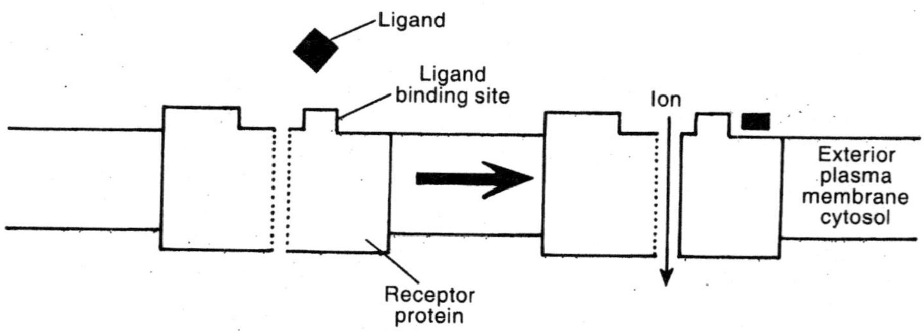

Fig. 7.6: Ion-channel receptors

plasma membrane and bind to specific receptors in the cytoplasm or nucleus. The receptor hormone complex initiates biological activities through transcription and translation. Intracellular receptors are subdivided into following categories—

(a) **Cytoplasmic receptors** : When receptors found in the cytosol are called **cytoplasmic receptors.** The cytoplasmic receptors are the receptors, which are in the process of synthesis and delivery to the plasma membrane or formed by the internalization of the cell membrane. Internalization is any change in the membrane that brings receptors into the cytoplasm from plasma membrane by the processes like pinocytosis.

(b) **Nuclear receptors :** These intracellular receptors are found on the surface of nuclear membrane. The steroid hormones exert their action on target cells after bindings to specific receptors which are ligand-inducible transcription factors localised primarily within the nucleus. The steroid receptor complex controls the synthesis of specific proteins primarily by altering the rate of transcription of specific genes.

(c) **Mitochondrial receptors** : The receptors located on the inner mitochondrial membrane are also called intracellular receptors. The thyroid hormones appear to bind with those high affinity receptors of mitochondria and to affect the synthesis or action of some mitochondrial enzymes.

HORMONE ACTION THROUGH INTRACELLULAR RECEPTORS AND GENE MODULATION

It is apparent that some hormones, mainly steroids, enter into the target cells to work on their nuclei. These hormones can themselves penetrate the plasma membrane as they are diffusible through the lipid matrix of the cell membrane. On entering the cytoplasm, the hormone binds with a specific receptor protein and is carried to the nucleus where it activates directly the appropriate genes to induce the synthesis of specific proteins (enzymes) that are responsible for the actions of the hormone.

The physiological processes regulated by hormones result from interaction of the hormone with specific constituents of the cell, referred to as **receptors.** All peptide hormones, as well as non-peptide neurotransmitters, act on membrane receptors. Stimulation of membrane receptors leads to activation of cyclizing enzymes, which initiate the production of a cyclic nucleotide, either cAMP or cGMP. These and other so called second messengers of hormone action generally activate one or more specific protein phosphorylation events within the cell. Addition of a phosphate group to a protein, an enzyme, for example, by a phosphoprotein kinase may result in its activation.

First messenger and second messenger concept : Most of the hormones as first messenger molecules, exert their effects on cellular metabolism by binding to receptor on the cell surface and activating a membrane associated enzyme that in turn elaborates an intracellular **second messenger.**

According to Southerland et al, the hormone molecule that is released into the blood stream, where it is free to interact with membrane receptor on target cells, is recognised as the **first messenger** of intercellular communication. The intracellular molecules that are generated following the binding of first messenger to the membrane receptors which convey the intracellular enzymatic action, gene expression, synthesis of proteins, etc. are called second messenger cAMP, cGMP, inositol phosphate, Ca^{++} or H^{+} ions, enzymes, etc. act as second messenger.

Second messengers are small molecules or ions that relay the signals from one location in the cell, such as from the plasma membrane to the interior of the cell, initiating a cascade of changes within the receiving cell.

Third messenger Concept : Recently increasing evidence shows that Ca^{++} acts as a third messenger since many cell functions are regulated by Ca^{++}—cAMP metabolism, cell motility, endocytosis, exocytosis, axonal flow, muscle contraction, neurotransmitter release etc. Calcium binding proteins can modulate cell metabolism. Calmodulin, the calcium binding proteins are widely distributed in tissues and the calmodulin acts as a "receptor" for Ca^{++} in order to become physiologically active. Now this active calcium must first bind to calmodulin or other calcium binding protein such as troponin of muscle.

Each steroid hormone has its own specific intracellular receptor. The effects of steroid like hormones are mediated by specific receptors that belong to a superfamily of transacting "Zinc finger" proteins. Steroid hormone and thyroid hormone molecules can diffuse through the plasma membrane of the targe cells. The hormones like progesterone, estrogen, testosterone, thyroid hormones etc. perform their action through intracellular receptors.

The hormone diffuses through the plasma membrane and encounter with the specific site of hormone receptor in the target cell and leads to the formation of **hormone receptor**

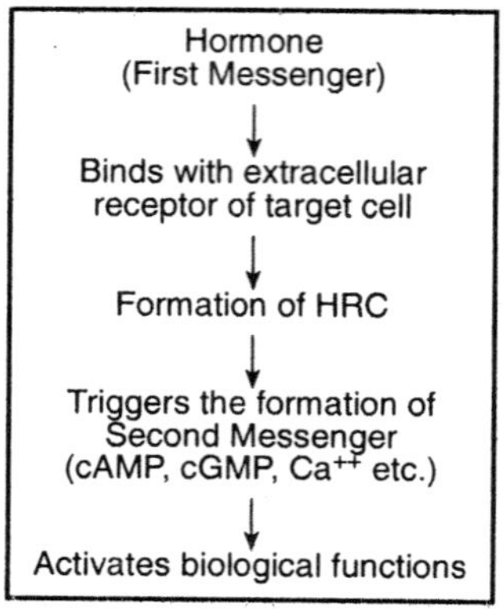

Fig. 7.7: Hormone receptor complex (HRC)

complex (HRC) [Fig. 7.7]. If the intracellular receptors do not bind to the specific hormone, then the receptor molecules remain in inactive state with poor affinity. The following hormones produce the HRC during their actions.

The classical model of steroid action involves its binding to intracellular receptors that are members a superfamily of ligand induced transcription factors. The HRCs then modulate the expression of target genes by binding to specific DNA sequences, the so-called hormone-response elements (HREs). There is increasing evidence for rapid, actinomycin-D-and cycloheximide-intensive effects of some steroid hormones. For example, in rat, short term exposure to the gonadal steroid progesterone is associated with rapid changes in behaviour and this effect occurs in the absence of new protein synthesis [Fig. 7.8].

Free testosterone enters the target cells by the process of diffusion. Some testosterone is reduced to Dihydrotestosterone (DHT) and NADPH by reductase. Both testosterone and NADPH bind to specific receptors of the target cells and produce the testosterone receptor complex.

Again estrogen diffuses in the target cells of uterus, fallopian tube, mammary gland etc and binds to intracellular estrogen receptor to form the estrogen receptor complex (ERC).

Hormone action through membrane receptor : The protein hormones are usually lipophobic or hydrophilic in nature and the molecular weight of these hormones is usually greater than steroid hormones. The protein hormones cannot pass through target cell membrane, thus bind to specific receptor protein on the plasma membrane. Now the HRC acts as **first messenger** and exerts the formation of second activating intracellular signal molecules for biological action, is called **second messenger**. In respect to biological functions of protein molecules there are different categories of second messengers

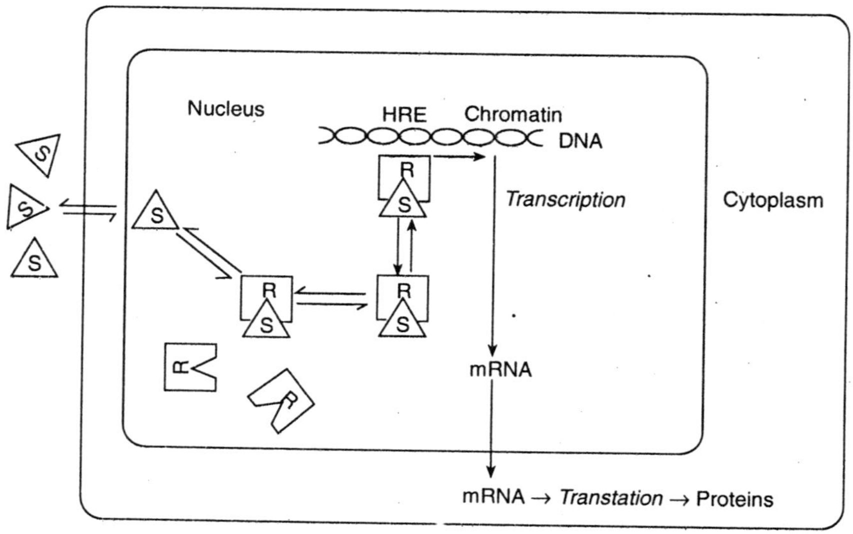

Fig. 7.8: Mechanisms of steroid hormone action

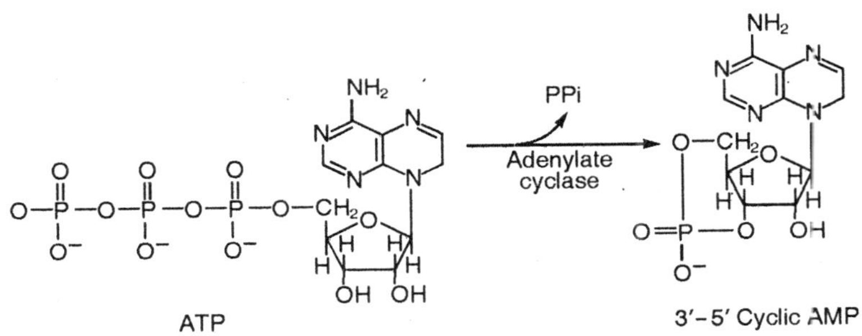

Fig. 7.9: Structure of cAMP

like, **cAMP** (for FSH, LH, Glucagon, ACTH, epinephrine etc), **cGMP** (for acetylcholine), **Phosphatidyl Inositol** (for vasopressin, GnRH, TRH etc), Ca^{++} (for calcitonin) and **Calmodulin** etc.

cAMP AS SECOND MESSENGER

cAMP is synthesised by a membrane bound enzyme known as Adenylate cyclase (AC) from ATP.

Transduction Pathway :

1. Signal transduction by cAMP is mediated by a protein called GTP binding protein or the G-protein.

2. When Gs stimulatory hormone binds to its specific receptor, Gs protein complex is stimulated.

3. Stimulated Gs replaces GDP on its α subunit by GTP, which becomes detouched from the β and γ subunits and moves towards AC on the membrane.

4. Gsα-GTP complex activates AC which produces cAMP from ATP. After this activated Gsα becomes inactivated by its internal GTP system which hydrolyses GTP into GDP and Pi.

> **Note :**
>
> **Adenylate cyclase : AC** is a large **transmembrane protein.** Its **catalytic domain** lies on the **cytosolic side** of the plasma membrane. At least **8 isoforms** of the enzyme are known in mammals. Most are regulated by **G-proteins** and **Ca^{2+} ions.** The enzyme is activated by receptors that activates the **stimulatory G protein** (Gs) and inhibited by the **inhibitory G-protein** (Gi). **AC** catalyzes the synthesis of **cAMP** from **ATP.**

(a) **Role of cAMP in cellular metabolism :**

1. Production of activated cAMP dependent protein kinase (cytosolic PKA) activates Phosphorylase Kinase by phosphorylation of the enzyme.

2. Active phosphorylase-kinase then phosphorylates inactive glycogen phosphorylase-b to active glycogen phosphorylase-a.

3. Both the phosphorylation reaction requires ATP and Ca^{2+} as cofactor.

4. In the last step active glycogen phosphorylase breaks down glycogen into Glucose-1-Phosphate. Hence it starts glycogenolysis.

(b) **Role of cAMP in Gene expression :**

1. cAMP activates protein kinase A (nuclear) by removing its repressor subunit (C-C, R-R).

2. Activated PKA now phosphorylates another cytoplasmic protein called cAMP Responce Element Binding Protein (CREB).

3. Phosphorylated CREB now enters into nucleus through nuclear membrane and binds to specific sites of DNA called CRE (cAMP Response Element).

4. After binding to CRE specific genes are become activated and by means of transcription form new mRNA, that can form specific proteins after translation into cytoplasm [Fig. 7.10].

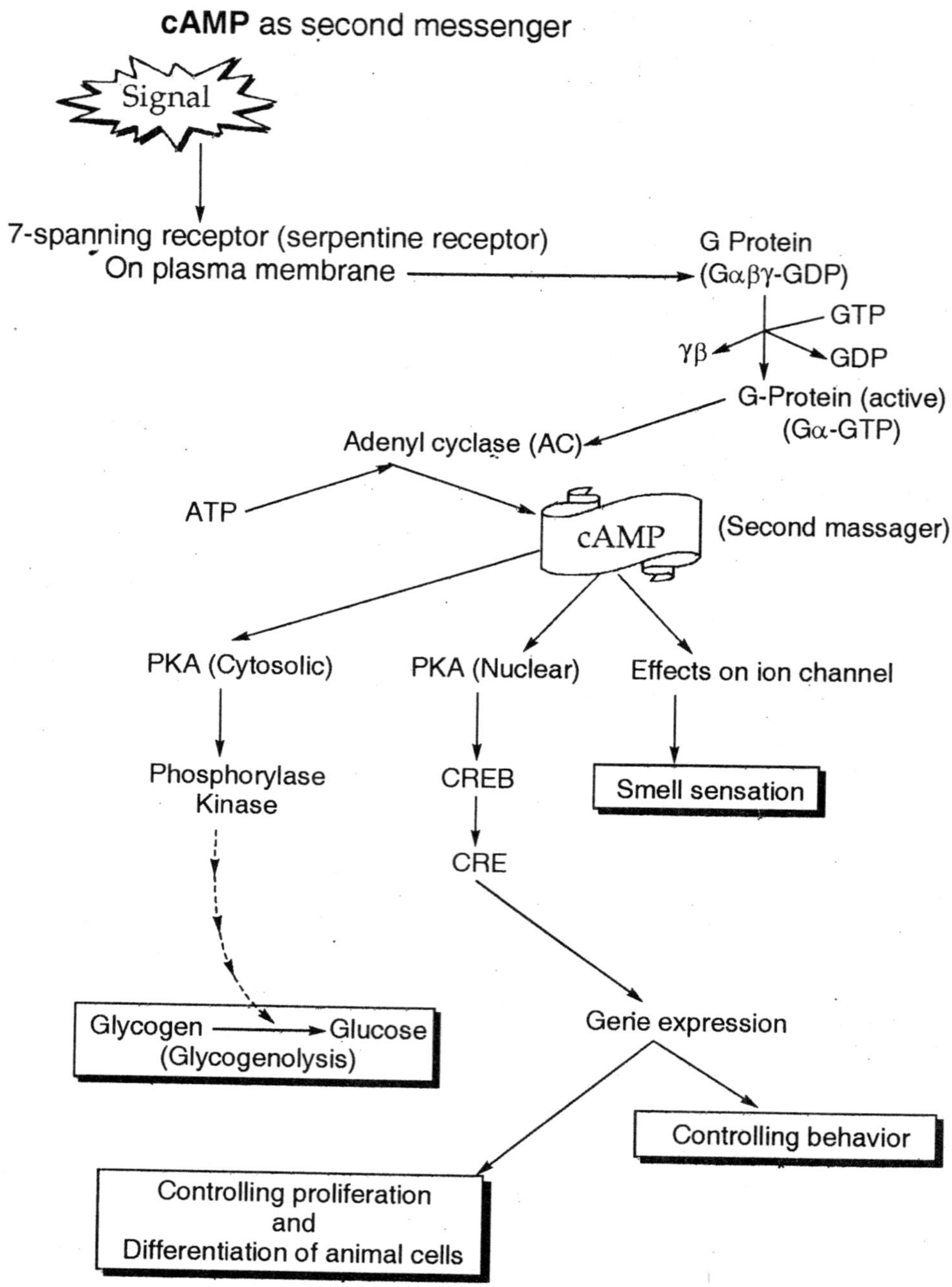

Fig. 7.10: cAMP as second messenger

Note : cAMP has also effect on Na^+-K^+ ion channels that cause smell sensation. The odorant receptors in the nasal passage contains Go protein which activates AC and produces cAMP.

ACTION THROUGH cGMP

G-protein stands for a guanosine nucelotide binding protein that activates the effector enzyme.

The heterotrimeric signal transducing G-protein is a kind of membrane bound (peripheral) regulatory protein composed of 3 subunits α, β of γ. It controls the activation of Adenyl Cyclase (AC) by GDP-GTP exchange and thus controls the **cAMP level** (2nd messenger) in the cytosol.

Discoverer : Alfred. G. Gilman and Martin Rodbell discover cGMP.

Types : It is mainly of two types—

(i) Stimulatory G-protein (Gs) :

Associated effector : Adenyl Cyclase (AC)

2nd messenger : cAMP (Increased).

Stimulatory G-protein links B-adrenergic receptors and some other GPCRS to Ac.

(ii) Inhibitory G-protein (Gi) :

Associated effector : Adenyl Cyclase (AC)

2nd messenger : cAMP (Decreased)

Inhibitory G-protein (Gi) is coupled to α-adrenergic receptors. These two types act co-ordinately according to the nature of stimuli.

Other major classes of Mammalian G-protein are :

Name	Associated Effector	2nd Messenger
1. Go4α	AC	cAMP (↑)
2. Gqα	Phospholipase C (PLC)	IP_3, DAG (↑)
3. Gtα	cGMP Phosphodiesterase	cGMP (↑)

Composition : The large heterotrimeric G-Proteins are mainly composed of 3 subunits α, β and γ; of which α is larger and functional.

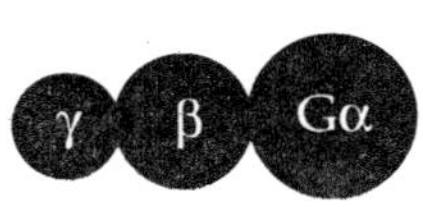

All the G-proteins have the same basic structure and mode of activation.

The α subunit contains a GDP molecule, but at the time of activation, GDP is replaced by GTP molecule. Gsα dissociates into Gβ and Gγ which are permanently bound together.

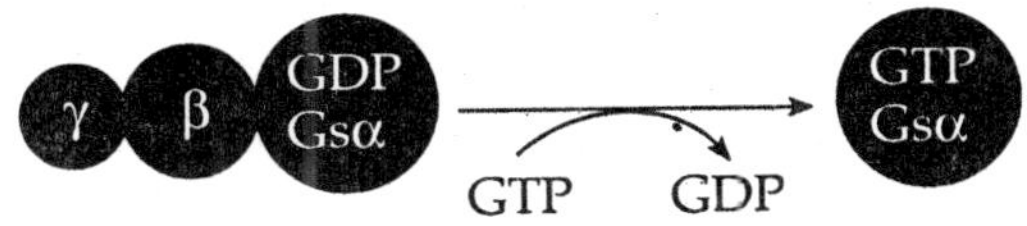

[N.B : There are two distinct classes of G-proteins—

(a) the large heterotrimeric G-proteins,

(b) the small monomeric G proteins [Ex. Ras].

Mechanism of Action: The mechanism of action of G-proteins depends upon the signal transmitted from the receptor. It also requires a plasma membrane receptor with seven transmembrane helical segments, (GPCR) or G-protein coupled receptor.

(1) When a hormone or any other stimulus binds to a site on the receptor deep within the PM, it promotes a conformotional change in the receptor intracellular domain that affects its interaction with the Gs on the cytoplasmic side of the membrane.

(2) The activated **β-adrenergic receptor** interacts with G_S, catalyzing replacement of bound GDP (on the α subunit) with GTP and converts Gs to its active form.

(3) As this occurs, the β and γ subunits of Gs dissociates from the α subunit as a βγ dimer and Gsα with its bound GTP moves in the plane of the membrane from the receptor to a nearby molecule of AC.

(4) After the binding of activated G-protein to AC it activates and synthesises cAMP from cellular ATP. This 2nd messenger (cAMP) then regulates cellular metabolism.

(5) After activation of AC, G protein becomes inactive and the monomeric form (Gsα) converts into trimeric form (Gsαβγ). The GTP of the α-subunit is again replaced by GDP [Fig. 7.11].

Remark : Disruption of G-protein signalling causes several human diseases. The bacteria *Vibrio cholerae* (which causes cholera) & *Bordetella pertussis* (causes whooping

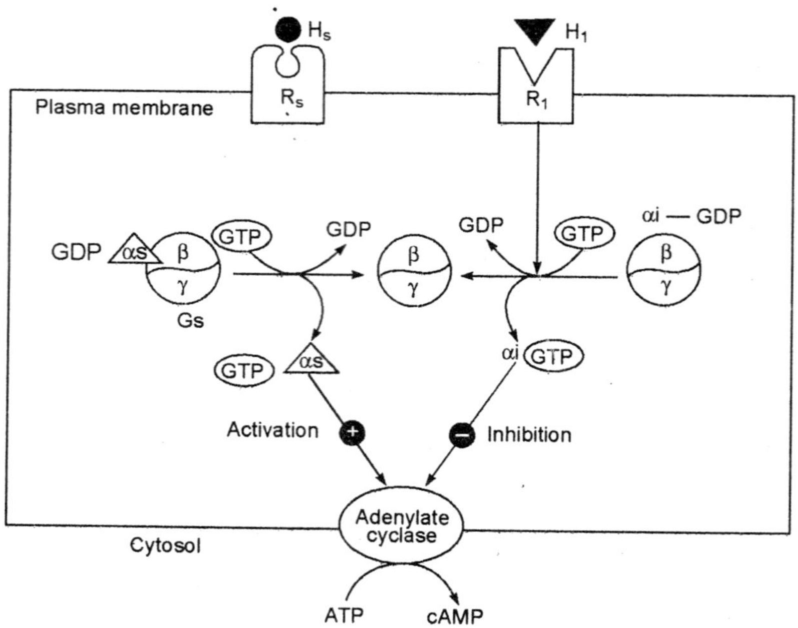

Fig. 7.11: Mechanism of G-protein mediated cAMP synthesis (S-Stimulatory; I-Inhibitory; H-Hormone; R-Membrane receptor, a, b, g-Subbunits of G protein

cough), both cause disease through their effect on heterotrimeric G-protein. Cholera toxin (CTX) always locks Gsα in active state.

Glycoprotein hormone : TSH, FSH, LH, etc. **Tyrosine containing hormone :** Epinephrine, Norepinephrine and Dopamine and Melatonin of Pineal gland.

ACTION THROUGH PHOSPHATIDYL INOSITOL (IP_3) AND DIACYLGLYCEROL (DAG)

IP_3 or Insitol 1, 4, 5-triphosphate : IP_3 is a short lived **chemical messenger**. It is water soluble and acts as **second messenger**.

Role : Many hormones like vasopressin, gastrin, GnRH, TRH, catecholamines stimulate cellular processes through activation of G-proteins which in turn activates a specific phospholipase that hydrolyses the phosphodiester bond of phosphatidyl inositol 4, 5-biphosphate (P/P_2) into two key metabolites, or messenger molecules, inositol 1, 4, 5-triphosphate (IP_3) and 1, 2-diacylglycerol (DAG). IP_3 diffuses through the cytoplasm and stimulates the ER via specific receptors on the membrane to release Ca^{++} ions into the cytosolic compartment of the cell. In muscle cells, these Ca^{++} ions bind to specific proteins that initiate contraction.

IP_3 which is released into the cytosol, mobilizes intracellular Ca^{++} from stores within the ER and possibly from transmembrane that helps in the transport of Ca^{++} ions into the cell.

During the initial phase of cell activation, two signals, the rise in DAG content of the plasma membrane and the rise in the Ca^{+} concentration in the cell cytoplasm, act synergistically to cause binding of protein kinase C (PKC) to the plasma membrane. The resulting association of PKC with the membrane leads to its conversion to a Ca^{++} ion-sensitive form [Fig. 7.12].

A wide variety of hormones and neurotransmitters like acetylcholine, norepinephrine (α_1), histamine (H_1), 5-hydroxytryptamine, vasopressin (V_1), substance P, angiotensin, pancreozymin-cholecystokinin, TRH, somatomedins, etc. bind to the respective

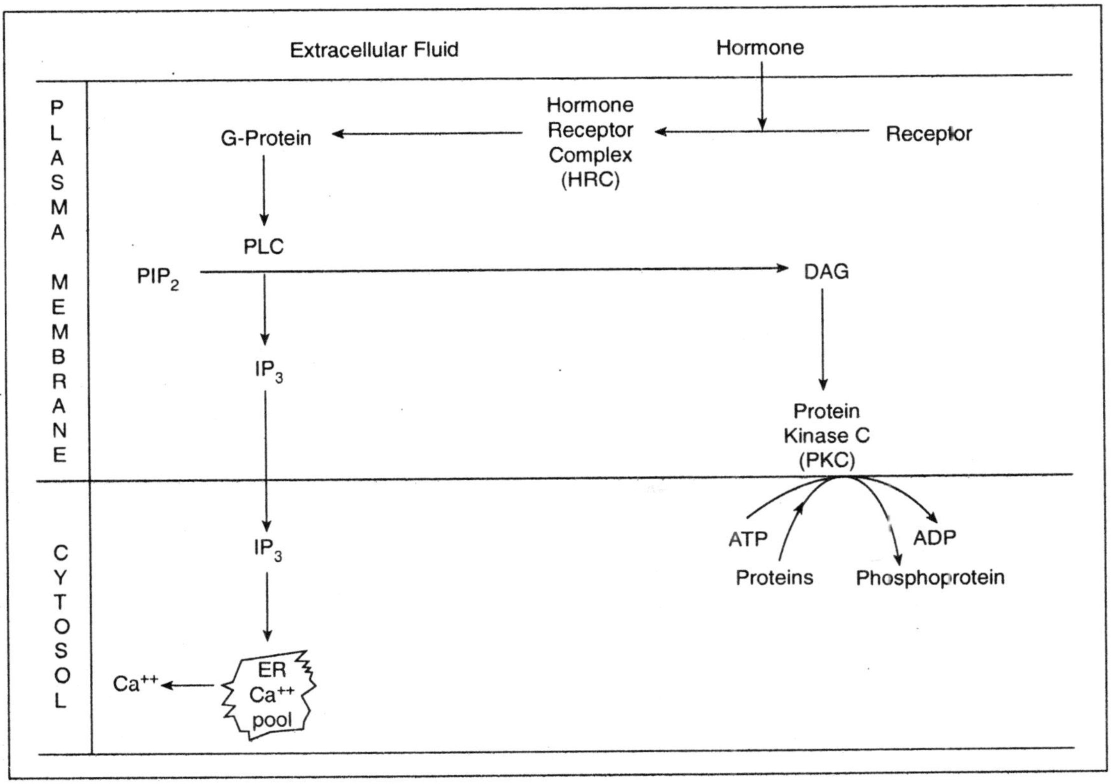

Fig. 7.12: IP_3 and DAG as second messenger

membrane receptor and lead to hydrolysis of membrane phosphoinositide-4, 5-phosphate by activating a phosphodiesterase yielding the two metabolites, **inositol-1, 4, 5-triphosphate (ITP)** and **diacylglycerol'** [Fig. 7.12].

These two compounds then function as two independent but parallel second messengers. DAG acts within the membrane to increase protein phosphorylation by activating C-kinase. ITP increases the intracellular Ca^{++} concentration. The two second messengers also influence a wide variety of other cellular processes such as the release of arachidonic acid (= **Prostaglandin** precursor, probably split off from the phosphoinositide), activation of guanylate cyclase (forming cGMP from GTP) and Na^+/H^+ exchange carriers. They control protein secretion and cellular growth and seem to play a role in short term memory, and many other cell responses.

• **Diacylglycerol (DAG),** being nonpolar, is retained in the membrane of the target cell, where it acts as a second messenger. DAG activates the membrane bound enzyme protein kinase C (PKC) which phosphorylates serine and threonine residues on target protein.

CALCIUM AND CALMODULIN AS SECOND MESSENGERS

Ca^{++} ions can act as secondary cellular messenger since they can diffuse into the cytoplasm and bind to various target molecules, triggering specific responses. The concentration of free calcium ions in the extracellular fluid is relatively very high compared with the concentration inside the cells. Ca^{++} exerts its effect by binding to specific calcium-binding proteins such as **calmodulin**, having binding sites for calcium. Under resting condition, the intracellular concentration of free Ca^{++} is low and most of the calmodulin is found in its inactive form. Increase in the concentration of free calcium, which enters from outside by stimulating the Ca^{++} pump or released from intracellular storage sites, favours binding of Ca^{++} to calmodulin. This Ca^{++} calmodulin complex now binds efficiently to a calcium-sensitive enzyme, thereby converting it from its inactive form to active form. Practically, calmodulin has no intrinsic activity of its own, after binding with calcium ion (each molecules of calmodulin has four calcium binding sites) it is activated and binds to various enzymes or effector molecules causing a change in their activities [Fig. 7.13].

• **Chemical messengers** are any substances produced by cells of endogenous or exogenous origin and that play a physiological role in the control of the activity of other cells, e.g., thyroxine, dopamine acetylaholine etc.

• **Catecholamines** : Catecholamines are amine derivatives of catechol compounds derived from the phenolic amino acid tyrosine. They include adrenalin or epinephrine, nor-adrenalin or norepinephrine and dopamine which function as neurotransmitters or neurohormones. These compounds are stored in adrenal medulla and some nerve endings (i.e., sympathetic postganglionic nerve endings).

Ca^{++} AS SECOND MESSENGER

In many cells Ca^{2+} serves as 2nd messengers that triggers intra-cellular responses like exocytosis, contraction of muscle, amoeboid movement etc.

Normally cytosolic Ca^{2+} is very low in concentration ($<10^{-7}$M). By the action of Ca^{2+} pumps in ER, mitochondria and PM concentration become raise. Changes in intracellular Ca^{2+} are detected by a special protein called calmadulin.

Transduction pathway

1. Calmodulin is an acidic protein with 4 high affinity of Ca^{++} binding sites.

2. When intracellular Ca^{++} raises to about 10^{-6}M, the bind of Ca^{++} to calmodulin occurs.

3. After binding there is a confirmational changes occur in calmodulin.

4. Altered conformational changes of CaM binds to G proteins to exert specific cellular function.

Example : Binding to troponin of thin filament of muscle triggers skeletal muscle contraction.

5. Direct inhibition of either Ca^{++}–ATPase or the Ca^{++}–Na^{+} exchanger or the Ca^{++}–H^{+}–ATPase of cell membrane decreases the active Ca^{++} extrusion from the cells.

6. Again direct opening of the ligand-gated Ca^{++} channels in the membrane increases the down gradient Ca^{++} diffusion from extra-cellular fluid (ECF) to cytosol. All such mechanisms lead to rise in cytoplasmic Ca^{++} concentration.

7. The rise in Ca^{++} level in target cells may modulate the activities of many enzymes like phospholipase,. guanyl cyclase, adenyl cyclase, PKC, calmodulin-dependent protein kinase etc [Fig. 7.13].

CALMODULIN (CaM)

Calmodulin (CaM) is a calcium-binding protein expressed in all eukaryotic cells. It can bind to and regulate a number of different protein targets, thereby affecting many different cellular functions. CaM mediates processes such as inflammation, metabolism, muscle contraction, intracellular movement, short-term and long-term memory, nerve growth and the immune response. Cam is expressed in many cell types and can have different sub-cellular locations, including the cytoplasm with organelles, or associated with the plasma or organelle membranes. Many of the proteins that CaM binds are unable to bind calcium themselves, and as such CaM acts as a

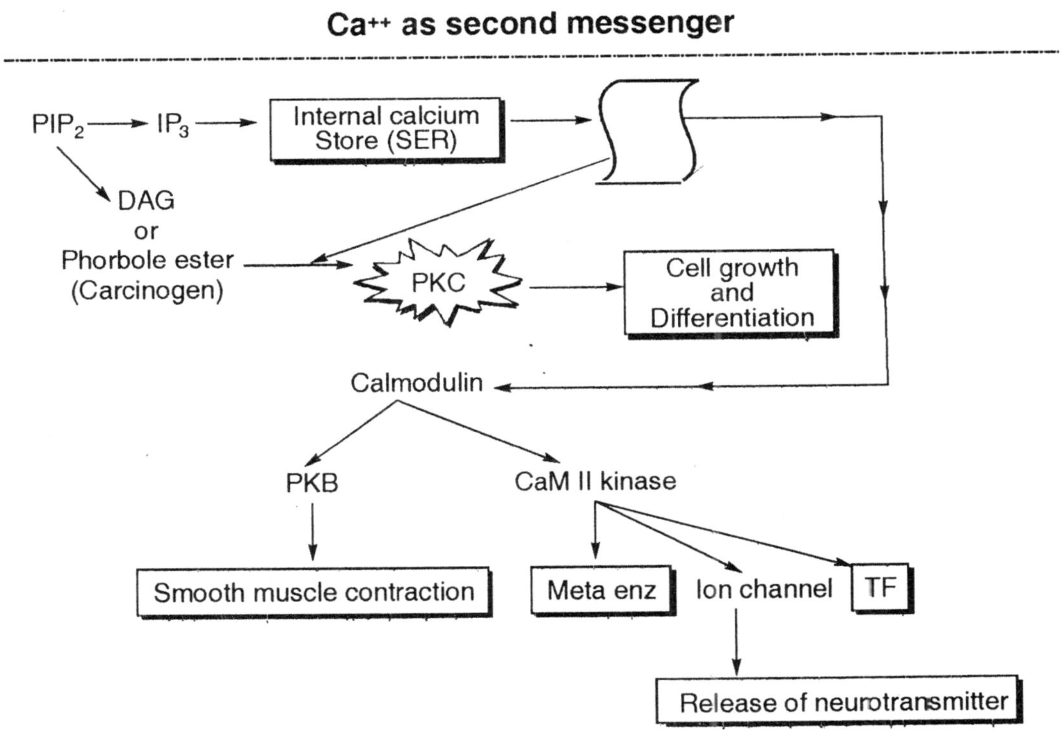

Fig. 7.13: Ca^{++} as second messenger pathway

calcium sensor and signal transducer. CaM can also make use of the calcium stores in the endoplasmic reticulum, and the sarcoplasmic reticulum. CaM undergoes a conformational change upon binding to calcium, which enables it to bind to specific proteins for a specific response. CaM can bind up to four calcium ions, and can undergo post-translational modifications, such as phosphorylation, acetylation, methylation and proteolytic cleavage, each of which can potentially modulate its actions.

Calmodulin is a small, acidic protein approximately 148 amino acids long (16706 Dalton) and, as such, is a favourite for testing **protein stimulation software**. It contains four EF-hand "motifs" or domains, each of which binds a Ca^{2+} ion.

Calmodulin can also bind to **edema factor toxin** from the **anthrax** bacteria.

PHOSPHOLIPID AS SECOND MESSENGER

Some GPCR [G-Protein Couple Receptor] are coupled with special kind of G-protein called G_q^+ follows the pathway of 2nd messenger system in which IP_3 (Inositol-triphosphate) and DAG (Diacylglycerol) act as second messenger.

Signal : Oxytocine, Auxine, Angiotensin-II, Platelet Derived Growth Factor [PDGF], Thyrotropin Releasing Hormone [TRH].

Transduction Pathway

1. When hormone binds to GPCR, G_q protein become activated by exchanging GDP to GTP.

2. GTP bound G_q is then bind to a membrane bound enzyme called phospholipase-C [PLC].

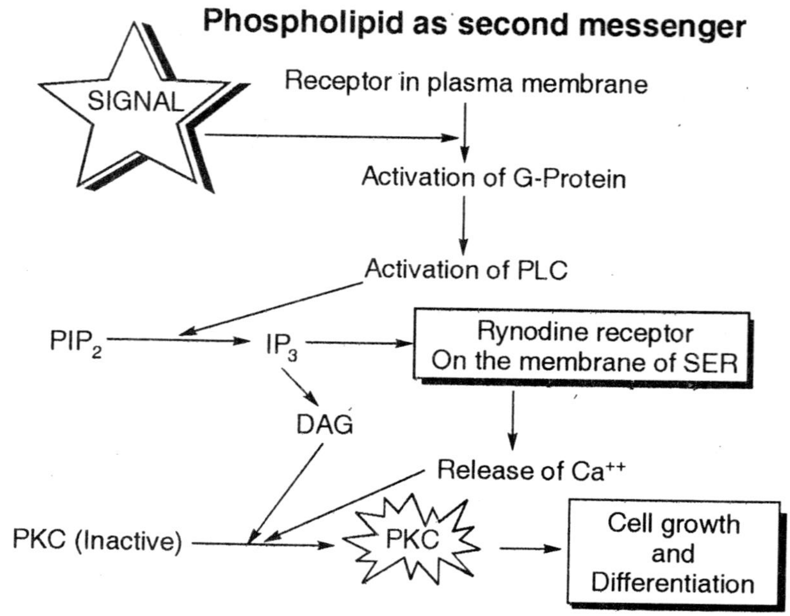

Fig. 7.14: Phospholipid as second messenger pathway

3. PLC become activated and hydrolyses a phospholipid called phosphatidyl-inositol 4, 5 biphosphate [P to IP_3 and DAG].

4. IP_3 releases to cytoplasm and binds to smooth membrane ER [SER] in specific receptor—ryanodyne receptor. But DAG remains in plasma membrane.

5. After binding of IP_3 calcium releases into cytosol [sequestered].

6. Released calcium is acting as **3rd messenger**. IP_3 and DAG act as 2nd messenger.

7. Calcium then binds to a specific protein and called Protein Kinase C [PKC] which already binds to DAG at plasma membrane.

8. PKC becomes activated to regulate growth and differentiation of cell.

- **CREB** (cAMP response element binding protein): cAMP regulates the rate of transcription of a number of genes, including those for hormones such as somatostatin and the glycoprotein hormones. These actions are mediated by CREB transcription factor. This protein is phosphorylated in response to cAMP.

Mechanism: Effect on gene expression

1. After inducing by hormone GPCR become activated, now stimulatory G protein (Gs) activates by exchanging GDP to GTP.

2. Activated Gs now touches membrane bound enzyme called AC (Adenylate cyclase).

3. Activated AC can transform ATP to cAMP. This cAMP now acts as 2nd messenger.

4. cAMP now binds to an enzyme called PKA (Protein kinase A) and activates it by removing repressor subunit (C-C, R-R).

5. Activated PKA now phosphorylates another cytoplasmic protein called cAMP response element binding protein (CREB).

6. Phosphorylated CREB now enters into nucleus through nuclear membrane and binds to specific sites of DNA called CRE (cAMP response element).

7. After binding to CRE specific genes become activated and by means of transcription form new m-RNA, that can produce

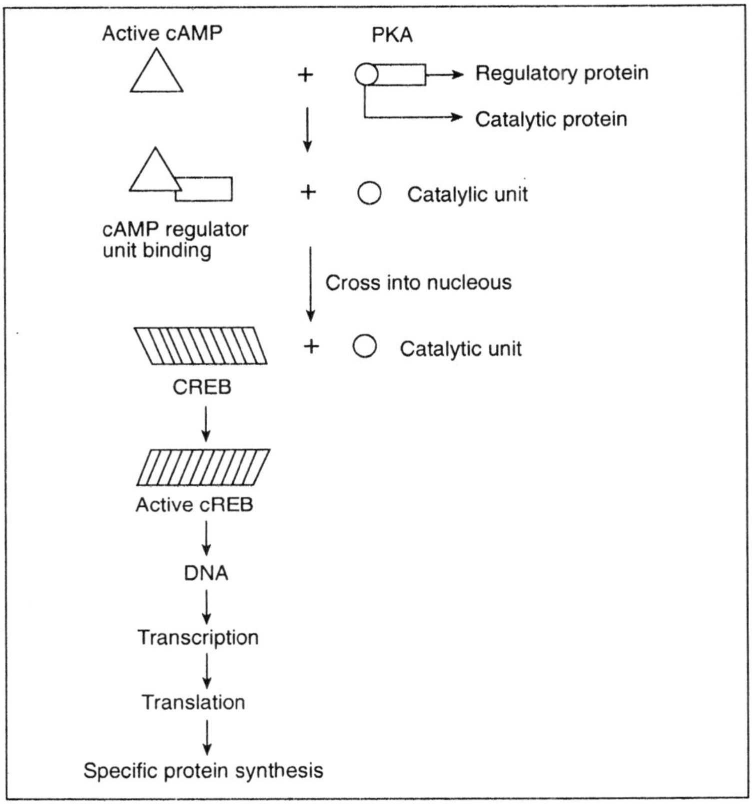

Fig. 7.15: Flow chart showing the gene expression of CREB

specific proteins after translation into cytoplasm [Fig. 7.15].

> **HRE (Hormone Response Element) :** It is a site on DNA where steroid hormone receptor can bind to activate specific gene. According to the name of the hormone different HREs are found with various DNA sequence; e.g., in case of estrogen the HRE is called as ERE and in case of glucocorticoid it is GRE.
>
> **CRE (cAMP Response Element) :** Specific sites on DNA to which CREB can bind to make the gene expression is called as CRE.

EICOSANOIDS AND HORMONE ACTION

Eicosanoids are compounds (including prostaglandins) that are derived from poly unsaturated fatty acids with 18-, 20-, or 22-carbon skeletons. Among tthese, archidonic acid (all-cis-5, 8, 11, 14-eicosatetraenoic acid) is the most important and abundant precursor for the various eicosanoids in humans. In other words, eicosanoids are paracrine hormone, substances that act only on cells near the point of hormone synthesis instead of being transported in the blood to act on cells in other tissues or organs. The derivatives of these substances include the prostaglandins, prostacyclins, leukotrienes and thromboxanes.

Hormone action : Eicosanoids are formed exclusively within the plasma membrane of cells and are derived mainly from arachidonic acid released from phospholipids by the action of phsopholipase A_2(PLA_2). Arachidonic acid is produced from the essential fatty acid, linolenic acid, by elongation and desaturation. Hormones and other stimuli (e.g. local hypoxia) may activate phospholipase activity and release arachidonic acid to serve as substrate for eicosanoid biosynthesis. This arachidonic acid may be used in one or more different pathways depending on the tissue concerned and type of external stimulus. In one pathway arachidonic acid is converted to unstable endoperoxide intermediates by a group of enzymes known as **cyclogenase system**. Depending on the action of other tissue specific enzymes, these intermediates may be converted to one of a number of related products (prostanoids) : Prostaglandin E_2 (PGE_2), Prostaglandin $F_2\alpha$ ($PGF_2\alpha$), Prostacyclin I_2 (PGI_2) or thromboxane A_2 (TXA_2). These fatty acid derivatives are ubiquitous in mammalian cells. They are produced by most cells, and are released with little storage. They are cleared rapidly from the circulation and are thought to act predominantly in a paracrine or autocrine fashion. They have mechanism

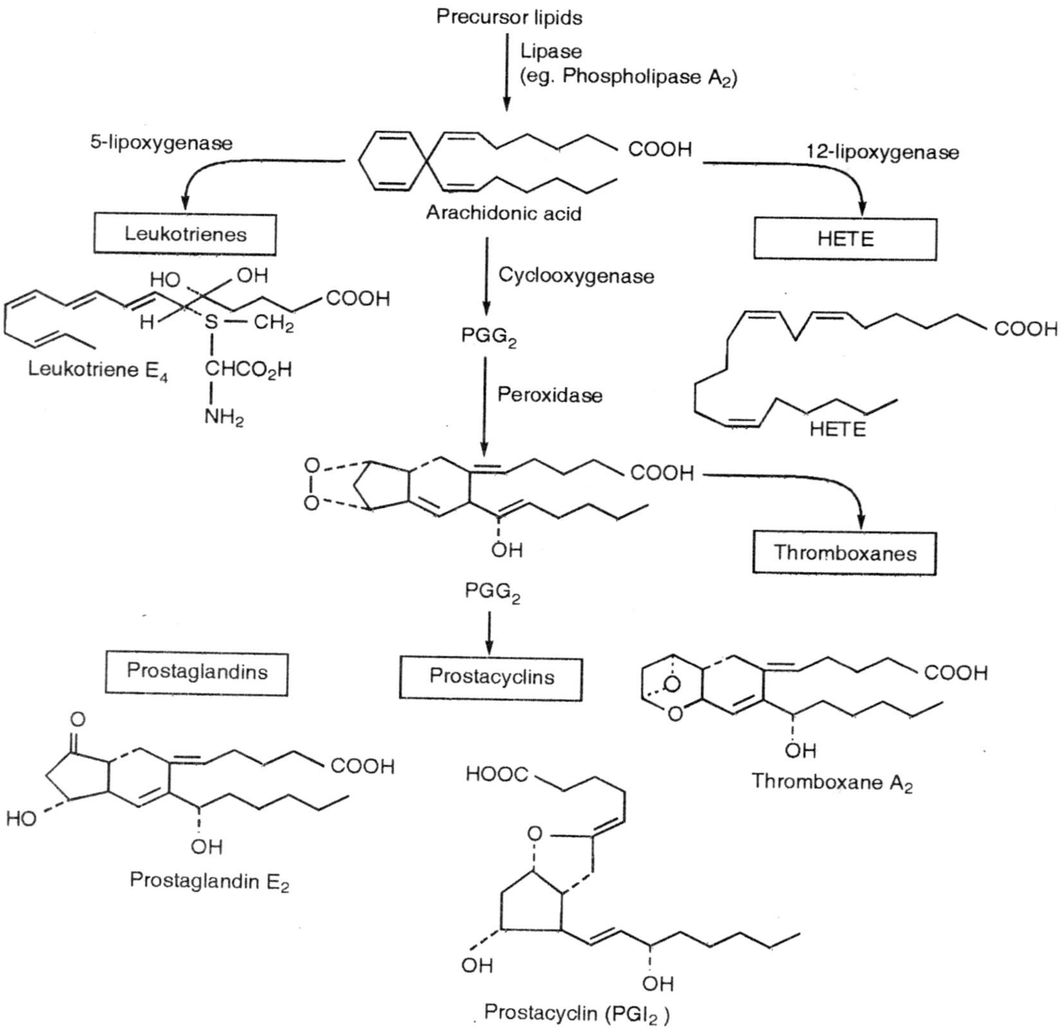

Fig. 7.16: General scheme of eicosanoid biosynthesis

of action that are similar to the hormones that act on the cell surface. Eicosanoid synthesis is frequently stimulated in response to hormones; thus these molecules serve as mediators of hormone action. For example, changes in prostaglandin synthesis are a common feature of hormones acting on the kidney. Eicosainoids can also regulate hormone release and actions. PGE compounds inhibit the secretion of growth hormone and prolaction (PRL) from anterior pituitary gland and of norepinephrine from sympathetic presynaptic nerve endings. Eicosanoids affect essentially every kind of cell in some way, including effects on homeostasis, smooth muscle contraction, Ca^{++} mobilisation, renal and reproductive function, injury, inflammation, immunologic, gut responses etc [Fig. 7.16].

Synthesis : Arachidonic acid is the most important and abundant precursor of various eicosanoids in humans and it is formed from linolenic acid (an essential fatty acid). Arachidonic acid precursor stores are found in membrane liquids from which it is released in response to various stimuli through actions of phospholipases. Phospholipase A_2 or both phospholipase–C and diglyceride lipase—catalyse the cleavage of esterified arachidonic acid. Phospholipase A_2 activity in vitro can be strongly inhibited by glucocorticoids.

Arachidonic acid can be cônverted to the endoperoxide prostaglandin H_2, which is the precursor to the prostaglandins, prostacyclins, and thromboxanes. For prostaglandin synthesis, cyclooxygenase (also called endoperoxide synthetase) converts arachidonic acid to the unstable endoperoxide, PGG_2 which is rapidly reduced to PGH_2. Cyclooxygenase is inhibited by aspirin, indomethacin and other non-steroidal anti-inflammatory agents. Depending on the tissue, PGH_2 can be converted to other prostaglandins (e.g. PGD_2, PGF_2, PGE_2) in reactions involving prostaglandin synthetases; prostacylins (e.g. PGI_2) in reactions involving prostacyclin synthetase, which is prevalent in endothelial and smooth muscle cells and thromboxanes [e.g. thromboxane A_2 (TXA_2)], which is prevalent in platelets and macrophages.

Importance : They are known to be involved in

(i) reproductive function;

(ii) inflammation, fever and pain associated with injury or disease in the formation of blood clots and the regulation of blood pressure;

(iii) in gastric acid secretion and in a variety of other processes important in human health or disease.

BIOSIGNALLING PATHWAY OF PEPTIDE HORMONE (INSULIN)

The ability of cells to receive and act on signals from beyond the plasma membrane is fundamental to life. These signals elicit appropriate responses, such as motion toward food or away from toxic substances or the formation of dormant spores in a nutrient-depleted medium. In all these cases, the signal represents information that is detected by specific receptors and converted to a cellular response which always involves a chemical process. This conversion of information into a chemical change, signal transduction, is a universal property of living cells.

Transduction Pathway :

It follows RTK receptor pathway with intrinsic kinase activity. Following is the sequence of transduction:

1. Insulin receptor binds insulin and undergoes autophosphorylation on its carboxyl-terminal Tyr residues at cytoplasmic domain.

2. Insulin receptor phosphorylates IRS-I (Insulin Receptor Substrate) on its Tyr residues.

3. SH2 domin of Grb2 binds to P-Tyr of IRS-1. Sos binds to Grb2.

4. Grb2 binds to Ras (small G-protein that binds to membrane). Ras is with GDP initially; but after binding of Grb2, GDP is replaced by GTP and Ras become activated.

5. Activated Ras bind and activates Raf-1.

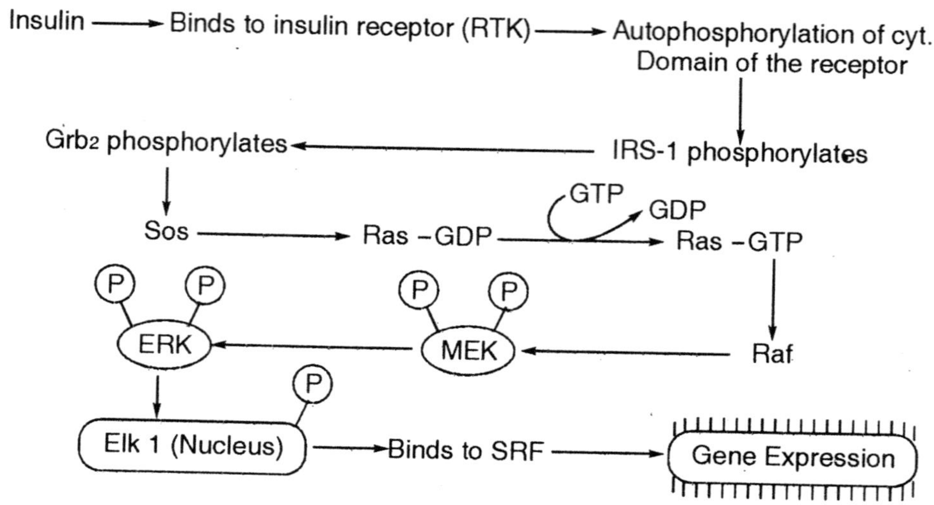

Fig. 7.17: Biosignaling pathway of peptide hormone (insulin)

6. Raf-1 phosphorylates MEK on its two Sos residues and activates it. It inturn phosphorylates ERK on its Thr- and Tyr residue and activates the protein.

7. ERK enters the nucleus and phosphorylates to activate transcription factors such as Elk1.

8. Phosphorylated Elkl binds to SRF to stimulate specific genes for transcription and translation needed for cell division [Fig 7.17].

Note : Ras is a G-protein activated by GTP binding and inactivated when the GTP-ase activity of the protein converts the GTP to GDP. Ras was originally described as an oncogene, and mutated or overexpressed. Ras molecules are extensively involved in human cancers. The normal cellular Ras is also involved in regulating a number of processes including cell growth.

JAK-STAT PATHWAY

Some receptor tyrosine kinase don't have kinase activity itself. That is why they have to recruit another protein for kinase activity. One of such protein is called as JAK (Janus-Kinase). Following is the transduction mechanism that follows such pathway.

- **Distinguish between PKA and PKC**

PKA	PKC
1. Activated by cAMP.	1. Activated by IP_3 and DAG.
2. It is formed of 4 subunits. (2 repressor, 2 catalytic subunit)	2. It is always monomer.
3. Repressor can be eleminated by the action of cAMP.	3. It becomes activated in the presence of Ca^{++} and DAG.
4. 2nd messenger comes from ATP.	4. 2nd messenger comes from PIP_2.
5. 2nd messenger forming enzyme is AC.	5. 2nd messenger forming enzyme is PLC.
6. Some PKA can enter into nucleus and by interacting with CREB regulates gene expression.	6. PKC cannot enter into nucleus but it can regulate growth and differentiation of the cell.

Signals : Growth hormone, prolactin, cytokine (developmental signals), erythropoietin (EPO).

Transduction Pathway :

1. When one of the above signal binds to RTK receptor they become dimerised into the plasma membrane (receptor cross stock).

2. After that soluble protein JAK binds to the cytoplasmic domain of the receptor.

3. After binding of the JAK cytoplasmic domain of Rik receptor becomes phosphorylated at several tyrosine residues.

4. A transcription factor called STAT (Signal Transduction Activators of Transcription) binds to JAK protein by SH_2 domain and becomes phosphorylated.

5. After phosphorylation STAT dimerises.

6. Dimerisation exposes a nuclear localisation sequence (NLS) that directs STAT towards the specific gene in nucleus.

7. STAT binds to specific gene and regulates the transcription.

8. On the other hand a second signal pathway is also triggered by auto-phosphorylation of JAK i.e. associated with aduptor protein called Grb_2 which inturn triggered MAP-Kinase pathway like that of insulin hormone mechanism [Fig. 7.18].

HYPOTHALAMIC-PITUITARY-TESTICULAR AXIS : AN OVERVIEW

This axis regulates the testicular function by the following two steps :

(1) **Hypothalamic Pituitary Leydig cell axis :** The hypothalamus releases and secretes GnRH (gonadotropin releasing hormone) into the hypothalamo-hypophysial portal blood. After reacting with the anterior pituitary, GnRH binds to the gonadotropes and stimulates the release of both LH and to a lesser

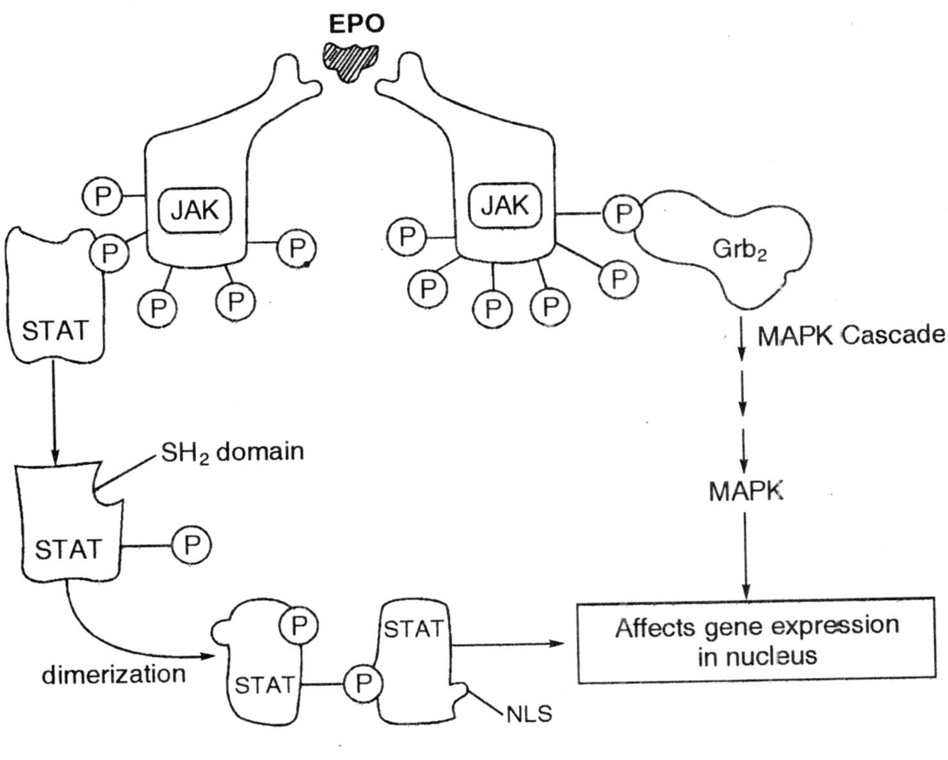

Fig. 7.18: JAK-STAT pathway

extent FSH into the general circulation. This LH from the general circulation is taken up by the Leydig cells of testis, where it binds to specific membrane receptors. It leads to activation of adenyl cyclase and ultimately results in secretion of testosterone. In turn, the elevation of androgens inhibits the secretion of LH from adenohypophysis via a direct action on the hypophysis and an inhibitory effect at the hypothalamic level. Both the hypothalamus and the hypophysis have testosterone and estrogen receptors. It is believed that DHT (dihydrotestosterone) inhibits LH pulse frequency and estradiol also reduces the LH pulse amplitude. So the major inhibitory effect of testosterone on the hypothalamus appears to be mediated chiefly by estradiol, which may be originated through the aromatization of androgen.

(2) **Hypothalamic-pituitary-seminiferous tubular axis :** After stimulation by GnRH, FSH (a glycoprotein hormone) secreted by anterior pituitary, binds to specific receptors in the Sertoli cells and stimulates the production of androgen binding protein, which is necessary for initiation spermatogenesis. It has been shown that the full maturation of spermatozoon appears to require not only the FSH effect but also the androgen. Practically, the major effect of FSH on spematogenesis may be through the stimulation of ABP formation, which allows a high intratubular concentration of androgen to be maintained [Fig. 7.19].

In addition, FSH stimulated Sertoli cells also secrete several other substances like inhibins A and B, GnRH-like peptide, transferrin, plasminogen activator, H-Y antigen. Of these, the inhibins can inhibit FSH release from the anterior pituitary without affecting LH surge. Inhibin is, therefore, probably a physiologic regulator of pituitary FSH secretion, possibly together with the gonadal steroids.

HYPOTHALAMIC-PITUITARY-OVARIAN AXIS—AN OVERVIEW

Pituitary gonadotrophin secretion is controlled by the hypothalamus, which releases pulses of GnRH into the pituitary portal system to reach the anterior pituitary gland. Endocrine changes from foetal life to puberty control of GnRH secretion is exerted by a 'hypothalamic pulse generator' in the acurate nucleus that is sensitive to feedback control from sex-steroids and inhibin. The portal vascular system connects the hypothalamus to the pituitary through which brain hormones are carried to pituitary. Any interruption in this circulation leads to a decline in gonadotropin levels and eventually to atrophy of the ovaries with failure of hormone release. The hypothalamus secretes GnRH that can regulate the secretion of both FSH and LH from the adenohypophysis.

In females FSH stimulates the granulosa cells to produce estrogen and the follicles to secrete inhibin. While LH appears to play a minor role until menarche when it triggers ovulation.

(1) Foetal life : The continuum of development between the foetus and the adult is well illustrated by the changes that occurs in the hypothalamic-pituitary-ovarian axis. Gonadotropins are found in pituitary glands and serum during the first trimester and those gonadotropins rise to plateau at mid-gestation. Serum concentrations of LH and FSH peak at mid-gestation and then gradually decrease until term. Hypothalamic GnRH content increases and the hypophysial-portal circulation achieves anatomic maturity. Early unrestrained GnRH secretion, stimulating pituitary gonadotropin secretion, followed by the appearance of factors that inhibit GnRH surge and decrease gonadotropin secretion after mid-gestation.

(2) Changes at birth : Plasma gonadotropin concentrations are inhibited, but with post-natal clearance of high circulating estrogen concentrations, negative inhibition is reduced and postnatal peaks of LH and FSH are measurable several months after birth. The episodic peaks of plasma gonadotropins may be found until 2 years of age and serum gonadotropin concentrations are suppressed during later years in normal childhood.

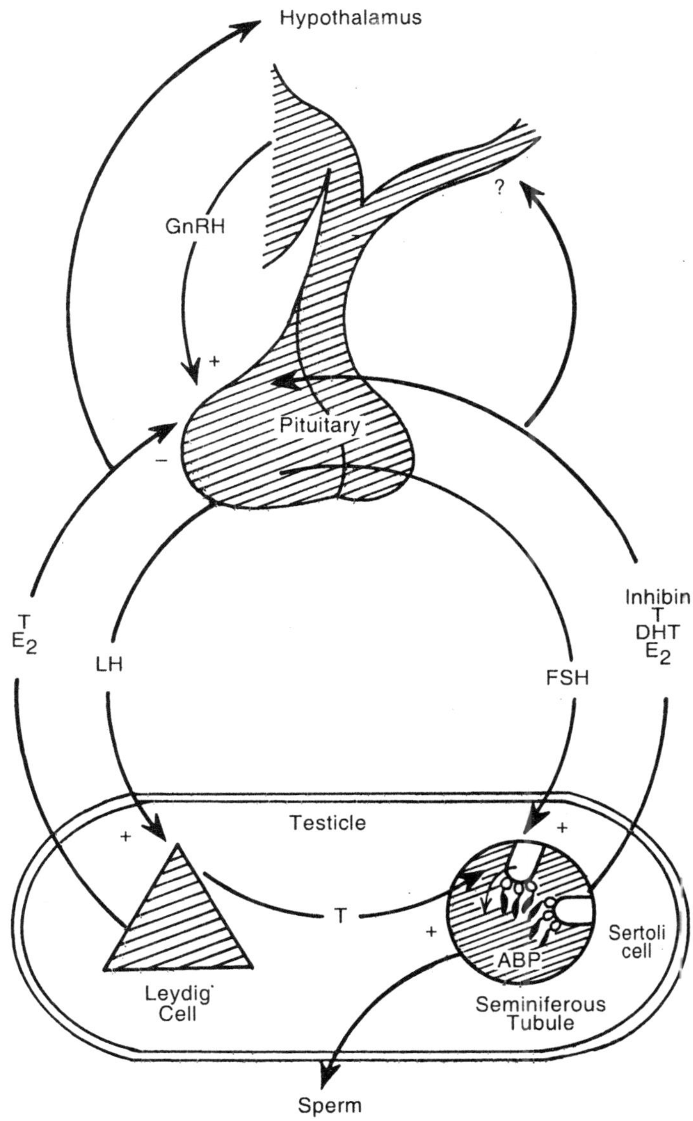

Fig. 7.19: Hypothalamic-pituitary-testicular axis

(3) Peripubertal gonadatropin increase : In prepuberty or early puberty, naltrexone, an opiate receptor antagonist, can completely suppress gonadotropin release as a consequence of its weak opioid effects while after mid-puberty the anti-opioid effects predominate and gonadotropin secretion increases. In peripubertal period, endogenous GnRH secretion increases in amplitude and frequency during the early hours of sleep. As puberty progresses, the peaks of LH and FSH occur more often during waking hours.

(4) Sex steroid secretion : Sex steroid secretion is correlated with GnRH secretion from hypothalamus. When gonadotropin secretion decreases in mid-childhood, gonadal activity decreases but ovaries can still be stimulated by FSH with resulting secretion of gonadal steroids. Most of the circulating estradiol is associated with sex hormone binding globulin (SHBG).

GnRH is secreted episodically about every 90-120 minutes in response to a CNS "pulse generator" [Fig. 7.20].

(5) Menarche : The last stage in hypothalamic-pituitary-ovarian development is the onset of positive feedback, leading to ovulation and menarche. After mid-puberty, estrogen can stimulate gonadotropin release.

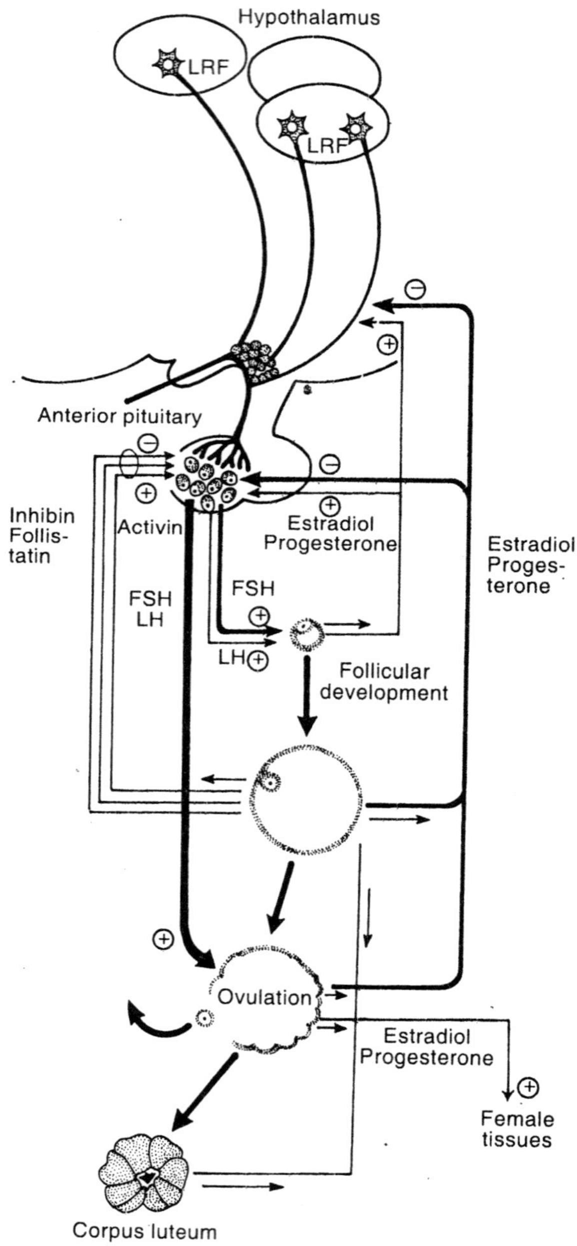

Fig. 7.20: Hypothalamic-pituitary-ovarian axis

The frequency of pulsatile GnRH release increases during the normal menstrual cycle and raises the ratio of LH to FSH surge. This stimulates the ovary to release estrogen and leads to the mid-cycle LH release that causes ovulation. Even if the mid-cycle secretion of gonadotropins is present, ovulation may not take place during the first menstrual cycles; 90% of all menstrual cycles are anovulatory in the first year after menarche. However, even the first cycle after menarche may be ovulatory and the girl may become pregnant prior to physical maturity. Menarche is closely correlated with a skeletal age of 13 years.

- **Note**

Spare receptor : A maximum biological response is achieved when only a small percentage of receptors is occupied. For example, maximal stimulation of steroidogenesis by Leydig cells of the testis takes place when only about 1% of LH receptors are occupied. The additional receptors are known as **spare receptors** and are considered to be fully functional. The role of this receptor reserve may be to increase the sensitivity of target cells to activation by low levels of hormone.

Long-loop and short-loop feedback mechanisms : When the target tissue hormones may undergo feedback at the level of pituitary or hypothalamus of the brain called long-loop mechanism. For example ICSH-RH of hypothalamus stimulates anterior pituitary for release of ICSH which in turn stimulates Leydig cells of testis for secretion of testosterone. Excess secretion of this hormone inhibits pituitary and hypothalamus by long-loop feedback mechanism.

In case of short-loop feedback mechanism high levels of tropic hormones sometimes inhibit the secretion of corresponding releasing hormones from hypothalamus through short-loop mechanism.

CHAPTER 8

Hormonal Regulation of Gametogenesis and Reproductive Cycles in Mammals

Reproduction is a significant physiological and vital phenomenon of organisms by which alike offsprings are produced, attain maturity and can thus maintain continuity of life. The process by which a fully developed organism produces a new individual of its own kind so as to maintain the continuity of the living race is known as reproduction. It is indispensable condition for preserving the species and is necessary to make up the losses that occur due to disease, predation, competition, starvation and other causes of death. Reproduction is always necessary to renew the genetic material which appears to have an inborn process of ageing

Like other higher animals, the human beings also reproduce by the process of sexual reproduction in which a female sexual cell or female gamete fuses with a male sexual cell or male gamete to form an embryo that finally develops into a baby. The male and female reproductive system of mammals consists of organs which are divisible into two groups—(i) **Primary sex organs** or **gonads** which produce the gametes and (ii) the **accessory sex organs** that are concerned with storage and transport of gametes, their fusion (fertilization) and development of the embryo. In addition to gametogenesis (formation of gametes), the gonads also secrete some hormones which are related to reproductive functions, these hormones are referred to as **sex hormones.** Hence, gonads are also considered as endocrine glands.

ROLE OF HORMONES IN SPERMATOGENESIS

Hormones are essential in the spermatogenesis from the spermatocyte stage through the spermatozoon, but not for earlier stages (**Lacy**, 1967, **Simpson et. al**, 1951).

Actions of testosterone on spermatogenesis :

(i) Transforms prophase stage of primary spermatocyte to metaphase stage of primary spermatocyte.

(ii) It is required for the transformation of immature haploid gametes (spermatids) to mature spermatozoa (**Blaquier et al.**, 1972, **Dyson et al.** 1973).

GnRH and its effects :

(i) Hypothalamus initially regulates the male reproductive physiology by releasing gonadotrophic hormone (GnRH). It is a peptide containing 10 amino acid residues. Practically, it is secreted by the neurons whose cell bodies are situated in the acurate nucleus of the hypothalamus.

(ii) GnRH is transported to the adenohypophysis via portal circulation and stimulates the release of the two gonadotrophic hormones, LH and FSH.

(iii) This GnRH is secreted intermittently a few minutes at a time once every one to three hours.

Actions of LH on spermatogenesis :

(i) Regulates androgen production by interstitial cells of the testis, synergistic with FSH in initiating androgen production.

(ii) It is required for maturation of spermatozoa; synergistic with FSH.

(iii) Participates synergistically with growth hormone in the growth of testis, ventral prostate and seminal vesicles (**Lostroh, A** : Regulatory mechanism of male reproductive physiology edited by **G. H. Spillman, J. J. Lobl, K. T. Kirton** 1976) via testosterone production as well as amplification of an organ response.

Actions of FSH on spermatogenesis :

(i) It is synergistic with LH in initiating androgen production (**Lostroh**, 1969).

(ii) It is synergistic with LH in development of spermatids in immature spermatozoa.

(iii) It stimulates formation of an androgen binding protein in testicular tubules.

(iv) Stimulates Sertoli secretion (**Tuna et al.**, 1975).

(v) A common mode of action suggests itself : FSH programs a target cell to respond to gonadotropin, the Sertoli cell to respond to FSH, the Leydig cell to respond to LH.

Actions of estrogen on spermatogenesis :

(i) Very little amount of estrogen is produced by the adrenal cortex in male.

(ii) Testosterone though in a little amount may also be converted into estradiol through aromatase activity within the testis.

(iii) Testosterone produced from testis is converted to either dihydro-testosterone or estrodiol affectinng many tissues [Fig. 8.1].

(iv) This estrogen plays an essential role in spermatogenesis.

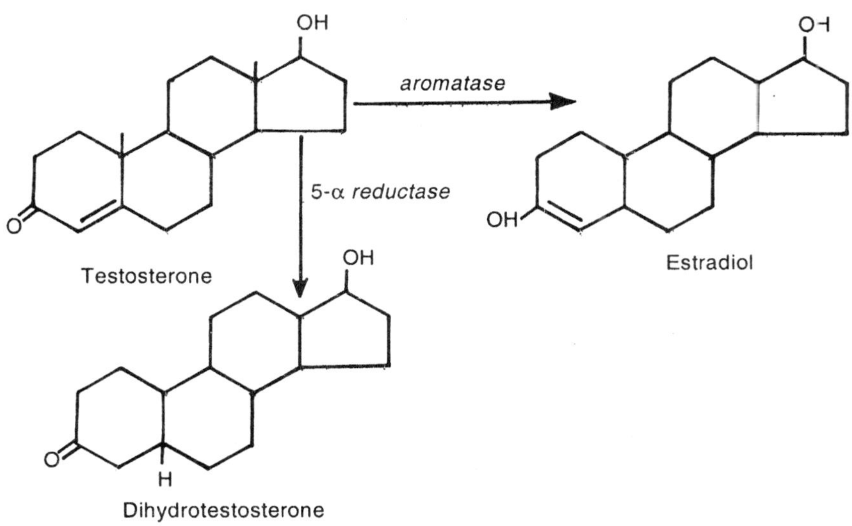

Fig. 8.1: Conversion of testosterone into estradiol.

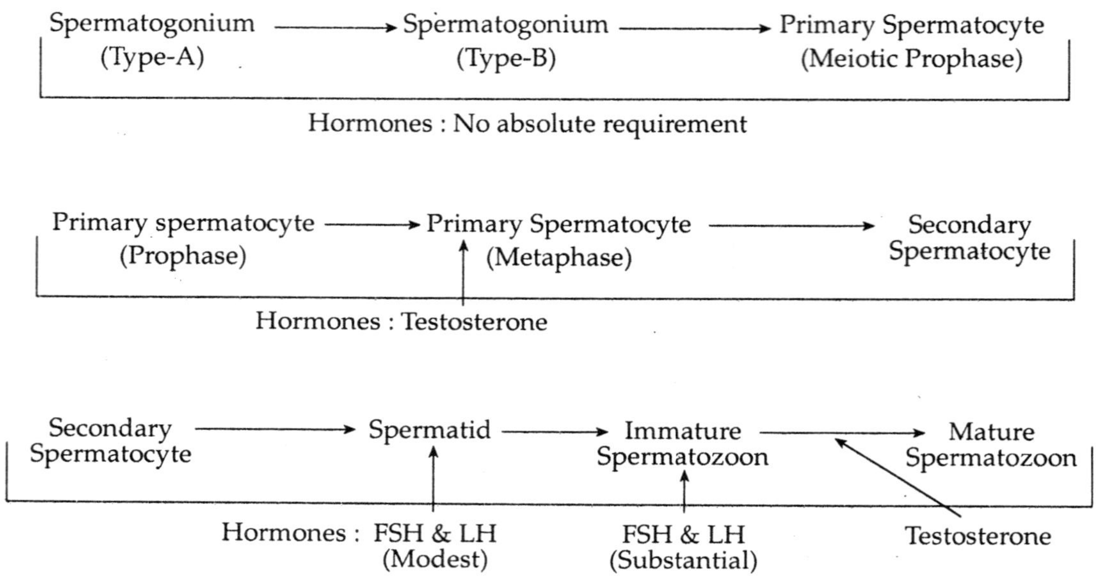

Fig. 8.2 Hormonal control of spermatogenesis encompases developmental stage rrom the prophase of meiosis through final maturation of spermatozoa; Testosterone is required throughout. LH stimulates testosterone production. FSH is synergistic with LH and in addition stimulates tubules and sertoli cells secretion (After Lostroh, A : Regulatory mechanism of male reproductive physiology. Edt. by **G. H. Spilman, J. J. Lobl, K. T. Kirton.** PP-13, Yr. 1976).

Duration of the process : Mammalian spermatozoa emerging from the testis must pass through the epididymis before they become fully matured.

In man autoradiographic studies reveal the presence labelled mid-pachytene spermatocytes after 16 days and immature spermatids after 32 days of injection.

The whole process of sperm formation probably requires about 64 days (**Heller** and **Clermont**, 1963) [Fig. 8.2].

Site of the process of spermatogenesis : All stages, with the exception of final maturation and activation of the spermatozoon, take place with the seminiferous tubules. Final maturation of the sperms takes place within the epididymis.

Feedback control : The process of spermatogenesis is periodically regulated by feedback mechanism.

(i) **Inhibin :** Inhibin is a peptide hormone produced by Sertoli cells. It controls the secretion of pituitary FSH. Pituitary FSH secretion normally is controlled by negative feedback by an inhibitory factor of Sertoli cell origin. Increased levels of inhibin secretion inhibits the FSH secretion and thus cylically regulates the process of spermatogenesis. (It has been shown that granulosa cells from the ovarian follicle also secrete inhibin that acts directly on pituitary cells from males or females to suppress FSH secretion).

(ii) **Androgen :** In adult human male there is a pulsatile release of ICSH about every one and half an hour. It has been shown that high androgen level in blood inhibits hypothalamus as well as ICSH cells of adenohypophysis and regulates the spermatogenic cycle by negative feedback mechanism [Fig 8.3].

HORMONAL REGULATION OF OOGENESIS

The functions of ovary and ovulation in vertebrates have been regulated by hormones of adenohypophysis. In mammals, the growth of the follicle and culminating in ovulation are controlled mainly by two gonadotrophic hormones of anterior pituitary gland. One hormone, the FSH (follicle stimulating hormone) induces ovarian follicular growth of female mammal. Another pituitary hormone, the LH (luteinizing hormone), acting alone, has little or no effect on ovarian size or follicular growth, but, when acting synergistically with a small dose of FSH, it elicits follicular maturation and undergoes ovulation.

Several nonsteroidal substances that may be important in the regulation of both intra- and extraovarian-processes have been found in follicular fluid. These substances include factors that can decrease (e.g., inhibin) or increase (e.g., activin) FSH secretion, modulate steroid secretion from granulosa cells, and delay the maturation of the oocyte in the developing preovulatory follicle (oocyte maturation inhibitor) [Fig. 8.6].

a little LH, stimulates the follicular growth along with the production of estrogen in the ovary. This estrogen now acts upon the pituitary to stimulate secretion of increased amounts of LH and LTH and to cause a decreased secretion of FSH.

The single dominant follicle then undergoes full development into a mature Graafian follicle, elaborating increasing amounts of estrogen, and ovulation is induced by a spike of LH secretion on day 13 (average 13th; ovulation takes place 12-16 days before the onset of the next menstruation). After exposure to rising estrogen levels for several days, the hypothalamus responds to a minute rise in progesterone levels by release of a pulse of GnRH. The resultant spike of LH secretion and the smaller rise in FSH secretion last only a few hours, but are sufficient to complete maturation of the follicle, and trigger ovulation within 6 to 18 hours.

Under such conditions, ovulation and formation of corpus luteum take place. The

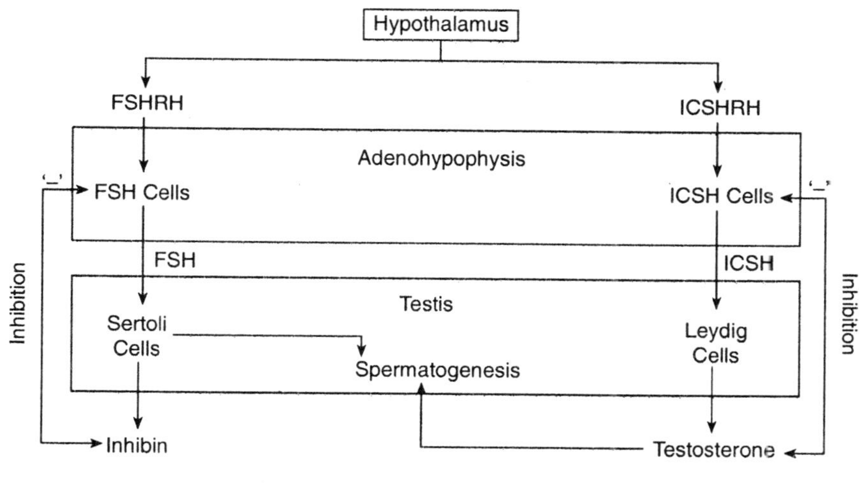

Fig. 8.3: Hormonal control during spermatogenesis

The hypophysis, in turn, is influenced by two ovarian hormones, namely the estrogen and progesterone. Interdependent chain reactions exist between the pituitary and ovarian hormones for the regulation of ovarian and other sexual activities of female mammal. Thus, the FSH with synergistic effect of

corpus luteum, which produces the progesterone, is activated and maintained by LTH. When the corpus luteum begins to regress, the amounts of ovarian hormones are reduced, with the result that the pituitary again produces FSH to initiate the ovarian cycle.

REPRODUCTIVE CYCLE

Reproductive cycle is a common phenomenon among animals, but in mammals, the period of sexual cycle is far more marked in the female than in the male. In some animals, such as those of the deer family there is a brief period of intense sexual activity at one particular season of the year and then a long period during which there is no sexual importance with the cessation of spermatogenesis. A brief period of pronounced sexual activity, when it takes place in the male, is called **rutting season.** This period always corresponds in time with the female period of strong mating impulse which breeds, known as **'period of heat'** and physiological activity as estrus. The females of most species will accept the male in copulation only during the estrus period. In cats the estrus period is accompanied by a period of restlessness and sexual receptivity.

During the reproductive life of a female, in non-pregnant state, the cyclical changes of the ovarian maturation and the concomitant changes in physiology and reproductive behaviour of the organism is called reproductive cycle. This cycle is related to the reproductive activities (but in male, there is no such cycle and the reproductive activity is maintained uniformly throughout the reproductive life). The reproductive cycle is influenced by rhythmic changes of neuro-endocrine system and reproductive organs. In mammals two kinds of reproductive cycles are recognised—**estrus cycle** and **menstrual cycle**.

A. ESTRUS CYCLE

The reproductive cycle of mammals other than primates is referred to as **estrus cycle.** The word estrus is derived from the latin word, means "in a frenzy". The estrus cycle is a conspicuous period when the ovulation occurs and the animal is said to be **'in heat'**. In other words, the occurence of ovulation is conveyed to the male, the female sends out some external signals and seeks the company of the male. In mammals this period of sexual activity by the females is called as **'heat'** or **'estrus'.**

At regular interval of ovulation, when the non-primate female is physiologically and psychologically conditioned to receive the male, it is known as estrus cycle. This cycle is marked not only by the changes in the intensity of the sex urge, but by changes in the lining of the vagina and uterus, which prepare the latter to receive a fertilized egg. The uterine lining becomes softer and thicker and its blood vessels and glands increase in number and size. These processes reach their height a short time after ovulation, and if fertilization and the embedding of a fertilized egg do not occur, the lining gradually reverts to its original condition. The females repeat the cycle at intervals that vary species to species.

Types : Estrus cycle is of three kinds—

(i) **Monoestrus :** When the wild animals have one estrus cycle in a year or season, the condition is called monoestrus; e.g., elephant, bear, bat, etc.

(ii) **Diestrus :** When two reproductive periods occur in a year, they exhibit diestrus condition; e.g., cats and dogs.

(iii) **Polyestus :** When more than two reproductive cycles occur in year, they exhibit polyestrus condition. Female rats and mice have these cycles as frequently as every five days; the guineapig every fifteen days and the cow every three weeks.

Among mammals the estrus cycle of Monotremata is not clearly recognised (**F. Griffith**, 1978).

Phases of estrus cycle : The different phases of estrus cycle are briefly described below :

(i) Proestrus phase (preparatory stage) : This phase of the estrus cycle is referred to as the "building up" phase or 'follicular phase'. The proestrus phase is characterised by the following features—

(a) **Vaginal epithelium :** In vagina, the surface epithelium is underlain by the newly cornifying layers. The epithelial cells proliferate and this is caused by estrogenic hormones secreted by the maturing follicles. The vaginal smear shows a large number of nucleated cells, broken off from the proliferating vaginal epithelium.

(b) **Uterine change :** The uterine wall or endometrium is going to increase in thickness, i.e., it becomes congested and secretes a clear sanguinous fluid. Vascularity is gradually increased and the uterus becomes very contractile.

(c) **Ovarian change :** In the ovary, follicles grow rapidly and the corpora lutea of previous cycle become completely degenerated.

In normal white albino female rats, proestrus lasts for 8-12 hours. Sexual desire is not developed. Both FSH and estrogen levels are gradually increased at peak [Fig. 8.4].

(ii) Estrus phase : This is the phase that occurs at the end of the proliferation phase. This is the period of desire only when the female will receive the male. This time of receptivity, immediately prior to ovulation is termed 'estrus' or heat. This phase shows the following characteristics :

(a) **Vaginal change :** The vaginal epithelium becomes much thickened. Mitosis occurs in the vaginal mucosa. The superficial layers become squamous and are fully keratinised. During late estrus, there are cheesy masses of cornified cells with degenerated nuclei in the vaginal lumen with a few leucocytes.

(b) **Uterine change :** Congestion of the uterine endometrium becomes maximum and the thickness of the uterine endometrium increases about 3-4 times than proestrus. The

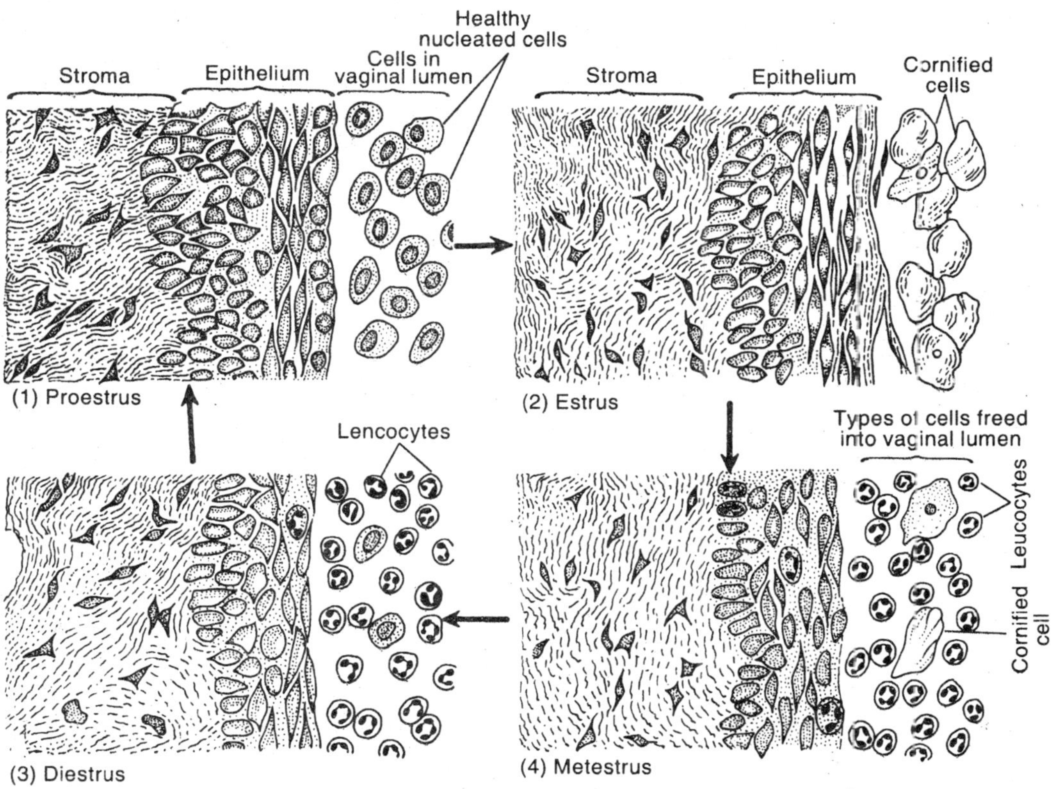

Fig. 8.4: Schematic representation of vaginal wall of white albino rat in different phases of estrus cycle

Table 1: Schematic outline of changes seen in the reproductive organs of rat during estrus cycle

Stage	Ovarian change	Histology of vaginal mucosa	Uterine change
I. Proestrus (12 hours)	Follicles are rapidly growing. Corpora lutea of previous cycle are degenerating.	Vaginal mucosa is slightly dry. Smear consists of epithelial cells only. It is the beginning of next heat. Cornified layer under surface layer of epithelium. Epithelium thick.	Uterus becomes distended with fluids increasing the diameters.
II. Estrus (12 hours)	Follicles are largest in size. Germ cells undergo maturation.	Vaginal mucosa is dry and lustreless. Smear consists of few cornified cells. Copulation is permitted. Cornified layer is well formed and on the surface epithelium is thick.	Reaches greatest distension and thinness of epithelium.
III. Early metestrus (15 hours)	Ovulation takes place.	As in stage II, but smear shows abundant cornified materials. Animal is not in heat. Cornified layer sheds and is finally completely detached.	Epithelium undergoes vacuolar degeneration.
Late metestrus (6 hours)	Young corpora lutea. Eggs are in oviduct. Follicles are smallest in size.	Vaginal mucosa is slightly moist. Smear consists of cornified cells and many leucocytes. Cornified layer gone, and epithelium is thin. Many leucocytes are found.	Some vacuolar degeneration is noticed but also regeneration is found.
IV. Diestrus (57 hours)	Follicles of various sizes. Corpora lutea continue to grow.	Vaginal mucosa is moist and glistening. Smear consists of leucocytes and epithelial cells. Epithelium is thin. No cornified layer yet. Some leucocytes are noticed.	Epithelium undergoes regeneration.

uterus enlarges and becomes distended owing to accumulation of luminal fluid. Much of such fluid is lost before ovulation. Vasculariy on the uterine endometrium has been increased. It has been observed that contractibility of smooth muscle has been increased in the uterine wall.

(c) **Ovarian change :** More than a dozen ovarian follicles grow rapidly in the ovary under the influence of FSH and complete maturation of Graafian follicle occurs. The ovulation takes place in late estrus and is preceded by histological changes in the follicle suggestive of early luteinisation. The vaginal smear of the estrus phase shows a large number of keratinised cells. Estrus is the period of maximum estrogen secretion and it is the period of heat, and copulation is permitted only at this time. In some animals (e.g., cat, rabbit) ovulation does not occur in absence of copulation [Table. 1].

This phase is characterised by high rate of running activity of the female albino rat. Other behavioural changes include quivering of the ears, lordosis or arching the back in response to approaches by the male. Sexual desire is increased at its peak and copulate with the male partner.

(iii) Metestrus phase : This is the luteal phase as well as ovulatory phase which occurs shortly after ovulation. It is the intermediate period between estrus and anestrus or diestrus. This phase is characterised by the following features :

(a) **Vaginal epithelium :** In vagina, the superficial squamous epithelial cells become shed entirely, and the leucocytes that invade the epithelium are apparent. The vaginal smear shows a large number of leucocytes along with few cornified cells.

(b) **Uterine change :** The uterine endometrium becomes proliferated. In this phase the uteri have reduced vascularity and contractility.

(c) **Ovarian change :** Metestrus is the functional development of the corpus luteum in the ovary. This occurs shortly after ovulation and the lining of the ruptured follicle begins to grow inward as the blood

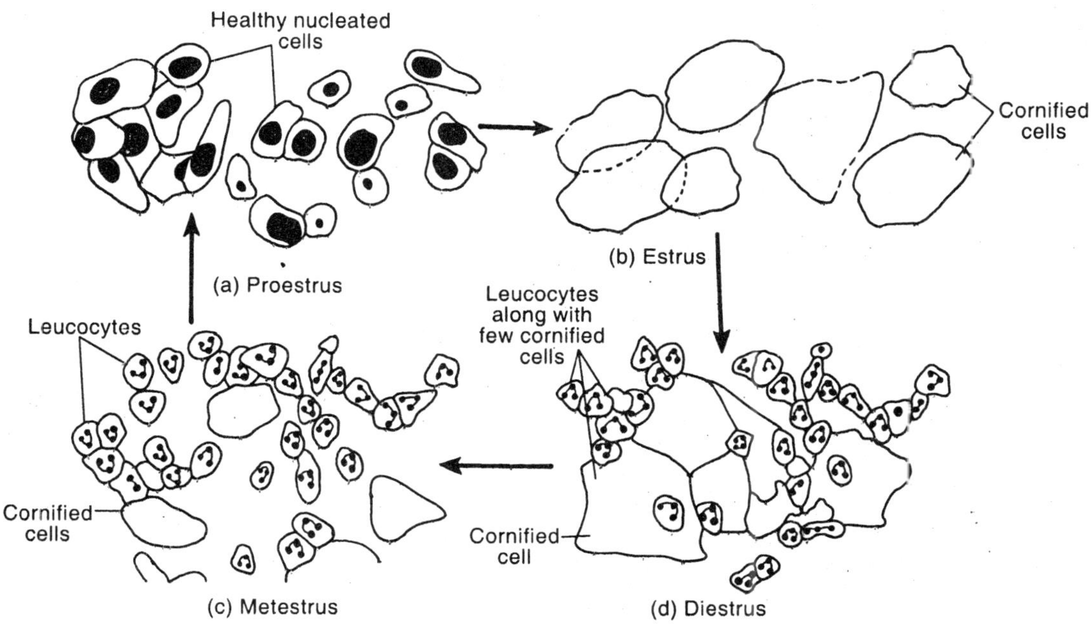

Fig. 8.5: Schematic changes of estrus cycle of white albino rat

vascular supply increases within the cavity. The cells lining the cavity, which have not been expelled, increase in size, multiply and become laden with fat droplets. The newly reorganised structure is called the corpus luteum. Small follicles of the ovary tend to appear.

During this period, there is a decrease in estrogen and increase in progesterone levels formed by the ovary. No sex desire occurs in female and the body temperature becomes normal.

(iv) Diestrus phase : This is the resting period of sexual inactivity. In monoestrus animals it lasts up to the next mating season, and is called **anestrus**. In polyestrus animals the resting interval is short up to the next cycle and is known as **diestrus.** Following metestrus diestrus starts which lasts 60 to 70 hours. In rats it lasts for 2-3 days. The characteristics are described below :

(a) **Vaginal mucosa :** The vaginal mucosa becomes very thin and some leucocytes migrate through it giving the smear consisting almost entirely of these cells. The vaginal smear consists of good number of leucocytes, a few epithelial cells and mucus.

(b) **Uterine change :** The uteri become reduced extremely and anaemic. They become slightly contractile and the endometrium shows regression.

(c) **Ovarian change :** In seasonal breeders the ovary becomes reduced in size. There is a functional regression of the corpus luteum.

In diestrus phase the body temperature becomes normal and it is the resting period without sexual desire. The estrogen and progesterone levels mainly regulate this phase.

Characteristics of the following :

- **Estrus (heat) :** It lasts from 9-15 hours. Under the influence of FSH, many ovarian follicles grow rapidly, uteri undergo progressive enlargement and become distended owing to the accumulation of luminal fluid. Vaginal smear shows cheesy masses of cornified cells with degenerate nuclei, and very few leucocytes may be observed. Ovulation occurs at this stage.
- **Sources of GnRH, TSH, Inhibin, Estrogen, Progesterone and Testosterone : GnRH**—Hypothalamus; **TSH**—Anterior pituitary thryrotrophs; **Inhibin**—Sertoli cells of ovary/Testis; **Estrogen**—Theca interna of ovarian follicle; **Progesterone**—Thecal cells of corpus luteum; **Testosterone**—Interstitial cells of Leydig.

Hormonal control of the Estrus cycle

The regulation is based on the hypothalamo–pituitary–gonadal axis and feedback actions of estrogen and progesterone. GnRH is secreted in episodic bursts (in pulses of high frequency) to stimulate secretion of FSH and LH, which then act on ovary. FSH level in blood is maximum in proestrus and estrus phases and thus helps in maturation and growth of the ovarian follicles.

During estrus phase the estrogen level in the blood becomes high and it acts to prevent a greater release of FSH by the hypophysis and to promote an augmented release of LH. It has been shown that regulation of LH and FSH secretion is dissociated during estrus cycle. Under the influence of rising titers of LH secretion ovulation is occured by the rupture of mature Graafian follicle and there is an immediate fall in the estrogen level under the strong stimulus of LH, the ruptured follicle cells change their characteristics to typical lutein cells, i.e., LH surge causes ovulation and the ruptured follicle becomes transformed into a pink coloured gland, the **corpus luteum**. So changes in the ovaries is the result of interaction of the gonadotrophins and ovarian hormones [Table 2].

Note that progesterone secretion commences before ovulation, and is an important component of the ovarian signal triggering the ovulation spike of gonadotropin. Even in species that ovulate spontaneously,

Table 2: Diagrammatic representation of hormonal control of different stages of the estrus cycle

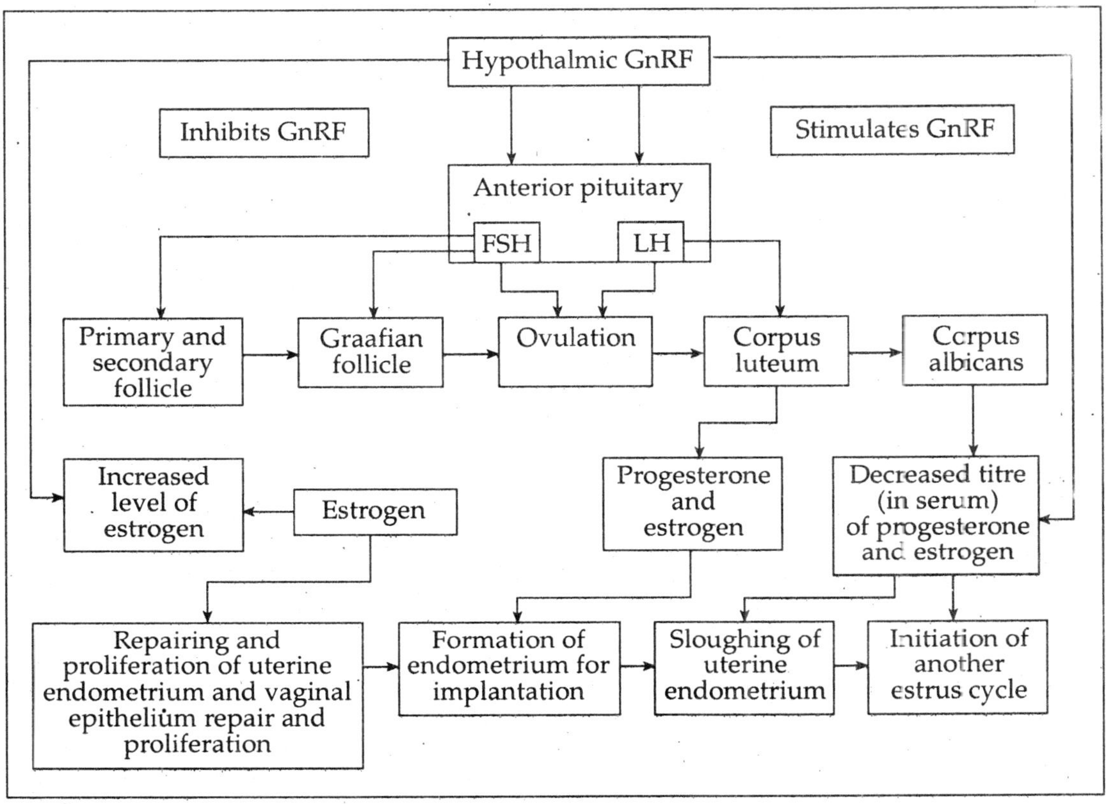

it has been shown that sexual receptivity precedes ovulation. In cow ovulation is spontaneous but it does not take place until 13 to 15 hours after the end of heat. The secretion of progesterone by the ovarian follicles of white albino-rat, guineapig and many other species coincides with the onset of sexual receptivity. Increasing production of estrogen and progesterone from the maturing corpus luteum results in falling gonadotropin levels by negative feedback suppression [Fig. 8.6].

In metestrus phase formation of corpus luteum is maintained by LTH or prolactin. If fertilisation does not take place progesterone level is withdrawn and the corpus luteum is converted into a scar like yellow body, **corpus albicans** during diestrus phase. In this phase all hormonal levels go down.

- **Lee-Boot effect** : It is one kind of pheromonal effects where the female mice housed with four or more other female mice may become pseudopregnant; that is the corpora lutea are maintained in the absence of mating.
- **Whitten effect** : The presence of a male mouse may cause shortening and synchronization of the estrus cycle of grouped female mice by pheromonal effect known as whitten effect. For example, if the female mice are housed in large groups, the incidence of anestrus increases. These findings suggest that female mice secrete one or more pheromones that affect the estrus cycle.
- **Vandenbergh effect** : The urine or bedding of a male mouse is the stimulus to synchronization and shortening of the estrus cycle. When the prepubertal female

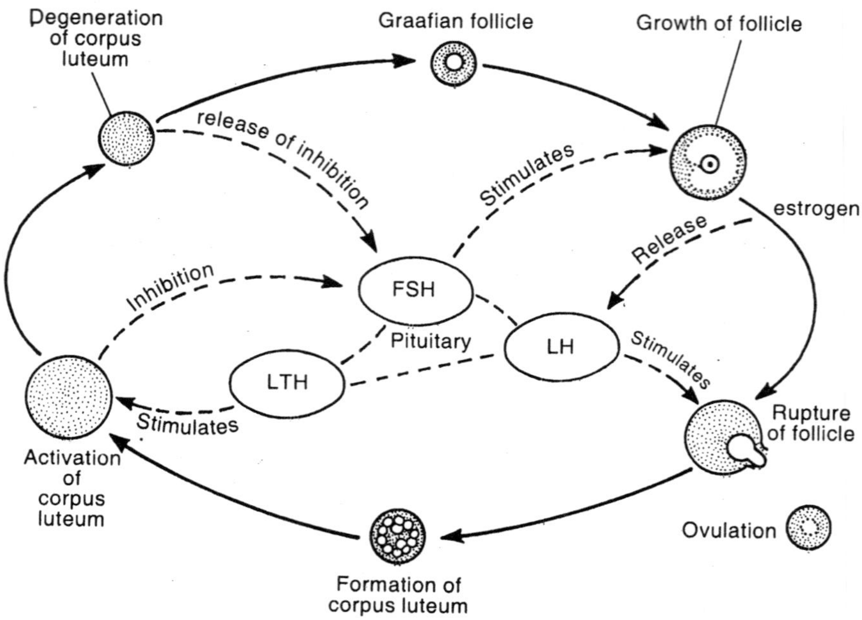

Fig. 8.6: Cyclic role of hormones in the regulation of oogenesis and ovulation in mammals (After Bodmer, 1968)

mice are reared in the presence of a male or its urine, the female mice attain first estrus several weeks earlier than if reared in the absence of the male. It has also been found that the odour (pheromone) of an adult female causes precocious testicular development of young males. Again, the development of testes is markedly retarded when the young males are reared with adult males.

- **Bruce effect :** The bedding or urine of the male is effective interminating pregnancy by pheromonal effect, called Bruce effect. Again if an impregnated female mouse is exposed to a strange male, pregnancy may be blocked; she will comeback to estrus within one week. The source of the male odour is unknown but may be derived from the preputial glands.

MENSTRUAL CYCLE

In most mammals, the endometrium (epithelium of the uterus) undergoes rhythmic cycle along with ovulatory and estrus cycles. Female primates including humans show periodic vaginal bleeding at regular intervals during their reproductive life except in pregnancy. This phenomenon of vaginal bleeding is known as **menstruation (or period).** The menstrual bleeding is due to disintegration and shedding of uterine mucosa (endometrium) causing rupture of blood vessels. **Cyclical discharge of blood, mucus and certain other substances from the uterus in the reproductive life of the females, at an average interval of 28 days (24-32 days) is called menstrual cycle.** It occurs every month from puberty to menopause. The menstrual cycle is characteristic of primates. It does not occur in other vartebrates. In mammals except primates, the female receives the male only during a definite period (heat period) in their sexual cycle. But in primates (menstruating mammals) copulation may be performed at any time during the sexual cycle. The menstruation has a duration of 3 to 5 days without any appreciable pain. Ovulation takes place about midway between the menstrual period following the commencement of the bleeding. The casting of endometrium can be considered as periodic preparation for fertilization of the ovum and pregnancy. If pregnancy does not occur, the hypertrophied mucosa breaks down and is discharged as **menstruation,** therefore, it may be described as the **'funeral of the unfertilized ovum'** or as the weeping of the uterus for the lost ovum. The end result is **menstrual flow.** It is made up of blood (30-40 ml) stripped of endometrium, mucus, leucocytes and an unfertilised ovum. The menstrual flow which comes out from the uterus clots promptly due to rapid formation of fibrin. If the blood remains in the uterus for sometime fibrin is deposited on

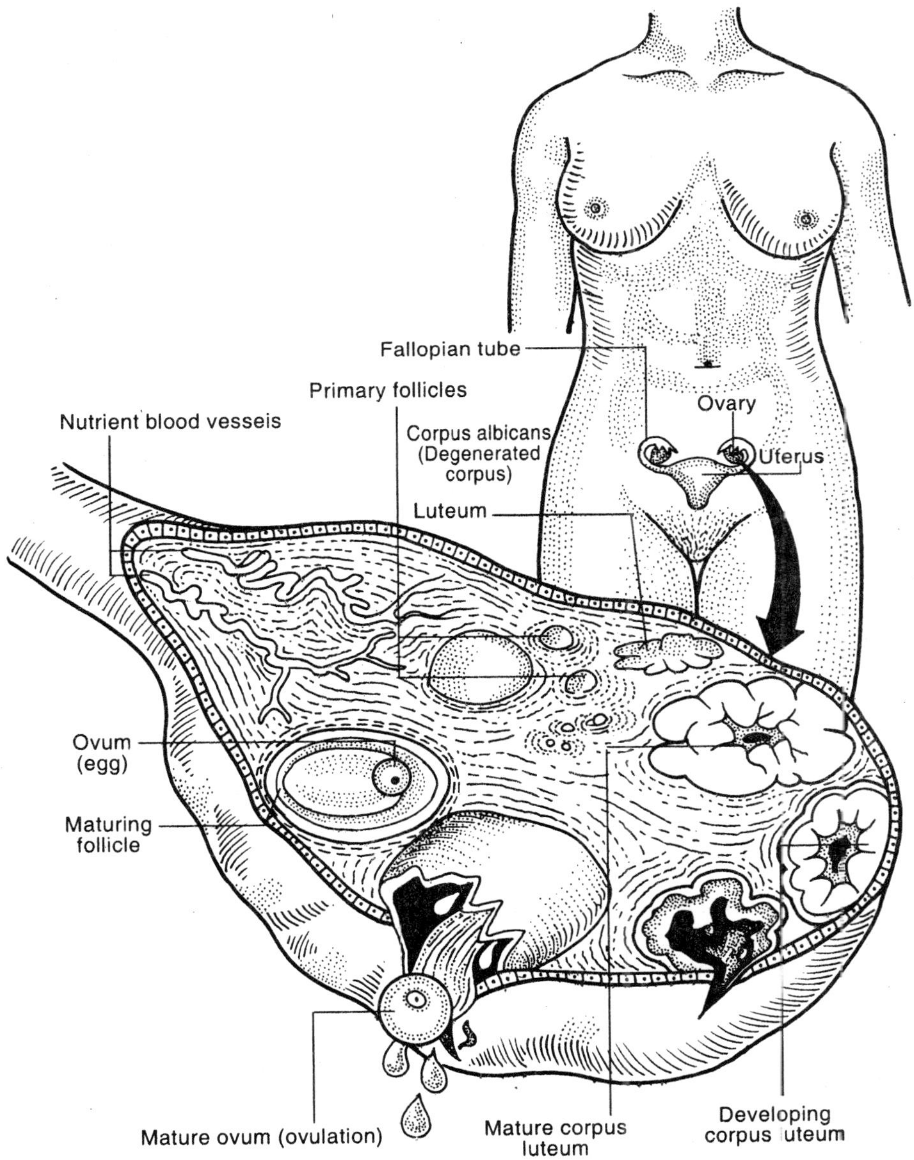

Fig. 8.7: Schematic diagram showing the site, structure and function of the human ovury

the endometrium and as a result there is partial clotting. Intra-uterine clots if retained for a longer period dissolves due to action of *plasmin*. The menstrual cycle is a monthly, rather 28-day (is usually of 28 ±4 days) cycle, duration of bleeding is 4 to 5 days and the amount of bleeding is 4 to 40 ml [Fig. 8.7].

• **Subdivision of the cycle :** The whole menstrual cycle is divided as follows— preovulatory part, ovulatory part and post ovulatory part.

(i) **Preovulatory part :**

(a) **Bleeding phase (Menstruation phase) :** 4 days; 1st to 4th day (may vary from 1 to 9 days).

(b) **Proliferative phase (Follicular phase) :** 10 days; 5th day to ovulatory day.

(ii) **Ovulatory part :**

(c) **Phase of ovulation (Body temperature becomes slightly increased during the time of ovulation) :** 14th day (it may vary).

(iii) **Post ovulatory part :**

(d) **Secretory phase (Luteal phase) :** 14 days; 15th to 28th day.

Copulation may take place at any time during the period of cycle.

• Phases of menstrual cycle

Menstrual cycle is usually divided into following four phases—

(1) Proliferative phase or follicular phase : This phase begins after the cessation of menstruation and continuess for about 10 days. In this phase, the pituitary secretes FSH which causes maturation of Graafian follicle in ovary (hence, the name follicular phase) and secretion of estrogen from it. The estrogen in turn initiates proliferation and growth of the uterine endometrium (hence, the name proliferative phase). This phase comprises the following characteristics—

(a) **Uterine change :** Immediately after bleeding has ended, the endometrium is less than 2 mm thick consisting of the remnants of glands and the stroma grows rapidly. Epithelial cells from the gland proliferate and cover the raw stromal surface. There is also growth of blood vessels. Uterine endometrium enlarges in diameter of about 4 cm thick.

(b) **Vaginal change :** Vaginal mucosa thickens from less than one to more than 2 mm and becomes more vascular. The vaginal mucous glands become enlarged and at the same time the vaginal epithelium becomes cornified.

(c) **Ovarian change :** The rapid follicular growth is occurred and as a result the immature follicles gradually mature into Graafian follicles [Fig. 8.8].

(d) **Other changes :** Small breast changes are observed during each menstrual cycle and ducts of breast grow to some extent. FSH assists in the growth of ovarian follicles and the estrogen level causes proliferation and thickening of the uterine endometrium. At the end of proliferative phase blood level of estrogen becomes very high which inhibits FSH secretion and causes LH surge from pituitary. In this phase no change in body temperature is seen. The estrogen hormone produces sex desire in female.

• **Menarche :** The onset of the first menstrual flow in the life of a girl is called menarche. Normally it appears between 11 to 13 years of age.

(2) Ovulatory phase : It is a very short period in the menstrual cycle. During this phase, the ovum is expelled out from the mature Graafian follicle and the process is called ovulation. It is characterised by the following features—

(a) **Uterine change :** No remarkable changes have been reported in the endometrium. Because by the late proliferative phase (i.e., before ovulation) the surface of endometrium is undulant and the uterine endometrium becomes thickened to about 5 or 6 mm. During this period endometrial crypts appear and the glands become tubu-

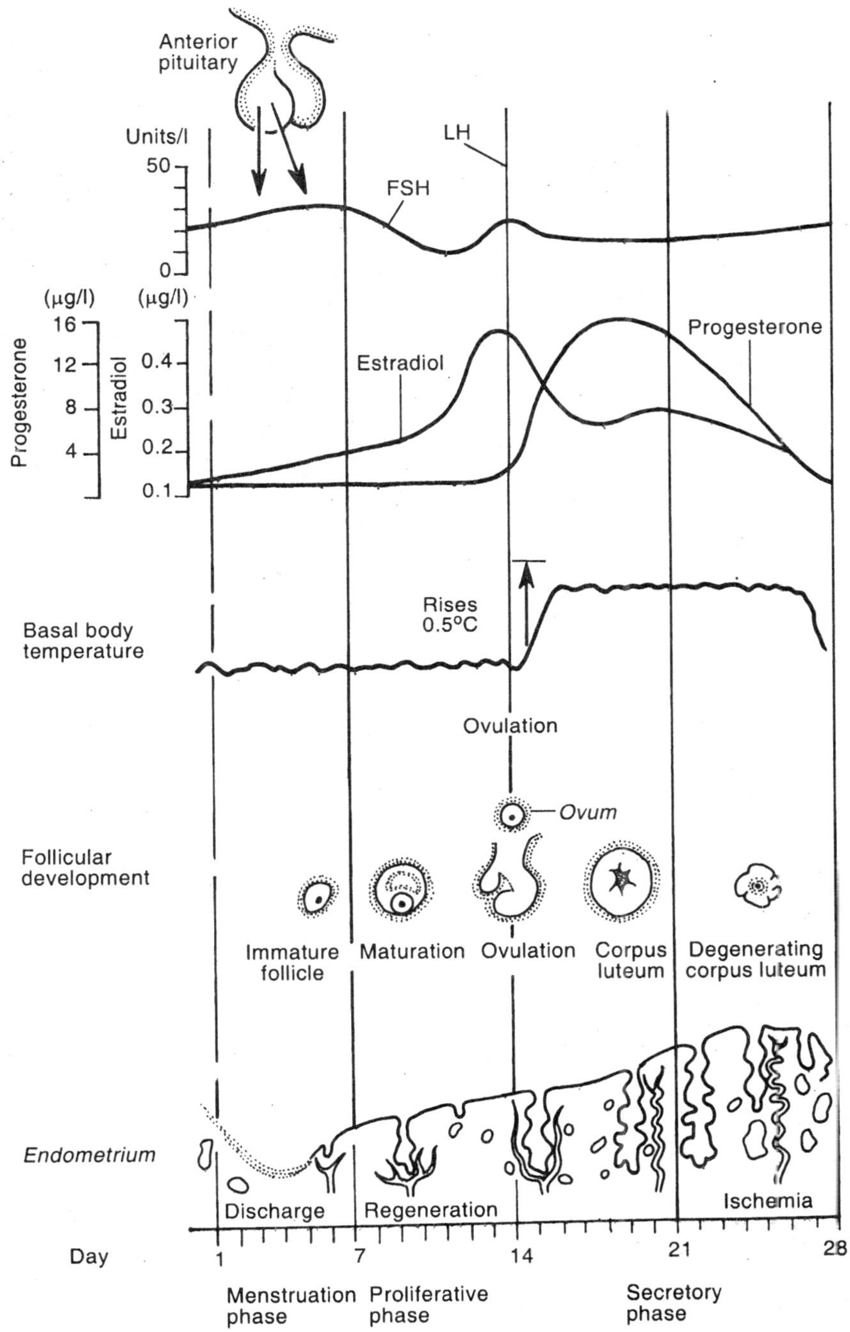

Fig. 8.8: Schematic representation during different phases of menstrual cycle

lar and tortuous. During this period there is also growth of blood vessels.

(b) **Vaginal change :** The vaginal epithelial cells become well developed and the vaginal glands are prominant. The basal secretory vacuoles appear beneath the nuclei of glandular cells.

(c) **Ovarian change :** The mature Graafian follicle of the ovary ruptures and ovulation takes place. Corpus luteum formation starts from the ruptured Graafin follicle [Fig. 8.9].

(3) **Luteal phase :** It is the phase where the corpus luteum is well formed. This phase lasts for about 13 to 14 days and is usually constant. Luteal phase starts after the ovulation and extends up to the next bleeding and is also known as **premeustrual phase** or **post-ovulatory phase**. It has the following features :

(a) **Uterine change :** During this period further thickening of the endometrium occurs to make the chance for implantation of

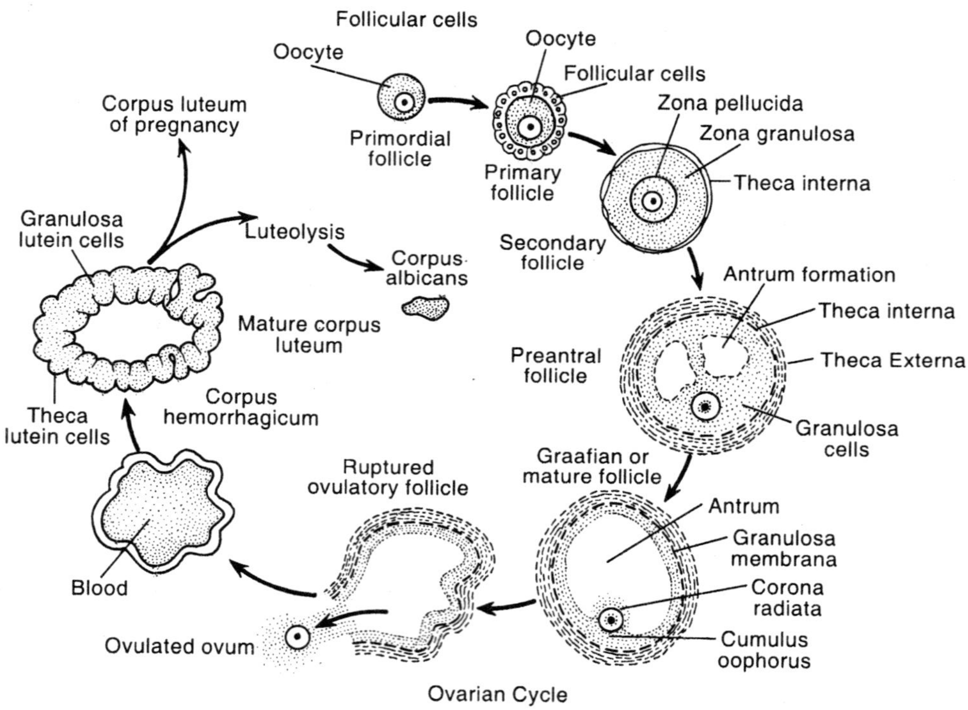

Fig. 8.9: Diagrammatic representation of ovarian cycle (in man)

(d) **Other changes :** The secretion of estrogen reaches maximum at the time of ovulation and such high level of hormone inhibits the secretion of FSH but stimulates the secretion of LH. This LH acting on sensitised follicle causes ovulation. Shortly after ovulation the basal body temperature rises by about 0.5 °C. During ovulation the cervical mucus is thin and watery. Sexual urge to mix up with the opposite sex is maximum.

a fertilized ovum. Vascular uterine crypts become well formed. The uterine glands increase in length and diameter and become more tortuous and are filled with mucus. The stromal cells proliferate, enlarge and stromal edema which was variable during the proliferative stage, also become prominant at this time and peaks on day 22.

(b) **Vaginal change :** During this phase proliferation of vaginal epithelium is also occurred and infiltration of leucocytes within the lumen is noticed.

(c) **Ovarian change :** Following ovulation corpus luteum grows from the ruptured Graafian follicle and this corpus luteum attains maximum size on the 19th day and lasts up to 27th day.

(d) **Other changes :** During this phase, both progesterone and estrogen are secreted in large quantities by the corpus luteum. It has been shown that the changes of luteal phase are largely due to progesterone and also estrogen. The blood capillaries in this phase dilate like sinus and exudation of clear or blood-stained fluid takes place.

Pregnanediol appears 2-3 days after ovulation, rises to maximum about one week before the period and falls 2 to 3 days before the menstrual flow starts. The estrogen level falls in the last phase.

Some growth of the alveoli in breast occurs; the breast may become temporarily tender and painful. Increased tendency to mix up with the male partner is seen.

(4) Menstrual phase : This phase is characterised by bleeding and shedding of the superficial part of the endometrium, leaving the basal layer intact. If pregnancy does not take place, desquamation and sloughing of the entire functional layer of the endometrium occurs and so this phase is also called **destructive** or **regression phase.** The menstruation occurs during the first 4-5 days (average) of this cycle. It has the following features—

(a) **Uterine change :** In this phase the endometrium shrinks without hormonal support and the coiled arteries become further coiled. There is also spasm of the arteries, causing stoppage of blood flow, which

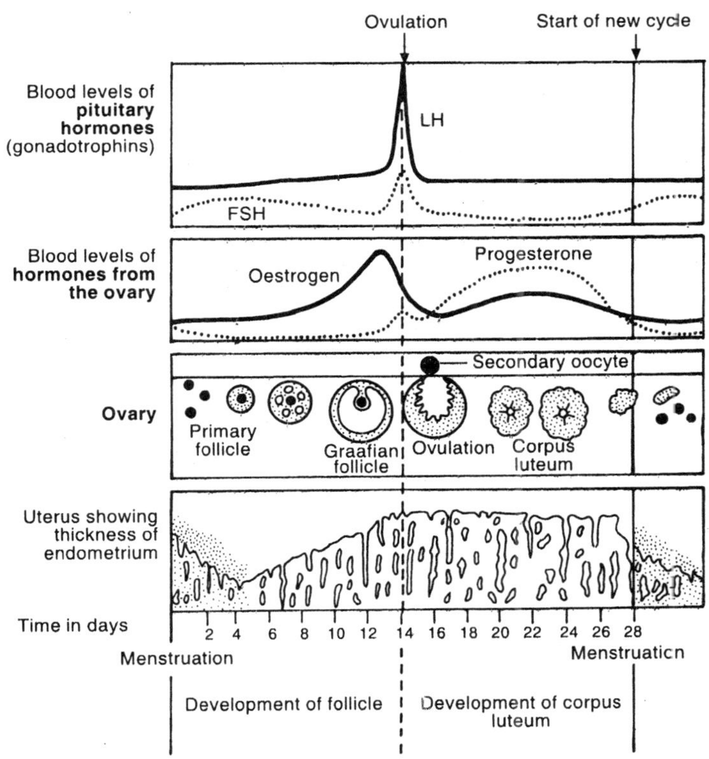

Fig. 8.10: Schematic representation of control of different hormone levels during ovulation and menstruation

leads to focal necrosis of the endometrium and haemorrhage. As a result sloughing of superficial endometrial tissue with pseudodecidual stroma and tortuous glands are shedded. The necrotic endometrium, together with extruded blood and much mucin, is cast off into the lumen of the uterus, when it passes to the exterior. As the uterus sheds bloody tears on being disappointed due to absence of pregnancy, the menstruation is also referred to as "weeping of the uterus".

(b) **Vaginal change** : No remarkable change is observed but the vagina contains the shedded superficial endometrial tissue, extruded blood and ruptured blood vessels, mucin etc.

(c) **Ovarian change** : During menstrual phase corpus luteum degenerates because of the absence of placental gonodotropins. The corpus is replaced by fibrous scar like tissue, called *corpus albicans*.

(d) **Other changes :** The blood shed in the uterus usually clots but due to presence of an enzyme called **fibrinolysin** in uterus, the clotted blood is liquefied, and it cannot coagulate again because fibrinogon is absent in it.

At the end of premenstrual period, blood level of progesterone reaches a peak which inhibits LH and LTH secretion from pituitary. As a result of this the corpus luteum is degenerated causing a sudden drop in progesterone secretion.

Irritation, mind disturbances, abdominal pain occur in this phase and there is no tendency to mix up with the male partner.

• The **cause of menstruation** is necrosis owing to cessation of blood flow. It may be due to (i) further coiling of the arteries, (ii) stretching of the coiled arteries and (iii) vasospasm of the arteries.

The menstrual blood contains prostaglandins which also cause contraction of myometrium. In abnormal situation where prostaglandin synthesis increases, there is severe spasm of myometrium leading to pain (Dysmenorrhoea) during menstruation.

• It is to be noted that the 1st day of menstruation is considered as the 1st day of menstrual cycle. So in each menstrual cycle, the bleeding phase continues from 1st to 4th day, the proliferative phase extends from 5th to 14th day and premenstrual phase extends from 15th to 28th day. Thus, missing of menstruation is the first sign of pregnancy.

INTRODUCTION TO HORMONES OF THE MENSTRUAL CYCLE

The female menstrual cycle is determined by a complex interaction of hormones. The predominant hormones involved in the menstrual cycle are gonadotropin releasing hormone (GnRH), follicle stimulating hormone (FSH), luteinizing hormone (LH), estrogen, and progesterone. GnRH is secreted by the hypothalamus, the gonadotropins FSH and LH are secreted by the anterior pituitary gland, and estrogen and progestin are secreted at the level of the ovary. GnRH stimulates the release of LH and FSH from the anterior pituitary, which in turn stimulate release of estrogen and progestin at the level of the ovary.

Gonadotropin releasing hormone (GnRH)

Gonadotropin releasing hormone (GnRH) is secreted from the hypothalamus in a pulsatile manner throughout the menstrual cycle. In order to proceed normally, GnRH must be released in pulses. On average, the frequency of GnRH secretion is once per 90 minutes during the early follicular phase, increases to once per 60-70 minutes, and decreases with increased amplitude during the luteal phase. GnRH induces the release of both FSH and LH; however, LH is much more sensitive to changes in GnRH levels.

Follicle stimulating hormone (FSH)

Follicle stimulated hormone (FSH) is secreted by the anterior pituitary gland and is essential for follicular growth until the antrum develops. FSH secretion is highest and most critical during the first week of the follicular stage of the menstrual cycle. FSH induces estrogen and progesterone secretion at the level of the ovary by activating aromatase and p450 enzymes and exerts negative feedback on GnRH secretion. FSH further induces the proliferation of granulosa cells and expression of LH receptors on granulosa cells.

Luteinizing hormone (LH)

Luteinizing hormone (LH) is secreted by the anterior pituitary gland and is required for both growth of preovulatory follicles and luteinization and ovulation of the dominant follicle. During the follicular phase of the menstrual cycle, LH induces androgen synthesis by theca cells; stimulates proliferation, differentiation, and secretion of follicular thecal cells; and increases LH receptors on granulosa cells. The preovulatory LH surge drives the oocyte into the first meiotic division and initiates luteinization of thecal and granulosa cells. The resulting corpus luteum produces high levels of progesterone and some estrogen.

Progestin

Progestin is secreted at the level of the ovary, primarily by luteinized follicles. Progestin levels increase just prior to ovulation and peak five to seven days post-ovulation. The first step in progestin synthesis requires p450 enzyme and the two circulating forms of progestin are progesterone and 17-hydroxyprogesterone. Progestins stimulate the release of proteolytic enzymes from thecal cells that ultimately prepare for ovulation. Progestins further induce migration of blood vessels into the follicle wall and stimulate prostaglandin secretion in follicular tissues (**A. Chatterjee**, 1980). During the luteal phase, progestins induce swelling and increased secretion of the endometrium.

Estrogen

Estrogen is produced at the level of the ovary and is crucial for the development of the antrum and maturation of the Graafian follicle. Estrogen is predominant at the end of the follicular phase, directly preceding ovulation. Estradiol, the most potent and abundant estrogen, is primarily derived from androgens produced by thecal cells. The androgens migrate from the thecal cells to the granulosa cells, where they are converted into estradiol by aromatase enzyme. Some estradiol can also be produced via de novo synthesis by thecal cells. The actions of estradiol include induction of FSH receptors on granulosa cells, proliferation and secretion of follicular thecal cells, induction of LH reeceptors on granulosa cells, and proliferation of endometrial stromal and epithelial cells. At low circulating levels, estrogens exert negative feedback on LH and FSH secretion; however, at very high levels estrogens exert positive feedback on LH and FSH secretion. Estrogen further induces proliferation of estrogen-converting granulosa cells and synthesis of estrogen receptors, establishing a positive feedback loop on itself. In the uterine endometrial cycle, estrogen induces proliferation of the endometrial glands.

Hormonal secretion during menstrual cycle

The menstrual cycle is regulated by the interactions of different hormones from hypothalamus, hypophysis and ovary. Several hormones are involved in the regulation of menstrual cycle. The **gonadotropic releasing hormones,** FSH–RH and LH–RH are probably identical : FSH/LH–RH or **gonadoliberin.** Gonadoliberin and **prolactostatin** regulate the release of the anterior pituitary hormones FSH, LH and

Differences between menstrual cycle and estrus cycle

Menstrual cycle	Estrus cycle
(i) Observed in all female primates except old world monkey.	(i) Found in non-primate mammalian female animals except monotremes and marsupials.
(ii) Occurs throughout the year in every month at an interval of average days.	(ii) Occurs once, twice or more in a year.
(iii) It is a bleeding type, i.e., characterised by vaginal bleeding.	(iii) Non-bleeding type, i.e., vaginal bleeding does not occur.
(iv) Copulation can occur at any time of the cycle.	(iv) Copulation usually occurs only during the 'estrus' (heat period) phase of the cycle.
(v) Sloughing of endometrium and bleeding occur.	(v) The disintegrating endometrium is absorbed.
(vi) Spiral arteries are well formed in endometrium.	(vi) Spiral arteries are extremely reduced in endometrium.

prolactin. This prolactin mainly influences the hypothalamus and the **mammary glands.** FSH and LH govern the ovarian hormones, i.e., primarily the **estrogenic** hormone, **estradiol** and the **gestagenic** hormone, **progesterone** [Fig. 8.10].

In the female, FSH/LH–RH or gonadoliberin is released in bursts at approximately 2-hourly intervals. A much faster rhythm or continual release considerably reduces the secretion of FSH and LH (infertility). Since the amounts of FSH and LH released, relative to one another, change continuously during the menstrual cycle, there must be other factors that influence their release. In addition to central nervous influences, estradiol plays a special role and this estradiol action in turn is modified by progesterone [Fig. 8.10].

During the **follicular phase** of the menstrual cycle the secretion of FSH rises whereas that of LH remains relatively low. On the 12th–13th day the estradiol production, enhanced by the action of FSH, leads to stimulation of the release of FSH and LH, which in turn stimulates the release of estrogen [Fig. 8.11].

Ovulation is induced by a spike of LH secretion on day 14. After exposure to rising estrogen levels, the hypothalamus responds to a minute rise in progesterone levels by release of a pulse of gonadotropin releasing hormone (GnRH). The resultant spike of LH secretion and the smaller rise in FSH secretion, last only a few hours, but are sufficient to complete maturation of the follicle and trigger ovulation within 6 to 18 hours. If this sudden rise in LH does not take place, or if it is too small, ovulation as well as pregnancy cannot occur (anovulatory infertility).

In the **luteal phase** or **premenstrual phase** of the menstrual cycle, the corpus luteum begins to form within the ruptured follicle under the influence of LH. Gonadotropins activate the corpus luteum and cause it to secrete progesterone and small amounts of estrogen.

Progesterone acting on the endometrium primed by estrogen, produces the luteal phase of the endometrial development which is of progestational character, i.e., the endometrium is prepared for nidation of the blastocyst formed (if) from the fertilized ovum. Prostaglandin E_2 is luteotropic in

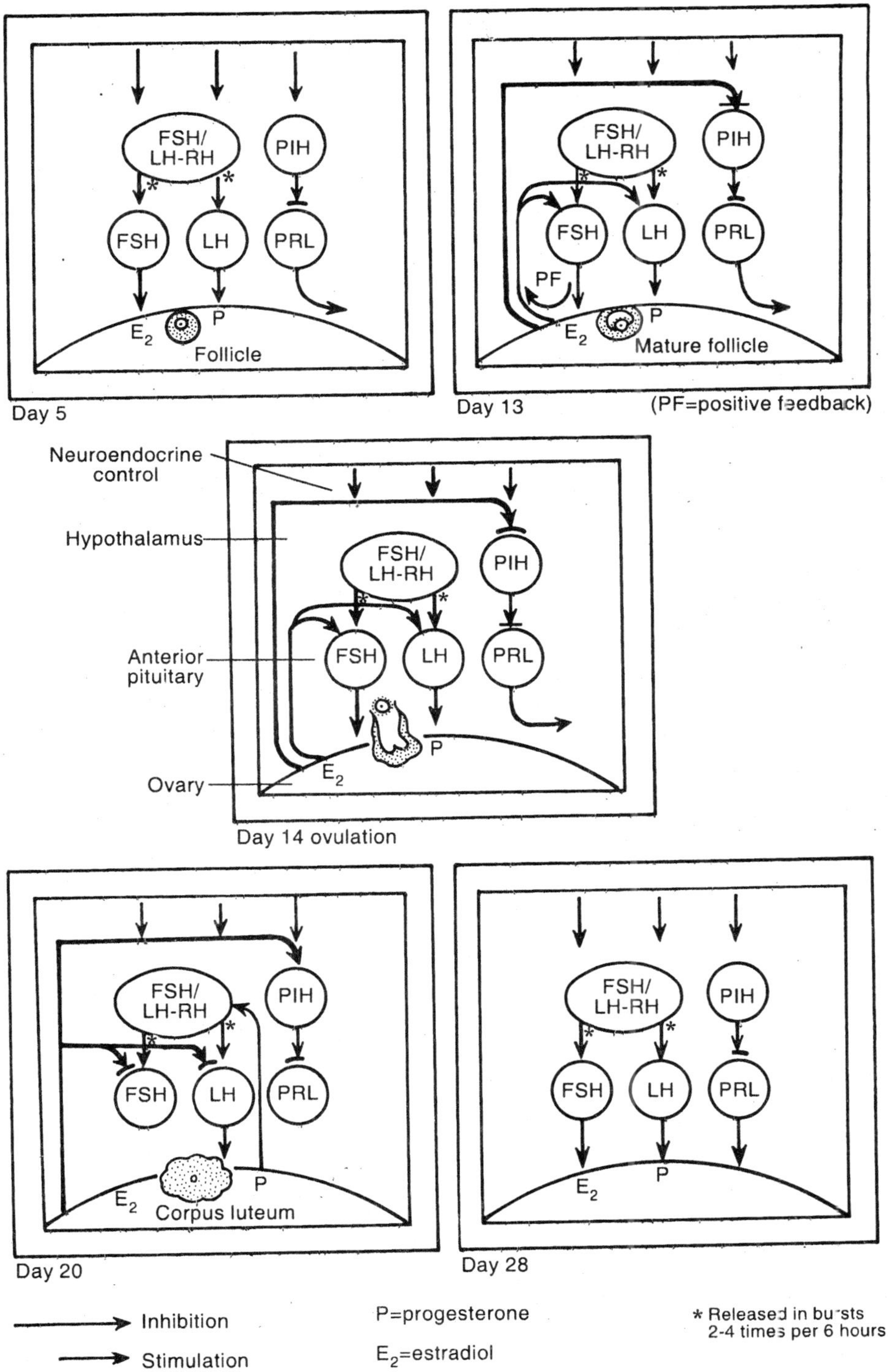

Fig. 8.11: Hormonal interactions during the menstrual cycle

isolated human corpus luteum cells and stimulates secretion of cAMP and progesterone.

Increasing production of estrogen and progesterone from the maturing corpus luteum (day 14 to 20) results in falling gonadotropin levels by negative feedback suppression, i.e., secretion of estrogen and progesterone drops towards the end of the cycle, and on the 26th day it sinks drastically, probably initiating menstrual bleeding.

• **Menopause** : It is the physiological cessation of menstrual flow in the life of a woman. It appears usually between 45 years to little under 55 years. At this stage, ovulation fails to occur and no estrogen or progesterone is formed by the ovary. The loss of estrogen and progesterone causes many physiological changes in the function of the body, such as—(i) Sex organs involute, (ii) **Osteoporosis** starts in the woman at an age about 55 years and progresses, (iii) FSH and LH levels in plasma (and urine) become high and psychologically there may be **depression,** (iv) In metabolism, the women's lipid profile alters and she becomes susceptible to atherosclerosis, (v) atrophy of breasts, uterus, uterine tubes and ovaries, (vi) in cardiovascular system hot flushes can appear and hypertension is common.

• **Pseudopregnancy** : It is the condition in which the persistance of functional activities of corpora lutea is observed in absence of mating in female. Pseudopregnancy may be induced in certain species of laboratory animals like rat, rabbit and mice in their estrus stage by electrical vibration of glass-rod or by mechanical means. In those species the onset of next estrus or 'heat' is delayed and changes alike pregnancy have been found to occur even when the female has not been fertilised. These include changes in the uterus and mammary glands. Activity of corpus luteum is very high and is prolonged in such animals. The vaginal smear shows a large number of leucocytes along with keratinised cells.

• **Puberty** : The onset of reproductive life is called puberty, i.e., it is the transitional period when a sexually immature boy or girl becomes sexually mature. It is the time when the gonads of both sexes develop both endocrine and gametogenic functions. Pubertal changes appear earlier in the girls than boys. The usual age of onset lies between 12 and 15 years. Puberty changes ultimately impart the physical features to the individual, characteristic of his/her sex. In girls, the limits of reproductive life are very sharp and begins with the first appearance of menstruation and ceases with menopause. In boys the limits of reproductive life are not so sharp and its beginning and termination are gradual and indefinite.

WHAT IS GRAAFIAN FOLLICLE?

A mature ovarian follicle in which the oocyte attains its full size and the surrounding follicular cells are permeated by one or more fluid-filled cavities; also called *secondary follicle, vesicular ovarian follicle*. It measures about 10 to 12 mm in diameter, that ruptures during ovulation to release the ovum. Under the influence of the follicle-stimulating hormone from the adenohypophysis, one ovarian follicle ripens into a Graafian follicle during the proliferative phase of each menstrual cycle.

A follicle, which enlarges and then regresses without proceeding to ovulation; occurs normally in animals as waves of follicles developing and regressing during estrous cycles and sometimes during pregnancy; occurs also in seasonally anestrous females. If the Graafian follicle instead of going on to ovulation, degenerates, there is death to the ovum being replaced by a ring of hypertrophied thecal cells. Such degenerating follicle undergoes fibrosis and are called **atretic follicle.** Follicular atresia can be a disease when it occurs at a time when the female should be coming into estrus but is on an inadequate diet, or suffering from a debilitating primary disease. The effect is a failure of the animal to come into estrus and to be fertile.

Structure: The cells of the ovarian follicle are the oocyte, granulosa cells and the cells of the internal and external theca layers.

(i) Oocyte

Each month, one of the ovaries releases a mature egg, known as an oocyte. A follicle is an anatomical structure in which the primary oocyte develops. The nucleus of such an oocyte is called a *germinal vesicle.*

(ii) Granulosa cells

Granulosa cells within the follicle surround the oocyte; their numbers increase directly in response to heightened levels of circulating gonadotropins or decrease in response to testosterone. They also produce peptides, involved in ovarian hormone synthesis regulation. Follicle-stimulating hormone (FSH) induces granulosa cells to express luteinizing hormone (LH) receptors on their surfaces; when circulating LH binds to these receptors, proliferation stops.

(iii) Thecal cells

The granulosa cells, in turn, are enclosed in a thin layer of extracellular matrix—the follicular basement membrane or basal lamina (*fibro-vascular coat* in picture). Outside the basal lamina, the layers, theca interna and theca externa are found [Fig. 8.12].

Development (Role of hormones) : The Graafian follicle is characterised by a large, fluid-filled antrum, and an eccentric oocyte.

At birth each oocyte is surrounded by a single layer of flattened epithelial cells, known as **granulosa cells;** the combined structure is called a **primordial follicle.** These primordial follicles lie mostly near the periphery (cortex) of the ovary but are separated from each other by stromal (connective) and interstitial tissue. Most primordial follicles remain in an arrested state, which may last until puberty or even menopause. Further

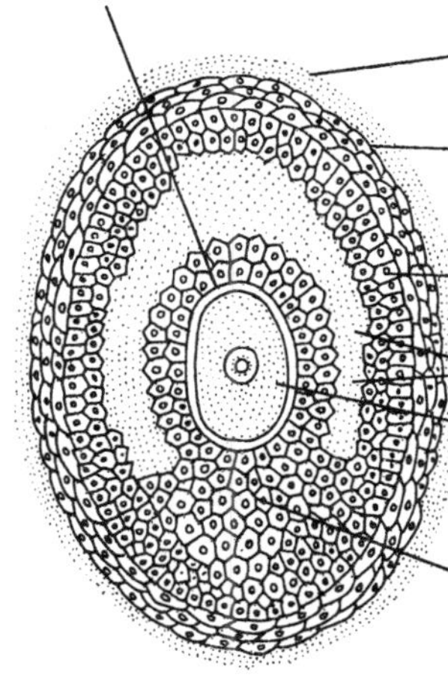

Fig. 8.12: Structure of Graafian follicle

development of a primordial follicle involves transformation of the follicular epithelial cells into a single layer of cuboidal cells surrounding the oocyte; the composite structure is referred to as a **primary follicle**.

Female gametogenesis starts at puberty due to pulsatile release of GnRH from the hypothalamus. GnRH causes secretion of FSH from the pituitary gonadotrophs and under the secretion of FSH, 6 to 12 primary follicles start developing at a time and converted into **secondary follicles.** During development of the follicle, the cells surrounding the oocyte (ovum) become cuboidal and are called **granulosa cells.** The ovum and the follicle gradually enlarge. Droplets of fluid appear between the cells, gradually run together and form a cavity (**antrum formation**) containing a fluid, called **liquor folliculi.** In this stage the follicle can be said as **Graafian follicle**. The cavity, thus fromed, separates the surrounding cells into two layers—the peripheral layer, called the **membrana granulosa** (multi-layered follicular granulosa), and the central layer—**discus proligerus** or **cumulus oophorus (ovaricus).** The innermost **cumulus cells** are disposed about the ovum in radial fashion, forming **corona radiata.** During the development of follicular oocyte, granulosa cells secrete a mucoid substance that forms the **zona pellucida** around the secondary follicle.

Before ovulation the growing secondary follicle is encapsulated by a sheath of tissue derived from the stroma, called the **thecal cells** or **tissue.** The thecal cells is histologically divided into two layers—the inner vascular layer, called **theca interna** or **tunica vasculosa** and outer fibrous layer, known as **theca externa** or **tunica fibrosa.** In this stage the Graafian follicle is not fully matured and it is matured only when the primary oocyte follows second meiotic division and leads to the development of secondary oocyte and first polar body.

This is the full maturation of the Graafian follicle and the ovum is discharged from the Graafian follicle as a secondary oocyte. The process of the rupture of the Graafian follicle to release the ovum is called **ovulation**. Early maturation of the follicle is chiefly controlled by FSH, but for full maturation both FSH and LH are necessary. During this time maturation of a single ovarian follicle produces increasing quantities of estrogen. The estradiol production of the follicle rises steeply from about the 13th day resulting highly increased release of LH that leads to ovulation.

The released ovum is enveloped by a membrane, the **vitelline membrane** which is again covered by a thick hyaline membrane, the **zona pellucida**. There is a narrow space in between the vitelline membrane and zona pellucida which is termed as **perivitelline space.** During the discharge of ovum from the Graafian follicle, several layers of epithelial cells from the **cumulus oophorus** adhere to the ovum. These epithelial cells are arranged radially over the zona pellucida to form the **corona radiata.** The Graafian follicle represents the final stage of follicular development before ovulation.

Function : The ovarian follicle has two major functions. It provides for the maturation and release of a fertilizable oocyte. It also forms the corpus luteum, which promotes and maintains implantation of the embryo. For these processes to occur, the follicle has to grow, ovulate, and luteinize. The transition of granulosa cells to luteal cells requires rapid changes in the expression of specific genes. In this transition, many genes expressed in granulosa cells are turned off, whereas the genes controlling terminal differentiation to luteal cells are induced. Of major importance are changes in the regulation of specific kinase cascades that regulate proliferation and differentiation as well as specific protease cascades that control the remodelling of the follicle during ovulation and formation of the corpus luteum.

OVULATION

The process of rupture of the Graafian follicle of the ovary to release the ovum (secondary oocyte) is called **ovulation**. The follicle of the ovary becomes fully matured in 12-16 days after the onset of the previous menses and measures about 10 mm in diameter. At the time of ovulation the follicle progressively and gradually migrate to the surface of the ovary. More **liquor folliculi** accumulates within the follicle and the pressure within it increases. The surface layer of the ovary undergoes necrosis and the enlarge follicle protrudes from the surface of the ovary. Due to increasing pressure the mature follicle ruptures. The tiny ovum, surrounded by the discus cells, is discharged and is carried out with the fluid and is subsequently drawn into the funnel-like free end of the fallopian tube. The ovum must be fertilized within 24-48 hours if conception is to result. For about 48 hours around ovulation, cervical mucus is copious, nonviscous and slightly alkaline. Following intercourse, sperms that are to survive, penetrate the cervical mucus and can remain viable there until the mucus character changes, approximately 24 hours following ovulation [Fig. 8.13].

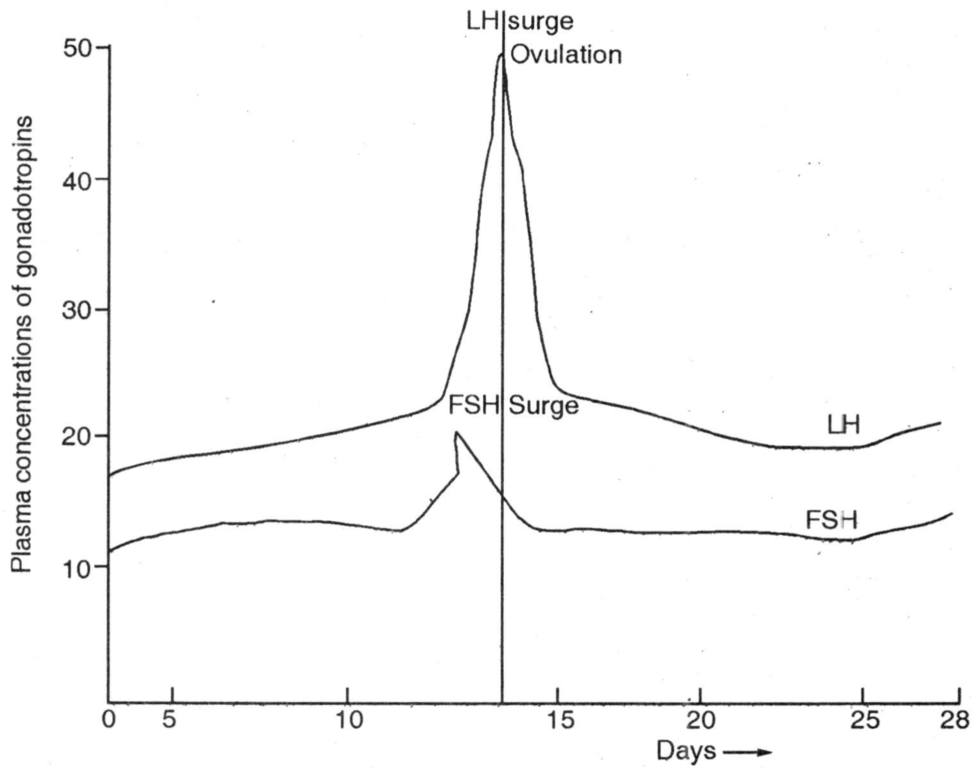

Fig. 8.13: Showing LH and FSH surge guring ovulation

Ovulation may also occur in any given cycle. An ovulatory cycle occurs frequently not only in adolescent girls but also in mature women. In anovulatory cycles the rise in basal body temperature does not occur. The time in ovulation in women can be simply determined by recording the body temperature before getting up in the morning. In the pre-ovulatory phase, the temperature is 36.3–36.8 °C (i.e., at the time of ovulation it increases by 0.3–0.5 °C) and the timing of ovulation is of value when it is desired to promote or avoid conception.

Types of ovulation : In mammals two kinds of ovulation are seen, (a) On the basis of the **presence or absence of Graafian follicle** or **stimulus.**

(i) **Spontaneous ovulation :** This type of ovulation occurs after the maturation of the Graafian follicle, e.g.; mice, rats, primate, etc. are the spontaneous ovulators.

(ii) **Induced or reflex ovulation :** This is where the ovulation is occurred by the stimulus in estrus phase like coitus, or cervical stimulation may induce to release of LH through hypothalamo-hypophyseal systems, e.g.; rabbits, minks, ferrets, cats, etc.

(b) On the basis of **maturation of the follicle** the ovulation is of two types—

(i) In **monotocous animals** at each heat period, one follicle usually develops more rapidly than others so that when it ruptures, only one ovum is released. Examples—horse and cow.

(ii) In **polytocous animals** at each heat period, several follicles develop and rupture during ovulation. Example—Carnivores.

• **Mittelschmerz** : In human female smoetimes there is a lower abdominal pain in the middle of the menstrual cycle, i.e. at the time of ovulation, known as **Mittelschmerz**. This is caused due to irritation of the peritoneum by the bleeding from the Graafian follicle after ovulation and it is common during ovulation following puberty.

Hormonal regulation of ovulation : Certain species have one or two estrus cycle per year, at which time ovulation and receptivity to the male coincide with the male's sexual interest in the female. In estrus cycle of non-primates ovulation occurs at estrus phase whereas in primates ovulation takes place at about the midpoint in the menstrual cycle. In rabbits, ferrets and cats, ovulation is the result of a compound neuroendocrine reflex which is initiated by the intravaginal tactile stimulation and involves the secretion of pituitary LH.

Ovulation occurs usually at regular interval in woman and it is a cyclical phenomenon. At about the time of ovulation other changes are : (i) an increase in urinary gonadotropins, (ii) an increase in number of large acidophilia squamous cells in vaginal smear, (iii) a peak in estrogen output just before ovulation, (iv) 3-4 days after ovulation a rise in pregnediol excretion. In anovulatory cycle none of these events take place.

A complicated reciprocal relationship exists between estrogen and progesterone of ovary and pituitary gonadotropic hormones like FSH, LH and prolactin. It is very difficult to assess the role of these hormones in the regulation of ovulation. The ovarian interstitial cells and the thecal cells of the follicle can make estrogen and this estrogen may indeed prepare the ovary for stimulation by gonadotropins.

The early preovulatory phase is characterised by a gonadotropin mixture (i.e.; FSH). As this FSH stimulates the ovary to produce more and more estrogen, information in ovaries is fed back to the hypothalamic centre which regulate composition of gonadotrophin recipe. Oestrogen and FSH together lead to the development of LH receptors on the granulosa cells, now LH also acts on the follicle. Then there is increased estrogen production which leads to a sharp rise of LH secretion. This LH surge is responsible for ovulation and the ovum is extruded from the ruptured follicle to the fallopian tube. After ovulation, the ruptured Graafian follicle becomes transformed into a pink coloured gland, the **corpus luteum** (i.e., the corpus luteum develops on the remnants of the ruptured follicle). It is a temporary gland producing both estrogen and progesterone. The progesterone causes inhibition of LH secretion. Inhibin is an ovarian peptide hormone which inhibits directly the FSH.

Prostaglandin (PG) is a steroid hormone which is secreted from the granulosa cells of the Graafian follicle. LH stimulates the production of prostaglandin and so the action of PG is LH mediated. The prostaglandin interacts with specific receptors on the surface epithelial cells of ovary. These PG receptors lead to the release of lysosomal enzymes which degrade the underlined tissues. PG also stimulates the contraction of smooth muscle cells of follicle to discharge the secondary oocyte and thereby helps in ovulation. It has been shown that the PG synthesis is inhibited by the introduction of indomethacin and threby blocks the ovulation in rats (**A. Chatterjee** 1980; **Erickson**, 1995). **Deg-root** and **Jameson** (2001) reported that the biosynthesis of PG fails to ovulate in case of female mice.

FSH stimulates ovary→ovary secretes estrogen—estrogen stimulates the release of **FSH**→LH→ovary secretes large amounts of estrogen→rising level of estrogen stimulates the release of FSH→LH→occurence of ovulation→development of corpora lutea begins and corpus luteum secretes estrogen and progesterone.

• **Spontaneous and induced ovulators :** Most mammals like man, ovulate at the end of a follicular phase. These are **spontaneous ovulators.** Certain mammals, like cats, rab-

The sequence of events by which copulation induces ovulation.

Copulatory stimulus

↓

Transmission of neuronal impulses from cervix to brainstem; activation of norepinephrine–secreting brainstem neurons

↓

Secretion of norepinephrine in hypothalamus by brainstem neurons, specifically activating hypothalamic neurosecretory cell that secretes GnRH

↓

Secretion of GnRH by hypothalamic neurosecretory cells into the hypothalamo–hypophyseal portal system.

↓

Transport of GnRH to anterior pituitary by blood flow in hypothalamo-hypophyseal portal system

↓

Greatly increased LH secretion into the general circulation by the anterior pituitary

↓

Surge in blood concentration of LH, exposing all tissues to elevated LH

↓

Response of key ovarian tissues to LH

↓

Ovulation

Fig. 8.14: Flow chart showing the schematic representation of induced ovulation

bits, minks, go through the follicular phase, but remain in a state of sexual receptivity where the follicles mature and the ova are released usually after copulation. After ovulation, there is a reflex release of LH that leads to ovulation after 12 to 48 hours. These are termed as **induced ovulators [Fig 8.14]**.

CORPUS LUTEUM

What is Corpus luteum?

The corpus luteum (**Latin** for "yellow body") is a temporary endocrine structure in mammals, involved in production of relatively high levels of progesterone and moderate levels of estradiol and inhibin A. It is colored as a result of concentrating carotenoids from the diet.

Structure and Development :

The *corpus luteum* develops from an ovarian follicle during the luteal phase of the menstrual cycle or estrus cycle, following the release of a secondary oocyte from the follicle during ovulation. The follicle first forms a corpus hemorrhagicum before it becomes a corpus luteum, but the term refers to the visible collection of blood left after rupture of the follicle that secretes progesterone. While the oocyle (later the zygote) traverses the Fallopian tube into the uterus, the corpus luteum remains in the ovary.

The corpus luteum is typically very large relative to the size of the ovary; in humans, the size of the structure ranges from under 2 cm to 5 cm in diameter. Its cells develop from the follicular cells surrounding the ovarian follicle. The theca cells lacked the aromatase enzyme that is necessary to produce estrogen, so the production of estrogen in granulosa cells indicate the presence of aromatase. Once the corpus luteum regressed the remnant is known as corpus albicans.

Fate:

The corpus luteum is essential for establishing and maintaining pregnancy in females. The corpus luteum secretes progesterone, which is a steroid hormone responsible for the decidualization of the endometrium (its development) and maintenance, respectively.

When egg is not fertilized

If the egg is not fertilized, the corpus luteum stops secreting progesterone and decays (after approximately 14 days in humans). It then degenerates into a **corpus albicans**, which is a mass of fibrous scar tissue.

The uterine lining sloughs off without progesterone and is expelled through the vagina (in humans and some great apes, which go through amenstrual cycle). In an estrus cycle, the lining degenerates back to normal size.

When egg is fertilized

If the egg is fertilized and implantation occurs, the trophoblast cells of the biastocyst secrete the hormone, human chorionic gonadotropin (HCG, or a similar hormone in other species).

Human chorionic gonadotropin signals the corpus luteum to continue progesterone secretion, thereby maintaining the thick lining (endometrium) of the uterus and providing an area rich in blood vessels in which the zygote(s) can develop. From this point on, the corpus luteum is called the **corpus luteum graviditatis**.

The introduction of prostaglandins at this point causes the degeneration of the corpus luteum and the abortion of the foetus. However, in placental animals such as humans, the placenta eventually takes over progesterone production and the corpus luteum degrades into a corpus albicans without embryo/foetus loss.

Function :

(a) Nourish and protect the egg cell

(b) Produce prolactin in the alveoli

(c) Produce progesterone and oestrogen

(d) Convert into hormone producing follicle after ovulation

(e) Stimulate ovulation.

LH SURGE

What is LH Surge?

There are three phases in menstrual cycle—follicular phase, ovulatory phase and luteal phase. In the mid cycle at the time of ovulation there is sudden increase in the level of LH with abrupt drops that initiates ovulation by increase follicular internal pressure, this situation is called as LH SURGE.

An increase in LH followed by the LH Surge

As the cycle comes closer to ovulation, at the end of the follicular phase, LH levels start to rise. FSH, or follicle stimulating hormone, causes the egg to quickly mature in preparation for the ovulatory phase when the egg is released from the ovary and subsequently into the fallopian tube. LH, or luteinzing hormone causes a gradual increase in estrogen. As you move from the follicular phase to the ovulatory phase, LH rebuilds the lining of the uterus. The uterine lining thickens and fills with blood and nutrients in preparation for egg implantation. This process occurs every month until an egg is implanted in the uterine lining or if not the menstrual bleeding begins.

Increased estrogen thins cervical mucus to help sperm travel toward the egg. Estrogen levels continue to gradual rise until they hit the tipping point that triggers LH surge. LH surge is a drastic increase in estrogen that forces the follicle to release the mature egg. When the egg releases into fallopian tube it is known as ovulation.

Can LH Surge be Tested?

There are currently over—the—counter urine tests called OPKs or ovulation predictor kits that measure LH surge in urine. According to test manufacturers, the OPK test results are 99% accurate. There are two forms of over-the-counter LH surge testing kits, commonly marketed as ovulation tests. The first measures LH in urine for seven days. Women need to calculate the correct seven days to use the kit based upon menstrual cycle and cervical mucus changes. Many women choose to use the calender method to track ovulation cycles and choose the best time to perform LH surge home testing.

The other option is a monthly testing kit that includes enough tests to measure LH for 20 consecutive days. Testing often begins one to three days after the menstrual cycle ends depending on the length of your menstrual cycle. If your menstrual cycle ends or your cycle lasts more than 35 days, wait two to three days before you start testing for LH surge.

Does LH Surge occur in All Women?

LH Surge does not occur in all women, but when LH does not surge there is often an underlying condition causing lower than normal LH levels. Some of the conditions that can contribute to lower than normal LH levels include **Kallmann syndrome, hypothalamic suppression** etc.

Alternatively, having higher than normal LH levels can also cause problems with LH surge and fertility. Common conditions that cause an abnormally high LH level include **premature menopause, Swyer syndrome and polycystic ovary syndrome.**

Hormonal regulation during pregnancy : When fertilisation of the ovum takes place (i.e., pregnancy occurs) corpus luteum goes on increasing in size. Then the adenohypophysis continues to secrete LH and this in turn ensures the activity of corpus luteum. The corpus luteum of pregnancy serves as an important source of estrogen and progesterone, so it is essential for maintenance of the pregnancy in the early stage. The continuous secretion of progesterone inhibits the FSH secretion and further ovulation and also inhibits the tendencies of the uterine muscles to contract. Note that progesterone secretion commences before ovulation. Luteinisation results from the action of LH.

Within 14 days of conception, the human chorionic gonadotropins (HCG) are secreted from the placenta, whose activities are similar to LH. The placental hormones replace LH from the anterior pituitary gland in maintaining the function of corpus luteum.

Increasing production of estrogen and progesterone from the maturing corpus luteum (days 14 to 20) results in falling gonadotropin levels by negative feedback suppression. Full maturation of the corpus luteum occurs at about day 21. Maintenance of the corpus luteum continues until day 26, when luteolysis commences and this luteolysis may be prevented by HCG produced by an implanting blastocyst.

The role of HCG is to rescue the corpus luteum, thereby prolonging its life-span by converting it into a **corpus luteum of pregnancy.** Plasma levels of HCG rise to their highest on about the 9th and 14th weeks of gestation and then begin to decline gradually, reaching a nadir approximately after 20 weeks of pregnancy. Luteal function begins to decline while circulating levels of HCG are at their peak.

It has been shown that luteal cell HCG receptors are similar to LH receptors, hence, they are known as LH/HCG receptors and either hormone may be used to study activation of cAMP formation and progesterone synthesis by luteal cells. These two hormones bind to the same receptor and elicit identical biological responses. The immediate response of target cells to the binding of LH or HCG is an increase in adenylate cyclase activity mediated by intracellular, membrane-associated G proteins.

In many mammals (rabbits, rats, etc. but not in primates) the pituitary gland is considered for the initial development as well as the survival of corpora lutea in the pregnant female. The pituitary hormone responsible for luteotropic action in these species is PRL.

Role of hormones of corpus luteum in menstruation : If pregnancy does not follow ovulation, the regression of the corpus luteum begins on 24th day of menstrual cycle and the process is known as **luteolysis**. This is the key point of the menstrual cycle and heralds the onset of the next cycle. Luteolysis is probably done by prostaglandins released by corpus luteum itself.

In the begining of the menstrual cycle theca interna of the vesicle or follicle secretes estrogen and mediated through the secretion of follicular fluid by the granulosa, sensitise the follicle to FSH secreted by the adenohypophysis. FSH initiates the maturation of only one follicle (very seldom, two), which has been primed by estrogen. The secretion of estrogen reaches maximum at the time of ovulation, and such high level of the hormone inhibits the secretion of FSH but stimulates the secretion of LH. Adenohypophysis begins to secrete LH and LTH in increasing amounts. LH acting on sensitised follicle causes ovulation and then together with LTH helps in the development of corpus luteum. Progesterone secretion starts—causing the pre-menstrual changes (luteal phase). But if fertilisation does not occur, the high level of progesterone inhibits the secretion of LH and LTH. This causes involution of corpus luteum, fall in progesterone secretion and dissolution of uterine endometrium. The hypertrophied endometrium breaks down and discharge as **menstruation.**

• **Atretic follicle :** If the Graafian follicle instead of going on to ovulation, degenerates, there is lost of ovum from the ovary and being replaced by a ring of hypertrophied thecal cells. Such degenerated follicles are called **atretic follicles.** The incideuce of follicular atresia may be affected by age, stage of reproductive cycle, pregnancy, lactation, season, etc.

Hormonal control of hypothalamic-hypophyseal system : Hypothalamus and hypophysis act as a single unit owing to their structural and functional relationship. The adenohypophysis is connected with the hypothalamus through the hypothalamo-hypophyseal portal circulation. This allows the hormones of the hypothalamus to reach pituitary, and probably the hormones of adenohypophysis can also reach the hypothalamus through the same route. The neurohypophysis is an extension of the hypothalamus and is mainly formed by the dilated ends of the axons of some hypothalamic neurones. Certain neurones of the hypothalamus secrete hormones, this is known as **neurosecretion.** The hormones synthesised in the nerve cells are not released into the synaptic cleft like the transmitter substances, but enter the blood directly.

The neurosecretory neurones of the hypothalamus synthesise hormones on the ER of the soma and pass then on to the Golgi apparatus where the hormones are incorporated into the granules. The granules are transported by **axoplasmic flow** to the nerve terminals. Oxytocin and ADH even reach the posterior lobe of hypophysis in this way.

Release of the hormone granules by excytosis occurs after an action potential reaches the nerve endings. This is accompanied by an influx of Ca^{++} into the nerve ending, as with the release of neurotransmitters. The duration of action potential in neurosecretory nerves is up to 10 times greater than in other nerves, to allow sustained release of the hormone.

The hormones of neurohypophysis, i.e., ADH and oxytocin, like those of the adrenal medullary hormones, i.e.; epinephrine and norepinephrine are released from the neuro secretory nerves directly into the systemic circulation. The releasing hormones (RH) for adenohypophysis are secreted from the neurosecretory neurons of the hypothalamus into a kind of portal blood system of adenohypophysis, where they bring about release (usually via cAMP) of the anterior pituitary hormones into the general circulation.

Regulation of the release of RH is accomplished by feedback via the plasma concentration of the tropic anterior pituitary hormones.

Release-inhibiting hormones (RH) exist for some of the adenohypophyseal hormones. The RH also pass from the hypothalamus to the adenohypophysis via the hypophyseal portal system. A reduction in the amount of RH released leads to an increased liberation of the corresponding adenohypophyseal hormone. For the normal secretion of some of the adenohypophyseal hormones in presence of additional hormones in the blood is essential, i.e., the release of STH requires the participation of glucocorticoids and thyroid hormone in addition to its own RH.

The following hormones are secreted by the adenohypophysis : STH, ACTH (acts on the adrenal cortex), TSH (acts on the thyroid gland), FSH and LH (act on ovaries and testes) and prolactin (acts mainly on mammary gland). The growth hormone, STH governs skeletal growth and other metabolic processes, usually with the mediation of somatomedins or growth factors (from the liver), as for example, in sulfate incorporation and in protein synthesis in cartilage. Somatomedins also inhibit the secretion of STH in the adenohypophysis (negative feedback).

Pro-opiomelanocortin (POMC) is the precursor polypeptide of ACTH and a lipotropic hormone in adenohypophysis. In the intermediate lobe of the hypophysis, the ACTH formed in this way is further processed to MSH, γ-lipotropin and β-endorphin. Their physiological significance is unclear.

Inhibin : It is a polypeptide hormone which is produced by the Sertoli cells of testis in male and its putative role is to control the secretion of pituitary FSH. High levels of inhibin reduces the FSH secretion and thus cyclically controls the spermatogenesis. It is postulated that inhibin production by Sertoli cells may be regulated by influences deriving from maturing sperms. FSH secretion from cultured anterior pituitary cells is inhibited when pituitary cells are co-cultured with Sertoli cells (but not spleen or kidney cells). Testosterone inhibits the secretion of LH by negative feedback; an inhibin has been postulated for the regulation of the release of FSH in the male. In female the ovaries secrete inhibin, both from Graafian follicle and corpus luteum. High level of LH stimulates the granulosa cells for secretion of inhibin, which leads to feed back inhibition of FSH from adenohypophysis. Thus, further growth of the ovarian follicle is inhibited.

NOTE

- **Blood testis barrier :** Within each testis there are almost 200m of seminiferous tubules, and these structures account for 80-90% of the testicular mass. The approximately 350 million androgen-producing Leydig cells, as well as the blood and lymphatic vessels and fibroblasts are interspersed between the seminiferous tubules. The seminiferous tubules are composed of Sertoli cells and germinal cells. The Sertoli cells line the basement membrane and form tight junctions with other Sertoli cells. These tight junctions prevent the passage of proteins from the interstitial space into the lumen of the seminiferous tubules, thus establishing a **blood testis barrier.** They divide the tubular epithelium into two compartments—a **basal one** containing spermatogonia and primary spermatocytes and an **adluminal one** containing secondary spermatocytes, spermatids and spermatozoa. It conserves certain products of Sertoli cells within the seminiferous tubule such as androgen binding protein.

CHAPTER 9

Hormonal Regulation of Carbohydrate, Calcium and Phosphorus Metabolism

Hundreds of reactions simultaneously occur within a living cell, in a well-organised and integrated manner. The entire spectrum of **chemical reactions, taking place in the living system,** are collectively referred to as **metabolism.** In broader sense, **metabolism** can be defined as the sum total of the physical and chemical processes occuring in the cells of a living organism.

The term **metabolism of a food substance** is meant by a series of specific biochemical reactions occuring within the living organism from the time of its incorporation into the cell or tissue till its excretion, of which some are concerned with tissue synthesis and others with tissue breakdown what are termed as **anabolism** and **catabolism** respectively.

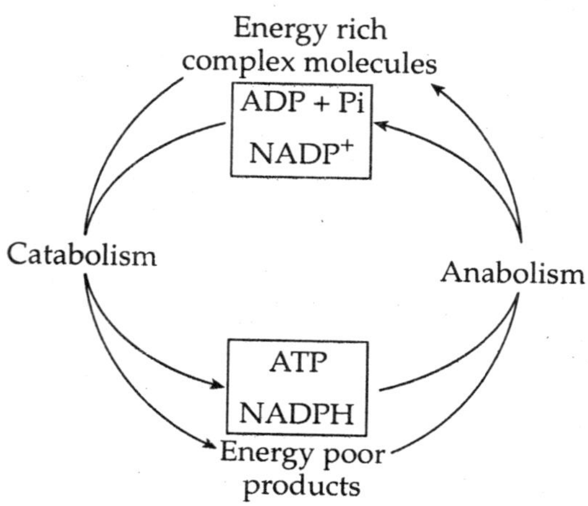

Fig. 9.1: An outline of catabolism and anabolism.

The degradative processes concerned with the breakdown of complex molecules to simpler ones, with a concomitant release of energy is called **catabolism.** The very purpose of catabolism is to trap the energy of the biomolecules in the form of ATP and to generate the substances (precursors) required for the synthesis of complex molecules, whereas the reactions which are included in the process of synthesis of larger protoplasmic molecules from lower ones for building up tissues are collectively known as **synthesis** or **anabolism** [Fig 9.1]. The anabolic reactions are dependent on the supply of energy (as ATP or GTP) and reducing equivalents (as NADPH + H^+).

A clear demarcation between catabolism and anabolism is rather difficult, since there are several intermediates common to both the processes.

REGULATION OF HORMONES ON CARBOHYDRATE METABOLISM

Glucose is the major source of metabolic energy in humans, the brain and the erythrocytes being totally dependent upon it for their energy. The glucose concentration in the blood (blood sugar level) thus plays a central role in energy metabolism. The blood sugar level is determined by the utilisation of glucose on the one hand and by its synthesis on the other.

Carbohydrate metabolism is chiefly constituted by glycogenesis, gluconeogenesis, glycolysis and glycogenolysis.

1. Role of pancreatic hormones

Glucose level of blood at any given time is always determined by the balance between the amount of glucose entering the blood stream and the amount leaving it. Liver takes an important role by allowing net uptake of glucose when the blood glucose is high and by allowing net release of glucose when the glucose level is low. Liver thus plays as a glucostat in maintaining a constant circulating glucose level by the relative activities of the above processes. These processes are not automatic but are manifested by the actions of different hormones.

(a) Action of insulin

The principal effect of insulin on carbohydrate metabolism is to increase the utilisation of glucose by most tissues and the most important effect is to increase the rate glycogen formation. It causes glucose transport across the cell membrane by increasing the permeability of cells. Insulin increases glycogen formation in liver and muscle by stimulating hexokinase and glycogen synthetase.

Physiological functions of insulin exerts following steps regarding carbohydrate metabolism.

(i) **Glycogenesis** is the process of glycogen formation from glucose (in the liver, renal cortex and muscle). Glycogenesis is important for the storage and for the maintenance of the blood sugar level. Glycogen stored in muscle is for the exclusive use of the muscle itself [Fig 9.2].

(ii) **Glycolysis** : Insulin and glucagon hormones are two important hormones,

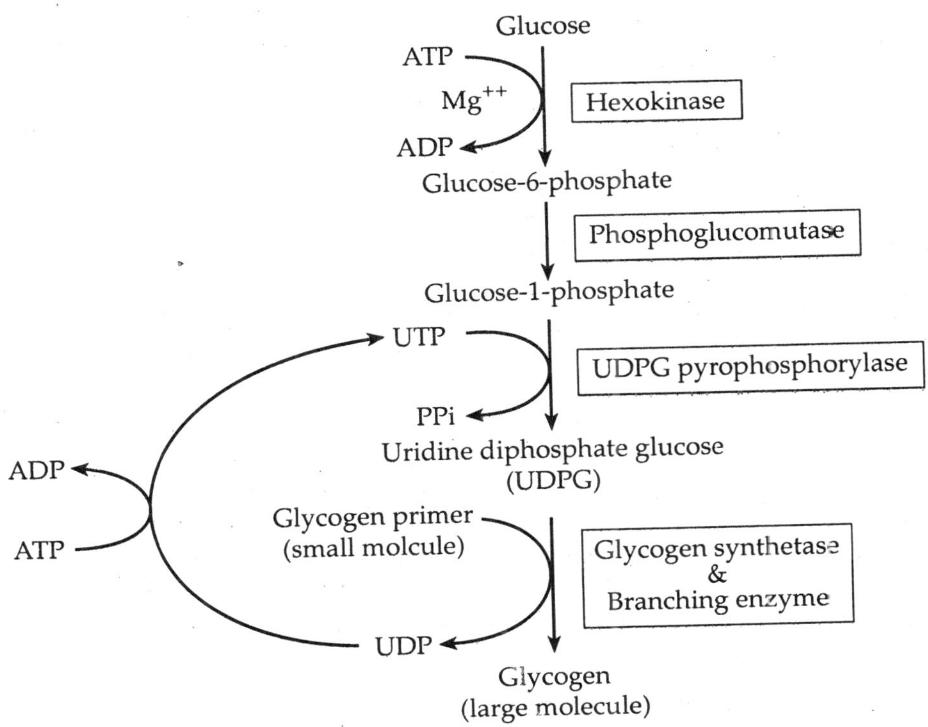

Fig. 9.2: Pathway of glycogenesis.

which greatly influence the overall carbohydrate metabolism. Insulin stimulates hexokinase and glucokinase which catalyse the conversion of glucose to glucose-6-phosphate. It also stimulates phosphofructokinase, which catalyses the conversion of fructose, 6-phosphate to fructose 1, 6-diphosphate. Glucagon stimulates liver glucose 6-phosphatase which is involved in the conversion of glucose 6-phosphate to glucose and also fructose 1, 6-diphosphatase involved in the conversion of fructose 1, 6 diphosphate to fructose-6-phosphate.

(iii) **Glycogenolysis** is the term given to the process by which glycogen is broken down to glucose, i.e., it is the reverse of glycogenesis. Glucagon is another important hormone which helps to conduct the process of glycogenolysis. Insulin inhibits breakdown of glycogen to glucose and depresses the release of glucose from the liver into the blood. In process of glycogenolysis, an enzyme, called phosphorylase, splits a terminal glucose residue of glycogen by adding a phosphate group at its C_1 position, producing glucose-1-phosphate. In the second step the glucose-1-phosphate is converted to glucose-6-phosphate by the enzyme phosphoglucomutase which transfers the phosphate group from C_1 to C_6 position of the glucose. Finally, the glucose-6-phosphate is hydrolysed by glucose-6-phosphatase to glucose and inorganic phosphate (ip).

(iv) **Gluconeogenesis** (in the liver and renal cortex) is the synthesis of glucose from non-sugars, i.e., from amino acids (from muscle protein), lactate (from the anaerobic glycolysis of muscle and erythrocytes) and glycerol (from the breakdown of fats).

Thus, glucose is normally formed from proteins and fats in the liver. But in diabetes the rate of neoglucogenesis is increased. In starving diabetic, dextrose/nitrogen ratio is nearly constant about 3.6 indicating that both sugar and nitrogen are derived from the source—the proteins. When insulin is given, both sugar and nitrogen excretion falls, indicating that formation of new glucose from proteins has been stopped.

In a reciprocal manner, gluconeogenesis in which carbon flows back into carbohydrate from lactate or pyruvate, is regulated at the steps catalysed by pyruvic carboxylase, fructose 1, 6-diphosphatase, glucose 6-phosphatase and glycogen synthetase. The regulation occurs at those reactions in glycolysis and gluconeogenesis that are unidirectional. Thus, glycolysis is not only the main pathway for glucose metabolism leading to the formation of acetyl CoA and oxidation in the citric acid cycle, but it also provides the principal pathway for the metabolism of fructose and galactose derived from the diet. It produces ATP in absence of oxygen because this allows skeletal muscle to perform efficiently when aerobic oxidation becomes insufficient and it allows tissues with significant glycolytic ability.

On regulation of blood glucose, the major function of insulin is to promote the storage of glucose (and amino acids) taken up in the food. The overall effect of insulin is thus **anabolic** (tissue building) and it lowers the **blood sugar level** by means of at least two different effects on the cell; (a) by raising the amount of glucose taken up by the cell, thus involving the cell membrane, and (b) by altering intracellular enzyme activity, one of the effects of which (in the liver and in muscle and fat tissue) is to increase lipogenesis and glycogenesis.

If the blood sugar level sinks below normal **(hypoglycaemia)** as a result of too much insulin or due to the lack of blood sugar raising factors, the consequences are voracious hunger, sweating and finally, due to glucose deficiency in the brain, hypoglycaemic shock (accompanied by loss of consciousness), which can rapidly cause death.

Factors influencing insulin secretion

The islets secrete insulin continuously. That the hormone is released continuously, is proved by the fact that the removal of pancreas is always followed by hyperglycaemia. In normal individuals about 50 units of insulin are secreted by the pancreas daily. Numerous factors influence the secretion of insulin. A pituitary trophic hormone exerts an important influence on the secretion of insulin through the effects of growth hormone, TSH, prolactin, and ACTH. It has been shown that excess sugar of arterial blood entering the pancreas controls the rate of insulin secretion.

(b) Role of glucagon

Glucagon is a peptide hormone with 29 amino-acids, produced in the α-cells of the pancreas. Like insulin it is stored in granules and released by exocytosis.

The main **stimuli for glucagon release** are hunger (hypoglycaemia) or a surfeit of aminoacids, although its release is also brought about by sympathetic stimulation via β-receptors or a lowering of the plasma concentration of free fatty-acids. Hyperglycaemia inhibits glucagon release. The effect of glucagon is to raise the blood sugar level, thus ensuring an adequate supply of glucose throughout the organism. The ways in which this is accomplished are : (a) by increased glycogenolysis (liver, not muscle) and (b) gluconeogenesis from lactate amino acids (protein breakdown = catabolism) and glycerol (from lipolysis).

The physiological function of glucagon on carbohydrate metabolism is discussed below—

(i) **Glycogenolysis in liver :** The process of breakdown of glycogen to glucose in the liver under the influence of glucagon is called glycogenolysis. In the first step, an enzyme phosphorylase splits a terminal glucose residue of glycogen by adding a phosphate group at its C_1 position, producing glucose-1-phosphate. In the second step, this is converted to glucose-6-phosphate by the enzyme phosphoglucomutase which transfers the phosphate group from C_1 to C_6 position of glucose. Finally, the glucose-6-phosphate is hydrolysed by the enzyme glucose-6-phosphatase to glucose and inorganic phosphate (ip). The significance of glycogenolysis is to maintain blood sugar level between two meals [Fig 9.3].

(ii) Glucagon causes breakdown of glycogen to lactic acid in muscle. The lactic acid is again converted to glucose by **cori cycle.**

(iii) Glucagon stimulates gluconeogenesis in liver [Fig 9.4].

(iv) **Inhibition of glycogenesis :** Glucagon suppresses glycogen synthetase which in turn inhibits glycogenesis in liver.

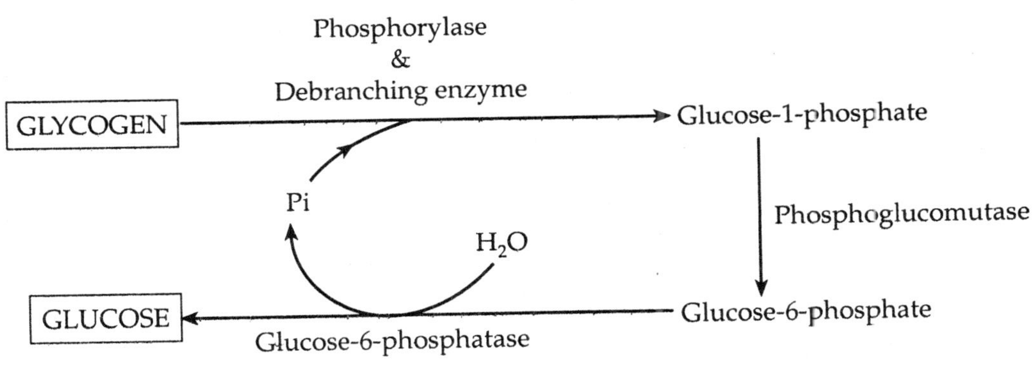

Fig. 9.3: Pathway of glycogenolysis.

Both insulin and glucagon control **glucose homeostasis.** Many factors like food

1. Glycogenolysis (liver—more active than adrenaline) → ↑ BSL

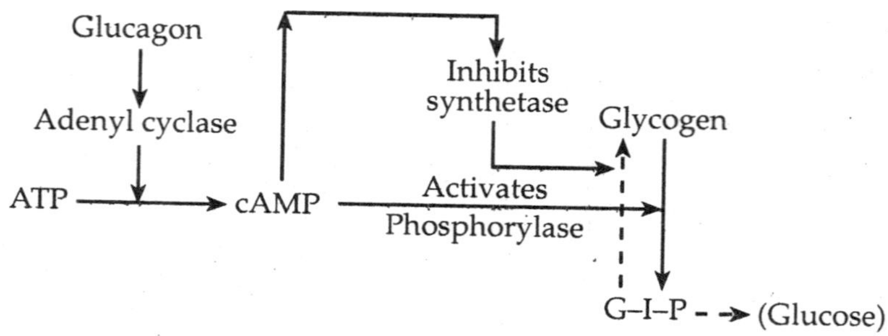

2. ↑Gluconeogenesis

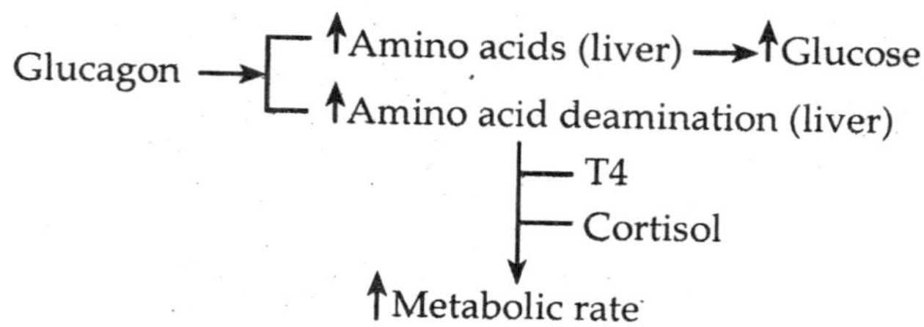

Fig. 9.4: Action of glucagon in muscle and liver.

intake, rate of digestion, excretion, exercise, psychological and reproductive states affect the circulating levels of glucose. The glucose levels may drop momentarily owing to muscular activity, especially if food intake is limited. The diminished level of blood glucose is in some way recognised by the α-cells of pancreas. These cells then release glucagon that acts on the cells of the liver to cause the release of glucose. Thus, the blood glucose level is brought back to normal. If, on the other hand, blood glucose is elevated, other pancreatic islet-cells, β-cells, release the insulin hormone. Now the insulin induces the uptake of glucose from the blood into the liver and other cells, so that the combined output of insulin and glucagon is a major factor in regulating glucose level [Fig 9.5].

Factors influencing glucagon secretion

Glucagon secretion is regulated by blood sugar level. Hypoglycaemia stimulates and hyperglycaemia inhibits the release of glucagon. This hormone is also secreted in

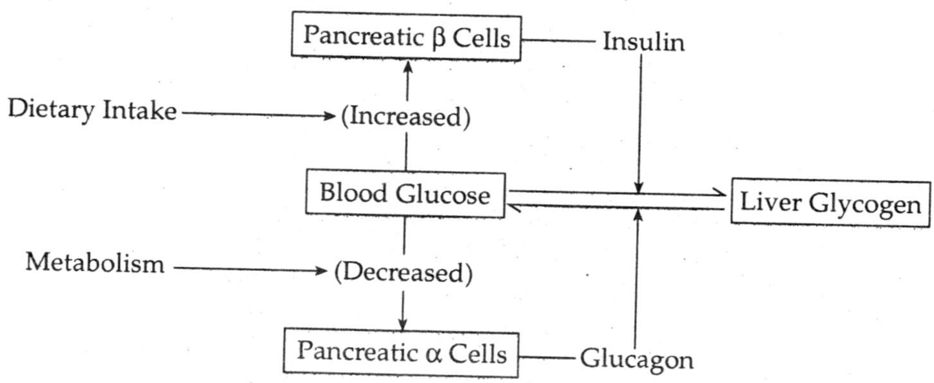

Fig. 9.5: Hormonal control of glucose homeostasis.

increased amounts during muscular activity. GH has been implicated as an agent capable of stimulating glucagon release. Pancreo zymin also stimulates the release of glucagon and this release is also accelerated by protein meals or amino acids. These amino acids also stimulate insulin, and hypoglycemic action is prevented by concomitant secretion of glucagon.

2. Role of anterior pituitary hormones

The anterior pituitary gland secretes hormones that elevate the blood sugar level by antagonizing the action of insulin. These hormones are growth hormones and ACTH. The growth hormones release is stimulated by hypoglycaemia. It increases glucose up take in muscles and also mobilizes free fatty acids from adipose tissue which themselves inhibit glucose utilisation. They also produce hyperglycaemia, which stimulate secretion of insulin causing β-cells to get exhausted.

ACTH enhances the release of free fatty acids from adipose tissues and inhibits glucose utilization. It also increases blood glucose level by stimulating the secretion of adrenal cortex hormones. The glucocorticoids are important in carbohydrate metabolism. They lead to neoglucogenesis by the increased protein catabolism in tissue and increased hepatic uptake of amino acids. They also inhibit the glucose utilisation in extrahepatic tissues. They are antagonist to insulin.

3. Role of thyroid hormone

Thyroxine accelerates hepatic glycogenolysis with consequent rise in blood sugar. This is due to increased sensivity to

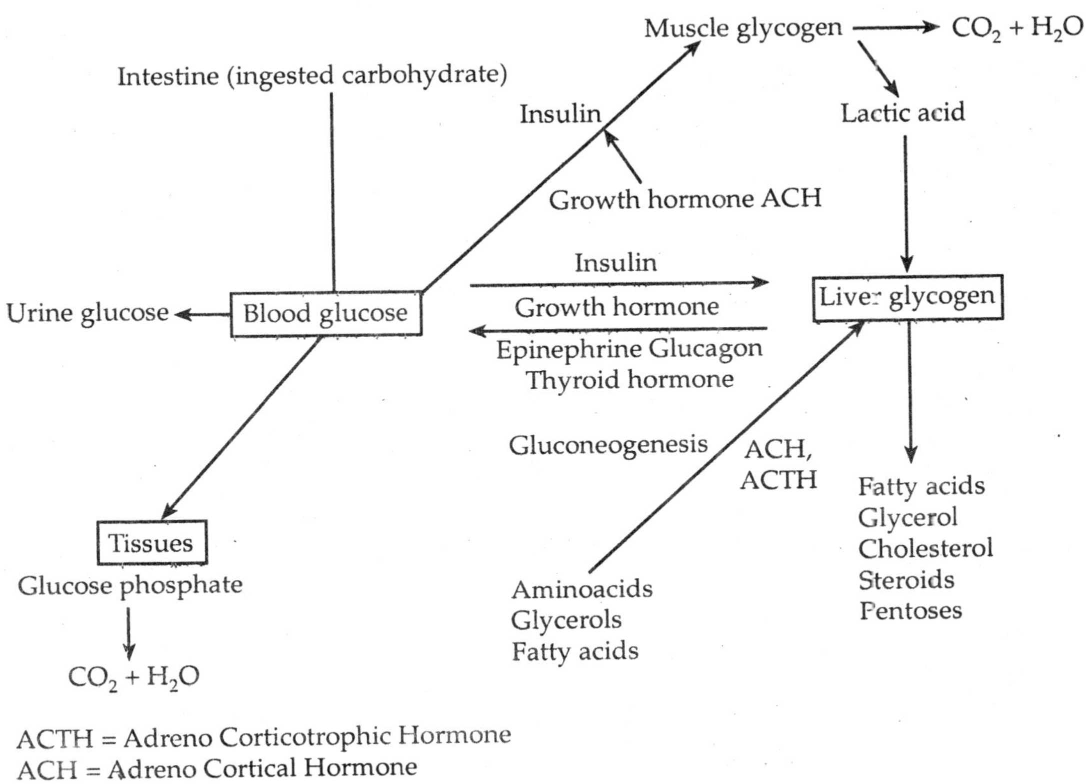

Fig. 9.6: Factors affecting blood glucose level in body.

epinephrine. Thyroxine also increases the rate of absorption of hexose from the intestine and accelerates gluconeogenesis [Fig 9.6].

4. Role of epinephrine

Epinephrine causes an increase in blood sugar and in blood lactate due to the acceleration of glycogenolysis in liver and muscles.

The hormones like epinephrine, norepinephrine and glucagon (in liver) activate adenylate cyclase to increase the production of cAMP. The enzyme phosphodiesterase breaks down cAMP. The hormone insulin also increases the phosphodiesterase activity in liver and lowers the cAMP levels [Fig 9.7].

The overall effect of hormones in glycogen metabolism is that an elevated glucagon or epinephrine level increases glycogen degradation whereas an elevated insulin results in increased glycogen synthesis [Fig 9.8].

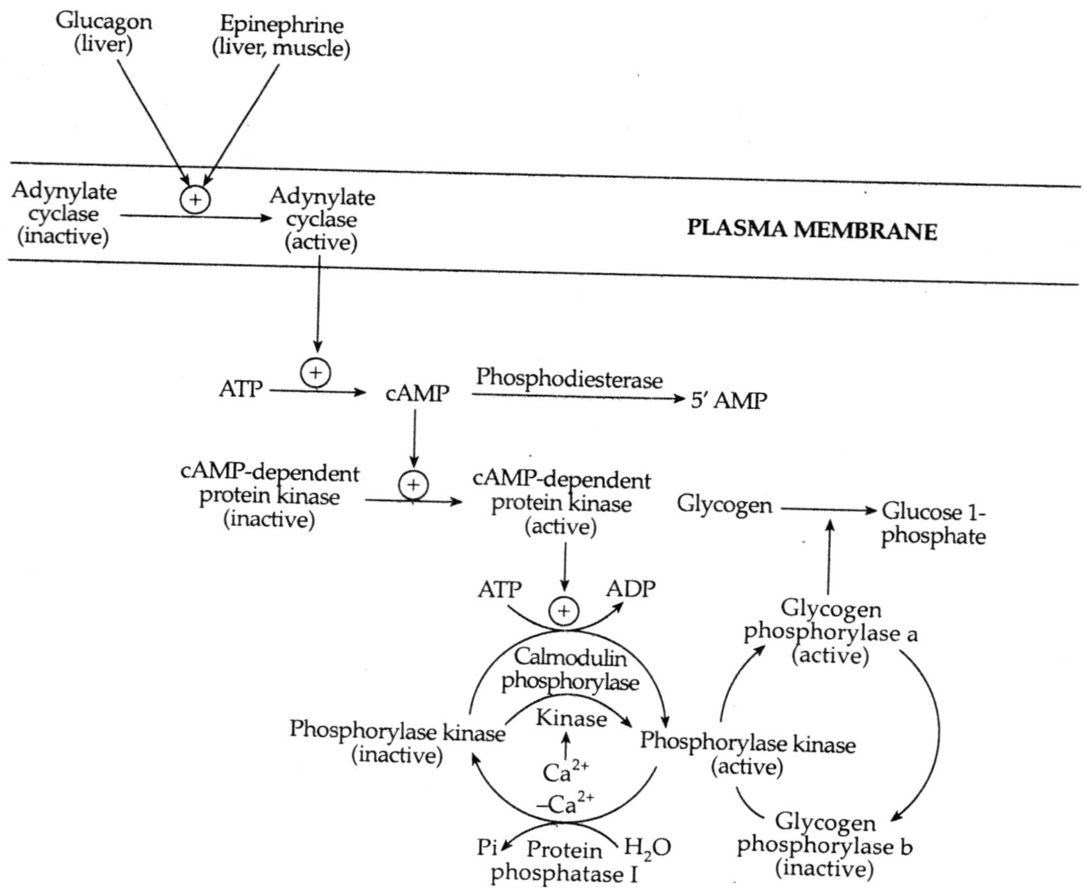

Fig. 9.7: Hormonal regulation of glycogen degradation (glycogenolysis).

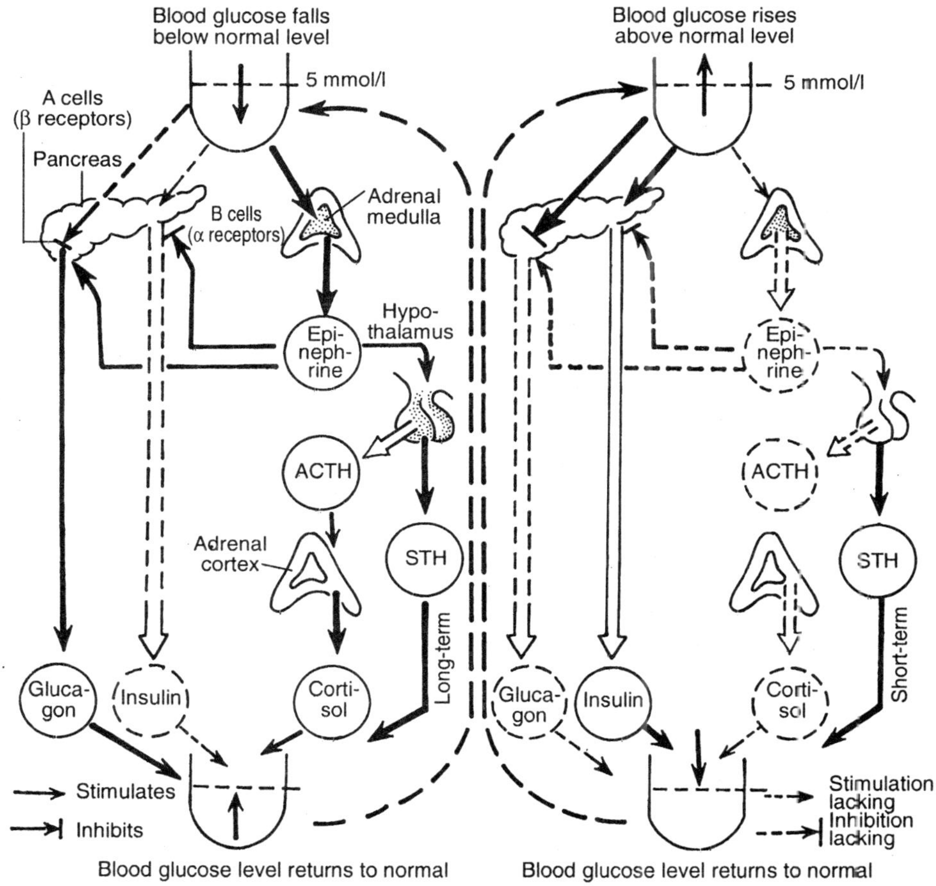

Fig. 9.8: Hormonal control of blood glucose level.

REGULATION OF HORMONES ON CALCIUM METABOLISM

Calcium is the most abundant among the minerals in the body. The total content of calcium in an adult man is about 1 to 1.5 kg. As much as 99% of it is present in the bones and teeth. A small fraction (1%) of the calcium, found outside the skeletal tissue, performs a wide variety of functions. The total Ca^{2+} concentration in the serum is normally 2, 3—2, 7 mmol/l (= 4.6 – 4.5 meq/l = 9.2 – 10.8 mg/dl). Calcium (Ca^{++}) plays a critical role in growth and in cell development and often acts as 'second messenger'. It influences membrane permeability, blood clotting, release of transmitter substances, muscular contraction and a whole series of enzyme reactions, etc. Intracellularly, Ca^{++} is often bound to special proteins (calmodulin, troponin). The Ca^{++} metabolism is mainly regulated by calcitonin (CT), parathyroid hormone (PTH) and vitamin D_3 (D hormone = calcitriol = [1.25 – $(OH)_2$ – cholecalciferol] : cholecalciferol (calciol = "Vitamin" D_3) [Fig 9.9].

1. Role of calcitonin (CT)

Calcitonin was reported in 1962 by Hirsch but the biochemical action of this hormone is not yet clearly known. Calcitonin is a peptide containing 32 amino-acids. It is secreted by parafollicular cells of thyroid gland.

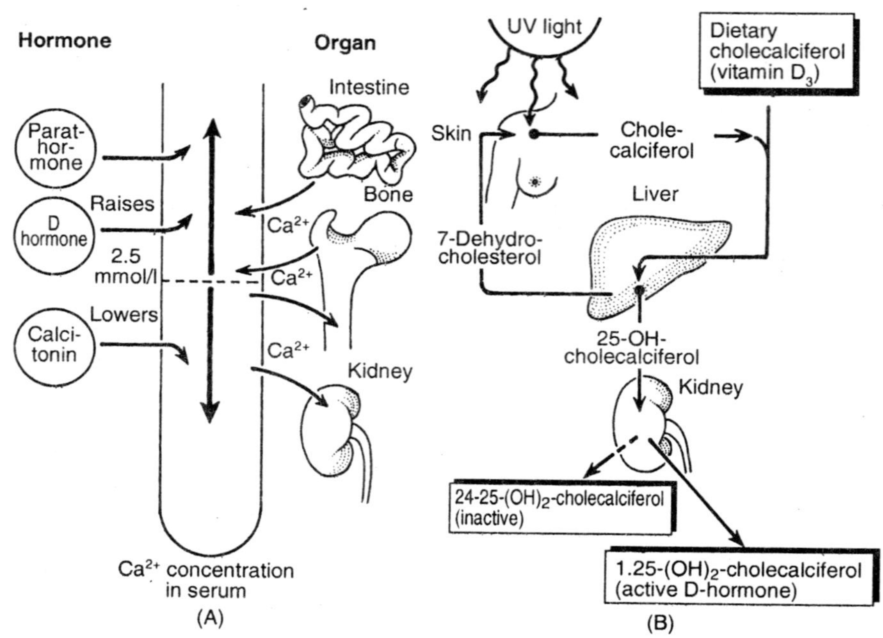

Fig. 9.9: (A) Influences on Ca^{2+} serum levels, (B) Synthesis of D hormone.

Mechanism of action of calcitonin

Calcitonin binds to a specific membrane receptor protein on the plasma membrane of osteoclasts (bone cells) and renal tubule cells and activates adenylate cyclase to liberate cAMP which acts as second messenger to produce the cellular effects.

Under normal condition calcitonin is released continuously and the secretion of CT is directly co-related with the plasma calcium level. Elevated blood calcium level enhances linear rises in calcitonin release, while fall in plasma Ca^{++} decreases its secretion. During calcium metobolism, the calcitonin acts on the following organs.

(i) **On bones :** Calcitonin exhibits two effects on bone, but both effects decrease plasma Ca^{++} levels. Firstly, on short term basis, calcitonin decreases Ca^{++} movement from the bone into the plasma of blood. Secondly, on a long term basis, calcitonin decreases the activities of osteoclasts, the rufflings and microvilli on their membrane, the activities of lysosomal hydrolases, alkaline phosphatase and pyrophosphatase in bones, collagen metabolism and hydroxyproline.

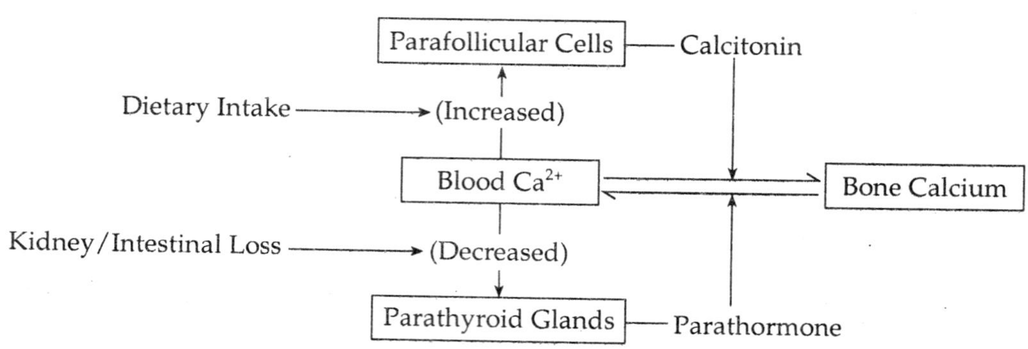

Fig. 9.10: Hormonal control of calcium homeostasis.

Calcitonin stimulates phosphate influx into bone cells and blocks the Ca^{++} mobilizing action of parathyroid hormone on osteoclasts rather than promoting bone synthesis by osteoblasts.

(ii) **On kidney :** Calcitonin enhances renal clearances of Ca^{++} and inorganic phosphate by decreasing their reabsorptions from the tubular filtrate in the thick ascending limb of Henle's loop and the distal convoluted tubule of kidney [Fig 9.10].

Calcitonin-sensitive adenylate cyclase is present in the kidneys but renal effects of calcitonin are not well understood.

2. Role of parathyroid hormone (PTH)

PTH is a peptide hormone and is formed in the ribosomes of the parathyroid glands. It is a single chain polypeptide, containing 84 amino acids. Its molecular weight is 95,000. Synthesis and release of the hormone are regulated by the Ca^{++} concentration in the plasma. If the plasma calcium concentration drops below the normal value (hypocalcaemia)more PTH is released into the blood, where as a rise has exactly the reverse effect.

Mechanism of action of PTH

This hormone binds to a membrane receptor protein on the plasma membrane of target cells like bone cells, renal tubular cells and intestinal cells and activates adenylate cyclase to liberate cAMP as second messenger. This, in turn, increases intracellular calcium that promotes the phosphorylation of proteins, which finally brings about the biological actions on three independent tissues—bone, kidney and intestine. The PTH effects on those tissues are all aimed to elevate serum calcium level.

PTH secretion is stimulated by hypocalcaemia and it works through three mechanisms to increase Ca^{++} levels :

- PTH stimulates the release of Ca^{++} from bone, enhancing **bone reabsorption.**
- PTH decreases urinary loss of Ca^{++} by stimulating **Ca^{++} reabsorption.**
- PTH indirectly stimulates Ca^{++} absorption in the small intestine by stimulating synthesis of 1, 25 $(OH)_2D$ in the kidney.

(i) **PTH effects on bone :** PTH has a **rapid effect** (occuring within minutes), whereby it stimulates osteoblasts to pump Ca^{++} ions out of the fluid surrounding the bone (which has a higher Ca^{++} concentration) and into the extracellular fluid (ECF). Over a longer time course, PTH stimulates bone reabsorption. Although PTH stimulates bone reabsorption, it is actually the osteoblasts that expresses PTH receptors. PTH stimulation of osteoblasts causes them to express a signalling molecule that activates osteoclasts.

PTH causes decalcification or **demineralization** of **bone,** a process carried out by osteoclasts. This is brought out by PTH stimulated increased activity of the enzyme, pyrophosphatase and collagenase. These enzymes result in bone reabsorption. Demineralization ultimately leads to an increase in the blood Ca level. The action of PTH on bone is quantitatively very significant to maintain calcium homeostasis. It must, however, be noted that this is being done at the expense of loss of Ca from bone, particularly in dietary Ca deficiency.

(ii) **PTH effects on kidney :** PTH increases the Ca reabsorption by kidney tubules. This is the most rapid action of PTH to elevate blood Ca levels. However, quantitatively, this is less important compared to the action of PTH on bone.

PTH has two important effects on the kidney that work to increase $[Ca^{++}]$ ECF. First, it decreases the loss of Ca^{++} ions in the urine by stimulating Ca^{++} reabsorption. **Reabsorption** is the term used to describe the transfer of substances from forming urine back into the ECF. **Filtration,** the first step in urine formation, is a non-specific process, whereby water and low molecular weight substances move by bulk flow from the plasma and into the forming urine. Reabsorption, which is performed by the cells of the kidney tubules, allows the recovery of those useful small molecules such as sugars, amono acids and Ca^{++} ions. As well as stimulating Ca^{++} reabsorption, PTH also inhibits phosphate reabsorption.

The other key effect of PTH on the kidney is to stimulate production of 1, 25-dihydroxy cholecalciferol [1, 25 $(OH)_2D$], the active form of vitamin D. Vitamin D_3 is synthesised in a photochemical reaction in the skin, in response to sunlight. Vitamin D_3 and a similar compound derived from plants are present in foods; collectively these are referred to as vitamin D. A constitutively active enzyme in the liver produces 25–(OH)D. The role of PTH is to stimulate the kidney enzyme, resulting in the production of 1, 25 $(OH)_2D$. This is extremely important for bone health and Ca^{++} homeostasis, because 1, 25 $(OH)_2D$ works in the small intestine to promote Ca^{++} absorption [Fig 9.13].

> **Note : In kidney disease,** in adequate amounts of 1, 25 $(OH)_2D$ are made. What happens is that Ca^{++} homeostasis is maintained at the expense of bone. [Ca^{++}] ECF drops because of a lack of Ca^{++} absorption from the diet. Hypocalcaemia stimulates high levels of PTH secretion; this is termed as **secondary hyperparathyroidism** because the problem that causes the hyperparathyroidism is in the kidney not at the parathyroid gland. Secondary hyperparathyroidism is treated by administering vitamin D and Ca^{++} supplements. The drug **cinacalcet** has recently been aproved for the treatment of secondary hyperparathyroidism. Cinacalcet is a calcimimetic drug that binds to the Ca^{++} receptor on cells in the parathyroid gland, inhibiting the secretion of PTH.

(iii) **PTH effects on the intestine :** In the intestine, Ca^{++} uptake is indirectly increased due to the stimulating effect of PTH on the formation of D hormone in the kidneys.

(iv) **Effect of PTH and CT on plasma calcium :**

The primary physiological stimulus for PTH secretion is a decrease in plasma calcium. The following figure exhibits the relationship between serum PTH concentration and total plasma calcium concentration. It is actually a decrease in the ionized calcium concentration that triggers an increase in PTH secretion. The net effect of PTH is to increase the flow of calcium into plasma, and return the plasma calcium concentration toward normal [Fig 9.11].

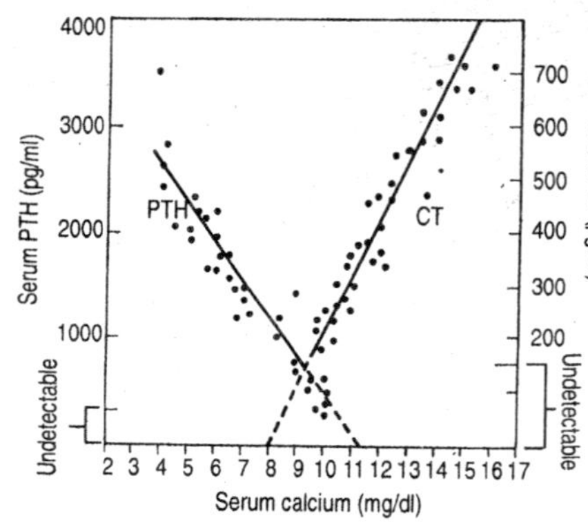

Fig. 9.11: Effect of changes in plasma calcium on parathyroid hormone (PTH) and calcitonin (CT) secretion. (Modified from Arnaud, CD, Littledike T, Tsao HS. Simultaneous measurements of calcitonin and parathyroid hormone in the pig. In Taylor S. Foster GV, eds. Proceedings of the Symposium on Calcitonin and C. Cells. London : Heinemann, 1969, p 99).

3. Role of Vitamin D_3

Vitamin D is also called sunshine vitamin. A metabolite of vitamin D_3 serves as a hormone in calcium homeostasis. The D vitamin, a group of lipid-soluble compounds derived from cholesterol, have long been known to be effective in the prevention of rickets. Vitamin D_3 can be provided by the diet or formed in the skin by the action of ultraviolet light on a precursor, 7-dehydrocholesterol, derived from cholesterol.

D hormone [= calcitriol = (1, 25 – $(OH)_2$–cholecalciferol) : Cholecalciferol (= calciol = "Vitamin" D_3) is formed in the skin by UV-irradiation (sun or UV lamps), from a precursor, 7–dehydrocholesterol, synthesised in the liver. In the absence of sufficient UV-irradiation the amounts of cholecalciferol produced are often inadequate and have to be supplemented via the diet. This is why the substance is termed vitamin. In the liver, cholecalciferol is transformed to 25–OH–cholecalciferol (= calcidiol) from which the active substance itself, 1, 25 – $(OH)_2$ – cholecalciferol, also known as D hormone or calcitriol.

Actions of Vitamin D_3

D hormone or calcitriol induces the synthesis of a specific calcium binding protein in the intestinal cells. This protein increases the intestinal absorption of calcium as well as phosphate. Thus, blood Ca-level is increased by calcitriol. Furthermore, calcitriol stimulates calcium uptake by osteoblasts of bone and promotes calcification or mineralization (deposition of calcium phosphate) and remodelling.

(i) **Action on bones** : The hormone involved in regulating plasma calcium is Vitamin D_3 (cholecalciferol). More precisely, a metabolite of Vit D_3 serves as a hormone in calcium homeostasis. The bones are the sites where cholecalciferol along with PTH and calcitonin interact to enhance or inhibit the resorption of calcium and phosphate into the blood. Vitamin D_3 increases the mobilization of Ca^{++} from bones to enhance serum Ca^{++} level. This mobilization is accelerated by PTH and inhibited by calcitonin.

(ii) **Action on kidney** : Vitamin D_2 and D_3 are by themselves relatively inactive. However, they undergo a series of transformation in kidney that convert them into powerful calcium regulatory hormones. The first step is found in the liver and involves addition of a hydroxyl group to carbon 25, to form 25–hydroxycholecalciferol (25 – OH D_3). Next 25, OH·D_3 is released into the blood, and it undergoes a second hydroxylation reaction on carbon 1 in the kidney. The product is 1, 25–dehydroxycholecalciferol or calcitriol. The reaction in the kidney is catalysed by the enzyme 1α–hydroxylase which is found in the tubule cells [Fig 9.12].

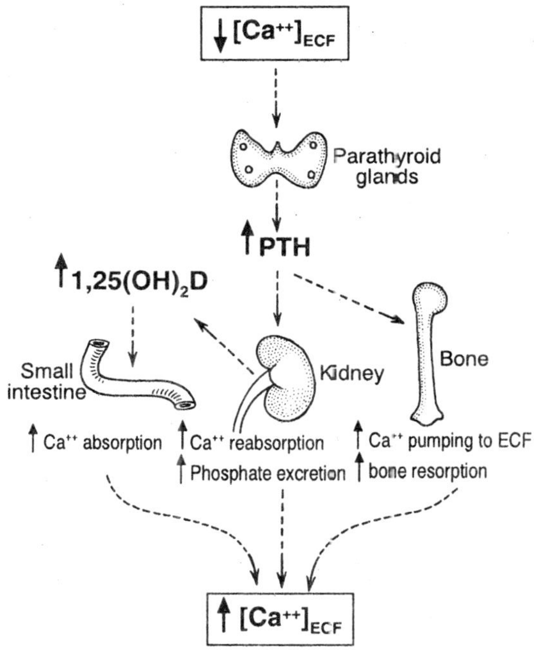

Fig. 9.12: Actions of Vit D_3 on bones and kidney.

(iii) **Action on intestinal mucosa** : Calcitriol (Vit D_3) enhances transepithelial Ca^{++} transport in the intestine by stimulating Ca^{++} entry, and the Ca^{++} uptake in the intestinal mucosa is increased with the help of calbindin D_{28}, by active transport mechanism.

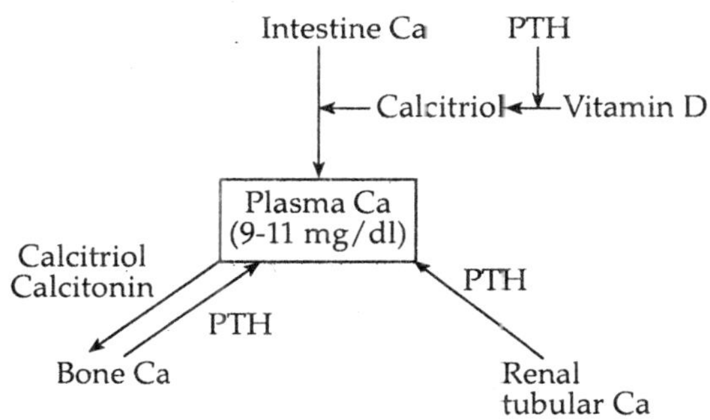

Fig. 9.13: Overview of calcium homeostasis (PTH—Parathyroid hormone).

Osteoporosis : This disease is characterised by demineralization of bone and loss of bone matrix resulting in the progressive loss of bone mass, shrinkage, distortion and increased birttleness of the bones. The elderly people (over 60 yr) of both sexes are at risk for osteoporosis. Here there is not only reduced 1, 25 $(OH)_2$ D_3 secretion, but also PTH plasma levels are diminished. Vitamin D deficiency is a real risk in old age. However, it more predominantly takes place in the postmenopausal women. Osteoporosis results in frequent bone fracture of the arm; vertebral crush, etc. are the major causes of disability among the elderly woman. Osteoporsis may be regarded as a silent thief.

The etiology is largely unknown but it is believed that several causative factors may contribute to it. The ability to produce calcitriol or 1, 25 $(OH)_2$ D_3 from vitamin D is inhibited with age, particularly in the postmenopausal women. Immobilized individuals tend to decrease bone mass while those on regular exercise tend to increase bone mass. It has been reported that osteoporosis is mainly a consequence of decreased ability to absorb sufficient dietary calcium. It may cause due to deficiencies of plasma PTH. Deficiency of sex hormones (in women) has been implicated in the formation of osteoporosis. Estrogen administration along with calcium supplementation to elderly women reduces the risk of fractures. Highly dietary intake of calcium is recommended to avoid this disease.

REGULATION OF HORMONES ON PHOSPHORUS METABOLISM

Phosphate plays a variety of important roles in the body, although its concentration is not as tightly regulated as that of calcium. Many of the factors involved in regulating calcium also affect phosphate.

An adult body contains about 1 kg phosphate and it is present in every cell of the body. Most of it (about 80%) occurs in combination with Ca in the bones and teeth. Phosphorus circulates in the plasma primarily as inorganic orthophosphate (PO_4). Nearly all plasma inorganic is ultrafilterable. In addition to free orthophosphate, phosphate is found in small amounts in the plasma in organic form, such as in hexose or lipid phosphates.

Endocrine control of phosphorus metabolism

Probably all the endocrine glands that are mentioned under calcium take part also in the phosphorus metabolism. The phosphate balance in the body is closely connected with that of Ca^{++}. Normally, the serum phosphate concentration amounts to 0.8-1.4 mmol/l (= 2.5 – 4.3 mg/dl). Calcium phosphate has a low solubility. If the product of the Ca^{++} concentration and the phosphate concentration exceeds a certain value (solubility product), calcium phosphate precipitates out of the solution. In the living organism, calcium phosphate is deposited, mainly in the bones, but in extreme cases in other part of the body as well.

(1) Action of calcitonin (CT)

(i) **On bones :** Calcitonin inhibits inorganic phosphate mobilization from bones into the blood and the effect is the decrease of phosphorus level in the blood.

(ii) **On kidney :** Calcitonin accelerates renal clearance of inorganic phosphate by decreasing the reabsorption from tubular filtrate in the ascending limb of Henle's loop and the distal renal tubule.

(2) Action of parathyroid hormone (PTH)

(i) **On bones :** It accelerates the mobilization of inorganic phosphate from bones into the blood.

(ii) **On intestinal mucosa :** With the help of vit D it enhances intestinal absorption of dietary phosphates.

(iii) **On kidney :** PTH decreases the transmembrane transport and reabsorption of the filtered inorganic phosphate. This enhances urinary excretion of phosphorus and lowers its plasma calcium levels.

It has been shown that if plasma calcium levels fall, PTH secretion increases; in turn, PTH promotes the formation of 1, 25 dihydroxycholecalciferol. In addition, enzyme activity increases in response to a decrease in plasma phosphate. This does not appear to involve any intermediate hormonal signals but apparently involves direct activation of either the enzyme or cells in which the enzyme is located. Both a decrease in plasma calcium which triggers PTH secretion and a decrease in circulating phosphate. In the renal proximal tubular cells, PTH increases the activity of mitochondrial mixed function oxidase, 25(OH)D_3, 1α-hydroxylase to enhance the renal formation of calcitriol (1, 25 $[OH]_2D_3$) which in its turn increases intestinal absorption of Ca^{++}.

Chapter 10

Hormone Mechanisms of Action in Thermoregulation, Osmoregulation and Excretion

TEMPERATURE HOMEOSTASIS

Homeostasis literally means "same state" and it refers to the process of keeping the internal body environment in a steady state, when the external environment is changed. The importance of this cannot be overstressed, as it allows enzymes, etc. to be 'fine tuned' to a particular set of conditions and so as to operate more efficiently. Much of the hormone system and autonomic nervous system are dedicated to homeostasis and their action is coordinated by the **hypothalamus.**

Thermoregulation or Temperature Homeostasis

One of the most important examples of homeostasis is the regulation of body temperature. Not all the animals can do this physiologically. Animals that maintain a fairly constant body temperature (birds and mammals) are called **endotherms,** while those that have a variable body temperature (all others) are called **ectotherms**. The animal kingdom can be broadly classified into two groups, depending on their body temperature. Those who can maintain their body temperature relatively constant in the face of wide variations of environmental temperature are known as **warm-blooded** animals or **homoiotherms,** whereas those whose temperature fluctuates with fluctuations of the environmental temperature are termed **cold blooded** animals or **poikilotherms.** All homeostatic mechanisms use **negative feedback** to maintain a constant value (called the **setpoint**). In the course of evolution, from poikilotherms to homiotherms, there exist another group who are known as **hibernants,** going into hibernation in winter, otherwise behaving like the warm-blooded animals in the remaining period. Hibernating mammals do not require an external source of heat to raise their body temperature to normal and can rouse themselves probably by activating their large stores of brown fat. Some mammals release hormones that reduce their setpoint to around 5 °C while they hibernate. This drastically reduces their metabolic rate and so conserve their food reserves, e.g., hedgehogs. Bats and humming birds reduce their setpoint everyday while they are inactive. They have a high surface area/volume ratio, so they reduce heat loss.

In humans, body temperature is controlled by the **thermoregulatory centre** in the

hypothalamus. It receives input from two sets of thermoreceptors in the hypothalamus itself to monitor the temparature of the blood as it passes through the brain (core temperature), and receptors in the skin (especially on the trunk) monitor the external temperature. Both sets of information are needed so that the body can make appropriate adjustments.

and heat loss (thermolysis). The body keeps its core temperature constant at about 37 °C by physiological adjustments controlled by the hypothalamus (thermostat centre) where there are neurons sensitive to changes in skin and blood temperatures. The temperature–regulating centres are found in the

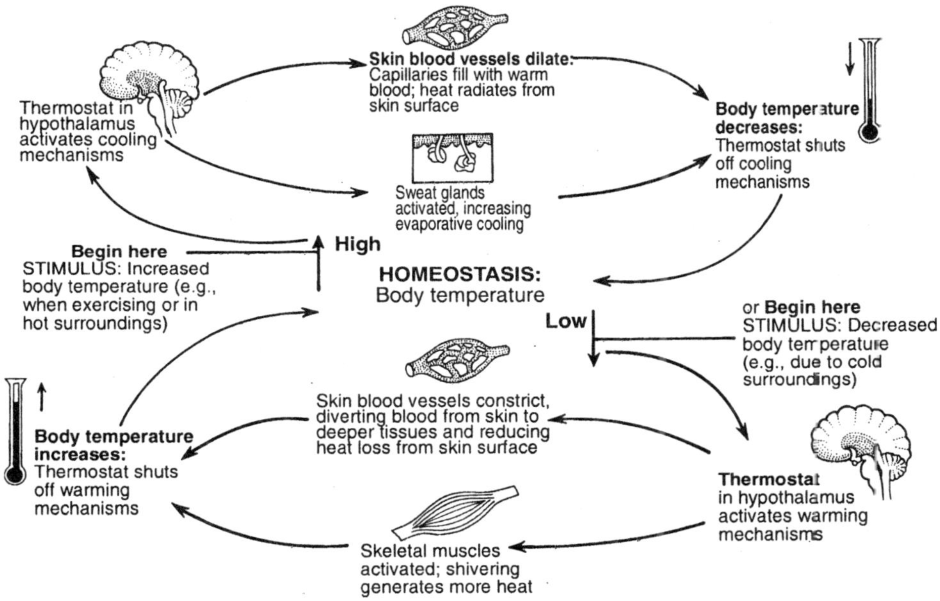

Fig. 10.1: Thermoregulation.

The thermoregulatory centre sends impulses to several different effectors to adjust body temperature [Fig 10.1].

Normal temperature

Oral 37 °F–99 °F or 36.11 °C–37.22 °C (average 98.4 °F or 36.89 °C). Axillary or groin temperature is 1 °F or 0.55 °C less while oesophageal temperature is 1 °F or 0.55 °C more.

Endocrine control of thermoregulation

Endocrine system is intimately related with the temperature homeostasis in mammals. Certain endocrine glands like pituitary, thyroid, adrenal glands, etc. also take part in heat production (thermogenesis)

anterior portion of the hypothalamus. This area receives imput from temperature receptors in the skin and mucous membranes (peripheral thermoreceptors) and from internal structures (central thermoreceptors) which include under the hypothalamus itself. The hypothalamic thermostat works in conjunction with other hypothalamic, autonomic and higher nervous thermoregulatory centres to keep the core temperature constant.

(i) Role of hormones in response to cold

The snow storm drops our skin temperature quickly. This stimulates skin cold receptors (increase in their activity) and cools the blood flowing into the skin. These signals are received by both the hypothalamic thermostat and higher cortical centres. The thermostat is also activated by the change in blood temperature. It initiates responses that promote heat gain and inhibits centres that promote heat loss. The activation of sympathetic centres results in several responses including :

(a) **Action of medullary hormones :**

(i) Epinephrine secretion from adrenal medulla increases thermogenesis. The hypothalamus is activated to initiate involuntary contraction of skeletal muscles causing shivering, which generates heat.

(ii) Norepinephrine secretion from sympathetic nerve fibres constricts vessels of integument.

(iii) Oxidation of brown fat increases thermogenesis.

(iv) Piloerection takes place which traps air close to skin.

(b) **Action of thyroid hormones :**

Again, when the environmental temperature decreases gradually, the hypothalamus releases TRH which activates the anterior pituitary gland to secrete TSH. This TSH induces the thyroid gland to liberate large amounts of T_3 and T_4 (thyroid hormones) into the blood. The thyroid hormone increases BMR which increases thermogenesis. So the hypothalamus sensors detect the warmth and diminish the heat producing and heat loss prevention responses.

(ii) Role of hormones in response to heat

When the body is exposed to heat (sun, fire, too much clothing), body temperature rises. Skin warmth receptors and blood convey these changes to the hypothalamic thermostat. The thermostat inhibits the adrenergic activity of the sympathetic nervous system, which regulates vaso-constriction and BMR, thus causing cutaneous vasodilation and reducing BMR.

Thyroxine takes part in regulation of normal body temperature. Less thyroxine secretion increases susceptibility to moderate cold. Thyroxine may cause catabolism of depot fat. The oxidative catabolism may lead to the formation of glucose by the process of neoglucogenesis and also there will be more production of heat. The thyroid gland is intimately related to thermoregulation as T_4 and T_3 influence the BMR in all cells. Hence, in **hyperthyroidism** condition temperature increases because the BMR is raised, there is increased oxygen consumption, the patient is hyperactive and adrenal function is enhanced. Hence body temperature is raised; the sufferer feels hot and does not like warm environments. Compensation takes the normal form of vaso-dilation and sweating, giving the classical symptoms of clammy, warm skin. The exact reverse is true for **hypothyroidism condition :** an inability to elevate core temperature to the desired set point leaves the sufferer cold and unhappy in cold environments.

(iii) Role of medullary hormones in response to heat production

Epinephrine is calorigenic and heat production is immediate but comes to normal level quickly. It enhances oxygen consumption and BMR.

Epinephrine stimulates liver glycogenolysis and may cause elevation of body temperature. Thermogenesis is affected by neoglucogenesis.

Again, the epinephrine along with norepinephrine activate lipase enzyme in adipose tissue and increase the formation of free fatty acids in blood after breakdown of triglycerides.

OSMOREGULATION

Osmoregulation term was coined by Hober in 1902 and it refers to the **collective activity of the variety of mechanisms used by organisms to control water movement and water volumes in the body.** According to him, osmoregulation implies the maintenance of an internal osmotic concentration different from that of the external medium. Along with this, it is also to be kept in mind that the distribution of ions also vary in the external and internal environment of an organism and also between the various compartments within the organism. The ionic differences which are essential for proper functioning of tissues and cells are controlled by various mechanisms which fall under the study of **ionic regulation.** Because of water and ionic regulations are inseparable activities in organisms, as such the term osmoregulation is now considered to include both activities.

Osmotic environment and animals

Generally the animals live in four sorts of environments. They are either marine, freshwater, terrestrial or brackish water dwellers. Each of these environments presents particular problems which are to be overcome by the animals living in them.

Aquatic animals can be categorised as below on the basis of their abilities to survive in different osmotic environments.

(a) **Stenohaline** (Greek *Stenos* = narrow, close; *halos* = salt) organisms have a limited tolerance to changes in the osmotic concentration of the external environment. Most animals fall into this category.

(b) **Euryhaline** (Greek *eurys* = wide, broad; *halos* = salt) forms are able to withstand a wide range of osmotic concentrations.

(c) **Osmoconformers** have an internal concentration which varies in parallel with changes in the external environment, i.e., animals who can adjust with changed medium by changing the osmotic concentration of the body fluid so that ultimately they become iso-osmotic to the surrounding medium. In fact, they are incapable of osmoregulation.

(d) **Osmoregulators** are those animals which maintain the osmotic concentration of body fluid at a constant state inspite of changes or no changes of the osmotic concentration of the medium.

(e) **Ionic conformers** regulate the concentration of inorganic ions and other solutes in their body fluids. They are called **ionic regulators.** The animals which possess little ability to regulate internal ionic concentrations are called **ionic conformers**.

Hormonal control of osmoregulation

The water potential of the blood must be regulated to prevent loss or gain of water from cells. Blood water homeostasis is controlled by the hypothalamus. It contains **osmoreceptor cells,** which can detect changes in the water potential of the blood passing through the brain. In response, the hypothalamus controls the sensation of thirst and it also secretes the hormone ADH, which is stored in the posterior pituitary gland and its target cells are the endothelial cells of collecting ducts of the kidney nephrons. These cells are unusual in that water molecules can pass only across their membranes via water channels called **aquaporins** rather than through the lipid bilayer. ADH cause these water channels to open. In addition to that cortisol, prolactin, growth hormone, thyroid hormone, etc. also play important role in osmoregulation.

(i) Action of cortisol and marine acclimation

Cortisols, produced by the interrenal tissue of freshwater teleost fish, improve their subsequent survival and capacity to maintain low levels of plasma ions after exposure to sea water. This effect is due to increases in the size and abundance of gill-mitochondrion-rich cells. The effect of exogenous cortisol generally requires several days to reach its peak, suggesting that the cell differentiation and proliferation are required for its complete action.

The release of cortisol from the inter-renal is primarily controlled by the ACTH, though other endocrine factors may also be involved. This ACTH production does not appear to be directly responsive to changes in external osmolality. The increase in cortisol during osmotic stress occurs in stenohaline and euryhaline fishes and may be part of a general stress response. Thus, the presence and regulation of cortisol receptors are also a critical component of osmoregulation.

(ii) Action of cortisol and freshwater acclimation

Cortisol is also involved in ion uptake, thus giving it a dual osmoregulatory function. Cortisol treatment in freshwater fish increases the surface area of gill mitochondrion-rich cells and the influx of sodium and chloride, affecting both renal and branchial functions.

Cortisol is also required to maintain water movement across the gut of freshwater eels. Cortisol treatment significantly increases the ion regulatory capacity of marine fish during exposure to low salinity and the ability of acid-resistant fish to maintain plasma sodium levels after exposure to acidic water.

So changes in circulating levels of cortisol also provide supporting evidence for a role of this hormone in ion uptake. Transfer of euryhaline species from sea water to freshwater results in short term increases in plasma cortisol. Again, transfer of several species of marine fish from high to low salinity results in increased circulating cortisol that remain elevated for few days to weeks.

(iii) Role of prolactin on osmoregulation

Prolactin has been shown to have sodium and chloride retaining activity in a variety of freshwater and euryhaline teleosts. It has been shown to affect chloride cells and promoting the morphology of ion uptake cells. Prolactin treatment also reduces ion and water permeability of the oesophagus and intestine, a response that normally occurs during acclimation to freshwater.

Both prolactin and cortisol are necessary for normal ion-regulation in freshwater. The two may even interact to control ion uptake. These two hormones together cause a greater elevation of plasma ions than either hormone alone.

(iv) Role of growth hormone (GH) and IGF-I

A major route of the osmoregulatory action of GH is through its capacity to increase circulating levels and local tisssue production of insulin-like growth factor-I (IGF-I). Exogenous treatment of IGF-I has been found to increase the salinity tolerance of rainbow trout, Atlantic salmon (*Salmo osalar*), and killifish (*Fundulus beteroclitus*). GH cannot directly increase gill NKA activity, whereas IGF-I can do.

In addition to the effects of exogenous hormones, changes in gene expression, secretion, circulating levels, and metabolic clearance rate of GH and IGF-I also provide evidence for the osmoregulatory actions of the GH/IGF-I axis in several euryhaline

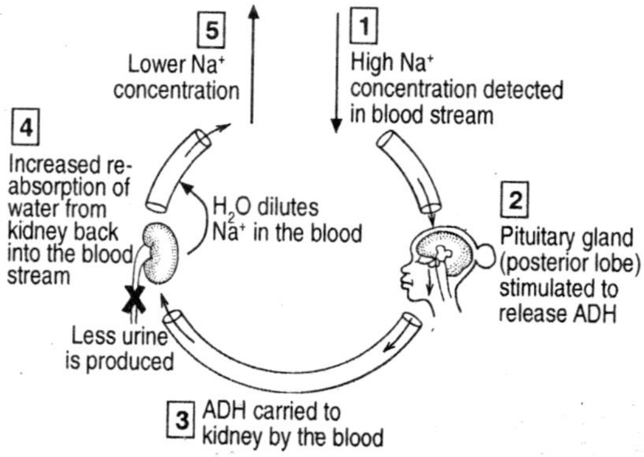

Fig. 10.2: Hormonal regulaton on excretion.

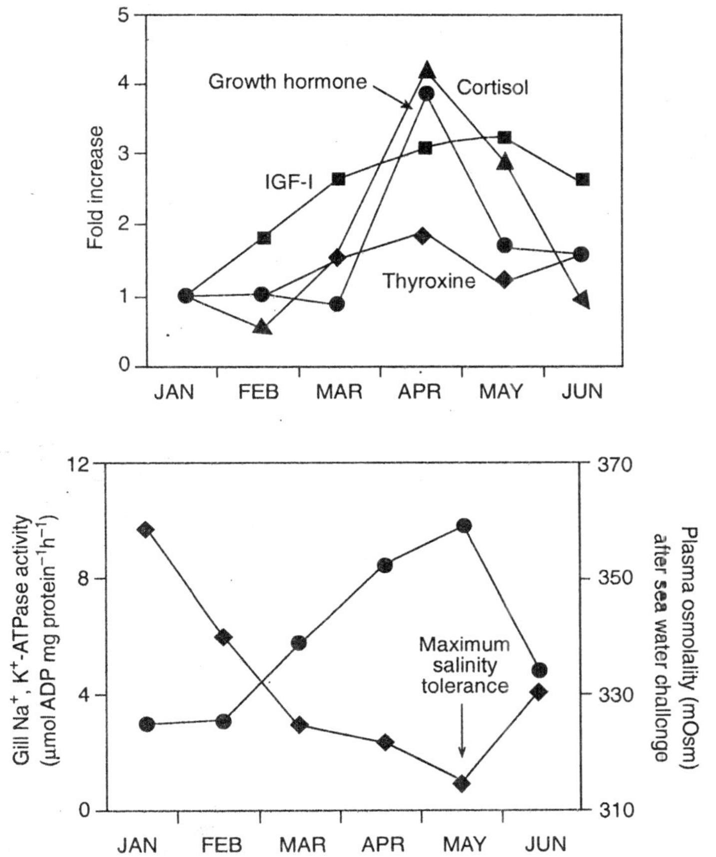

Fig. 10.3: Changes in plasma hormone levels, gill NKA activity, and salinity tolerance during the parr-smolt transformation of Atlantic salmon. Interaction among cortisol, growth hormone, IGF-I, and thyroid hormones results in physiological changes that are preparatory for sea water entry. Adapted from McCormick SD, Lerner DT, Monette MY, Nieves–Puigdoller K, and Bjornsson BTh (2009).

species. Plasma GH levels have also been found to increase in stenohaline freshwater fish following exposure to brackish water.

The GH/IGF-I and cortisol axis work together to regulate salt secretion in teleosts. Injection of GH and cortisol together increases gill NKA activity and salinity tolerance in salmonids and killifish to a greater extent than either hormone alone [Fig 10.3].

(iv) Role of thyroid hormones on osmoregulation

Thyroid hormones play atleast a supportive role in sea water acclimation, and may interact with both the GH/IGF-I and cortisol axis. Inhibition of the thyroid axis with thiomea in killifish caused increased plasma ions in sea water but had no effect in freshwater. T_4 treatment alone has no effect, but potentiates the action of cortisol on gill NKA activity in Tilapia, and the action of GH on gill NKA activity in salmon. Inhibiting the conversion of T_4 to T_3 interferes with normal and GH-induced sea water acclimation in trout. T_3 treatment increases the number of gill cortisol receptors in trout and salmon. Thyroid hormones thus appear to exert their influence on salt secretory mechanisms primarily through an interaction with cortisol and the GH/IGF-I axis.

HORMONAL REGULATION ON EXCRETION

The kidney tubule regulation of the salt and water in our bodies is the most important factor in determining the urine volume. Our urine is produced not only in order to eliminate many of the cellular waste products, but also to control both the amount and the composition of the extracellular fluid in the body. Controlling the amount of water and chemicals in the body is essential to life, and our body does so by producing various amounts of urine so that we can either excrete the "extra" water and chemicals (mainly sodium) or conserve the water and chemicals when they are in short supply. Therefore, the volume that we excrete everyday is a reflection of how much extracellular fluid and sodium our bodies have to spare. Too much water and salt in our bodies are dangerous. Therefore, the level of water and salts excreted in urine—the urine volume—is adjusted to the needs of the body.

Control of urine volume through hormones

(i) Role of ADH : The two endocrine glands that are concerned with the regulation of fluid balance within the body are the **pituitary gland** and the **adrenal gland**. The pituitary is insignificant in appearance but it packs an extremely powerful punch. The pituitary is actually two glands in one—posterior and anterior. Of the two, the **posterior pituitary** manufactures no hormones of its own, but stores two that are initially secreted in a part of the brain known as the **hypothalamus.** These hormones are **oxytocin** (a hormone responsible for stimulating labour at the end of pregnancy) and **anti-diuretic hormone** (ADH), which helps the body to retain its fluids. An anti-diuretic, on the other hand, is a chemical that inhibits urine formation. ADH produces its anti-diuretic effect by acting on the kidneys and causing them to reduce the amount of water they excrete. In this way, ADH is important in regulating the water concentration of body fluids, which ultimately helps to maintain an appropriate sodium concentration in the body. In fact, the sodium concentration in the extracellular fluid is the factor that either stimulates the pituitary to release ADH or to inhibit the release of ADH.

The release of ADH is regulated by hypothalamus. Apparently certain sensors in this part of the brain are sensitive to changes in the salt concentration of body fluids, particularly the blood. If for example, a person is sweating and losing large amounts of water, the sodium in the blood becomes more and more concentrated. The hypothalamus can sense this high concentration of sodium and it signals the posterior lobe of the pituitary to release ADH. This ADH is transmitted by the blood to the kidneys causing the kidney tubules to re-absorb more water into the blood stream to dilute the sodium. As a result of this effect, less urine is produced. This action conserves water in the body. The mechanism of action seems to be that the presence of ADH makes distal and collecting tubules in the nephrons more permeable to water. That is, water is moved more easily through the tubule membrane back into the blood and less urine is produced. For this reason ADH is referred to as the "water retaining hormone" [Fig 10.2].

If, on the other hand, a person drinks excess of water, the sodium in the body fluids including the blood becomes more dilute and the release of ADH is inhibited. The lack of ADH causes the distal and collecting tubules to become practically impermeable to water, and little or no water is reabsorbed from them back into the blood. Consequently, the kidneys excrete more watery urine until the water concentration of the body fluids returns to normal.

(ii) Role of hormones of adrenal cortex : The second set of glands that participate in the regulation of body fluids is the **adrenal glands.** The adrenals sit on top of each kidney like a cap and they generally look like pyramids. The central portion of this gland is termed the **adrenal medulla** and the outer part is the **adrenal cortex.** All of the hormones secreted by the adrenal cortex are **steroids** and these are also termed as **adreno corticosteroids.** Among the corticosteroids, the **mineralocorticoids** help to regulate the concentrations of extracellular electrolytes and the **glucocorticoids** influence the metabolism of carbohydrates, proteins and fats.

The aldosterone hormone of adrenal cortex stimulates K^+ secretion by the tubular cells latic in the nephron simultaneous to entrance in the cells as reabsorption of Na^+. An elevation in plasma K^+ concentration directly stimulates the adrenal cortex to increase its output of aldosterone which is an elimination of the excess K^+. Conversely, a decline in secretion and a corresponding decrease in aldosterone stimulate renal K^+ secretion [Fig 10.4].

Again, a rise in plasma K^+ concentration directly stimulates aldosterone secretion, whereas a fall in plasma Na^+ concentration stimulates aldosterone secretion by means of the complex renin-angiotensin pathway. Increased aldosterone secretion always promotes simultaneous Na^+ reabsorption and K^+ secretion. For this reason, K^+ secretion can be inadvertently stimulated as a result of increased aldosterone activity brought about by Na^+ depletion, ECF volume reduction, or a fall in arterial pressure totally unrelated to K^+ balance. The resultant in appropriate loss of K^+ can lead to K^+ deficiency.

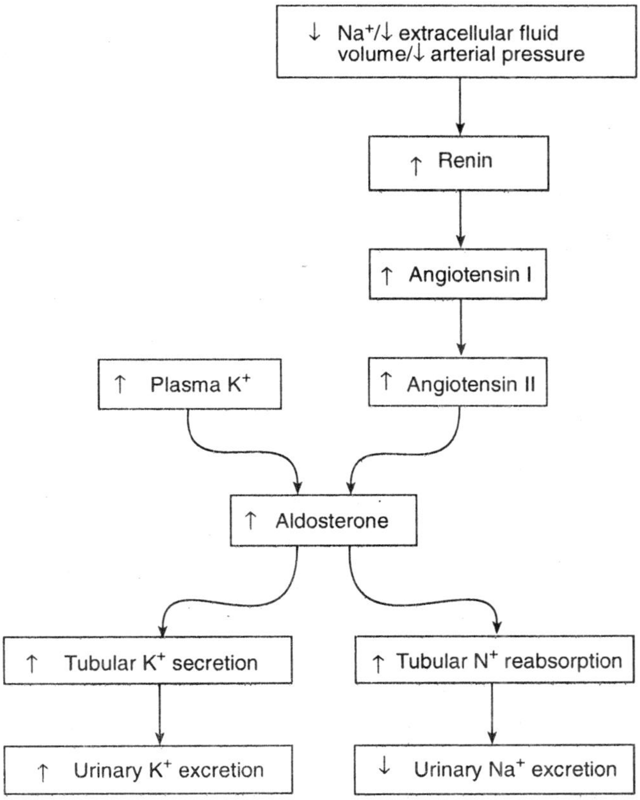

Fig. 10.4: Dual control of aldosterone secretion by K^+ and Na^+.

CHAPTER 11

Accessory Sex Organs

The primary reproductive organs of male and female are **testis** and **ovary** respectively. The sex organs or glands other than principal reproductive organs, which are involved in the transmission of gametes or the developing zygote from the place of their origin to perform various functions of reproductive process are termed as **accessory sex organs.**

IN MALES

In male the following accessory genital glands or organs are found—a pair of epididymis, a pair of vasa deferentia, a pair of seminal vesicles, a single prostate gland, a pair of cowper's gland and a single penis [Fig 11.1].

Epididymis

Each testis gives rise to numerous fine tubues which form together a hump around the testis known as **epididymis.** The epididymis is a crescent shaped structure that divides into three regions, namely **caput** (head), **corpus** (body) and **cauda** (tail). The caput is the largest and most cranial portion of epididymis. The corpus or body is narrow and runs along the medial border of the testis. The caudal part opens in the **ductus deferens.** The length of the epididymis varies in different mammals but generally it measures about 7.5 cm in length. The ventral part of it continues into vas deferens.

Histology : The epididymis consists of the efferent ductules and the duct of the epididymis and associated blood vessels, smooth muscles and connective tissue coverings. Practically the epididymis is lined by pseudo-stratified columnar epithelium. The columnar epithelium comprises of two types of cells—**principal cells** and **basal cells.**

(a) **Principal cells :** The principal cells vary from about 80 μm in height in the head of the epididymis to 40 μm in height in the tail. Numerous long and modified microvilli, called **stereocilia,** extend from the luminal surface of the principal cells.

(b) **Basal cells :** The small, round basal cells rest on the basal lamina. These are the stem cells of the duct epithelium and they are short columnar cells containing few cytoplasmic organelles. In addition, intraepithelial lymphocytes, called **balo cells,** are observed in the epithelium.

Functions :

(i) Acts as store house of sperms.

(ii) Helps in the maturation of sperms.

(iii) Acts as 'sperm exit' route from the testis.

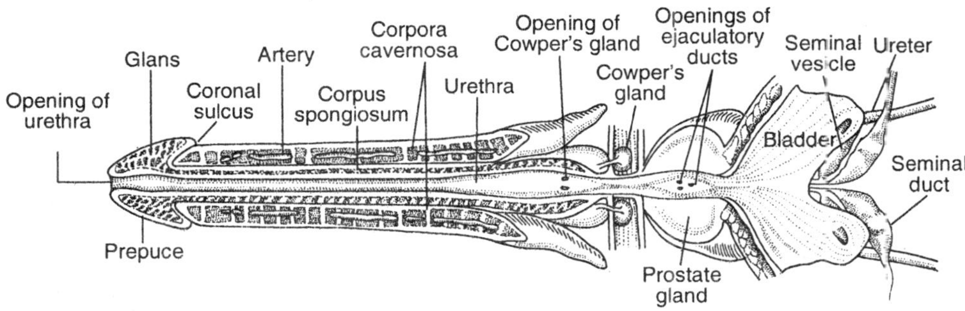

Fig. 11.1: A detailed view of the penis showing all its parts.

Vas deferens (Ductus deferens)

The ductus deferens is a direct continuation of the tail of epididymis. It ascends along the posterior border of the testis, arches over the ureter and continues medially to the base of the urinary bladder where it receives the seminal vesicle. Ultimately two ducts open into a median slit within the urethra. Each deferent duct is supported by a **mesoductus deferens** which extends through the spermatic cord as a separate fold of peritoneum. The terminal portion of each vas deferens enlarges to form the ampulla. The ampulla is joined there by the duct of the **seminal vesicle** and continues through the prostate gland to the urethra as the **ejaculatory duct.**

Histology : The ducts deferens is lined with a pseudostratified columnar epithelium like that of epididymis. The tall columnar cells have also long microvilli that extend into the lumen and the rounded basal cells rest on the basal lamina. The lumen of the duct does not appear smooth but it appears to be thrown into deep longitudinal folds.

The ampulla has taller, branched mucosal folds that often show glandular diverticula. The muscle coat surrounding the ampulla is thinner than that of the rest of the ductus deferens and the longitudinal layers disappear near the origin of the ejaculatory duct. The epithelial cells are provided with large numbers of yellow pigment granules. The wall of the ejaculatory duct have fibromuscular tissue instead of muscularis layer.

Functions :

(i) The proximal part of the vas deferens serves as the store house of spermatozoon.

(ii) In this storage part the sperms become motile after mixing with the secretion of accessory gland.

Seminal vesicle

Paired seminal vesicles are cylindrical, elongated and translucent sac like structures situated in close association with vas deferens and urethra, the free ends of which are bifid and sacculated. The seminal vesicles are the largest amongst the accessory glands. Each gland measures abcut 5 cm in length which is folded upon itself, the two seminal vesicles converge medially and open into the urethra by two separate ducts. The lumen of the seminal vesicles are filled up with a milky white fluid.

Histology : Histologically the wall of the seminal vesicles contains a mucosa, a thin layer of smooth muscle and a fibrous coat. The mucosa is thrown into numerous folds that increase the secretory surface area.

The pseudostratified columnar epithelium contains tall, non-ciliated columnar cells and short, round cells that rest on the basal lamina. The short cells appear identical to those of the rest of the excurrent duct system. These are the stem cells from which the columnar cells are derived. The columnar epithelial cells are non-ciliated and contain well apparent ribosomes, Golgi-bodies rER, yellowish lipochrome pigments and large secretory vacuoles in the apical cytoplasm.

Functions :

(i) The secretion of the seminal vesicles contains fructose which is used for the nourishment of the sperms.

(ii) The seminal fluid provides bulk of semen.

(iii) The seminal fluid also provides precursors for clotting of semen.

(iv) The seminal vesicles synthesize prostaglandins that stimulate the motility of sperms through the female genital tract after mating and help to flush sperms out of the urethra in male.

Prostate gland

The prostate is the largest accessory sex glands of the male reproductive system. It lies caudo-medial to the coagulation gland and its size and shape are compared to those of a walnut. This prostate gland consists of two pairs of lobes—large dorsal and small ventral, and the lobes are joined by isthmus. Each gland shows alveolations and it consists of 30-50 tubulo-alveolar glands. The ducts from the individual glands converge to open directly into the urethra. This prostate gland contributes about 15-30% of the total volume of semen. The secretion of the prostate gland comprises of prostatic acids, phosphatase (PAP), fibrinolysin, citric acid and prostate-specific antigen (PSA).

Histology : The prostate gland is covered by vascular capsule. It is composed by fibro-elastic tissue, plain muscles and mucosal glands. The prostate glands are tubulo-alveolar, containing a low cubical or pseudostratified columnar epithelium, highly folded upon itself. The secretory granules are found in the supra-nuclear portion of the epithelial cells. E.M reveals that epithelial cells possess luminal microvilli. Ribosomes and Golgi bodies are well developed.

Functions :

(i) The secretion of the gland increases the volume of semen.

(ii) The enzyme acid phosphatase of the prostatic fluid helps in nutrition of the spermatozoon.

(iii) The secretion lubricates the passage of urethra.

(iv) The fibrinolysin in the secretion serves to liquefy the semen.

Cowper's gland or bulbo-urethral gland

These are paired glands. Each gland is a small and pea-sized structure but lobulated tubuloalveolar gland. It is about 1 cm in diameter. The cowper gland is connected to the urethra by a single duct. The duct of each gland passes through the inferior fascia of urogenital diaphragm and joins the initial portion of the penile urethra.

Histology : The glands are compound tubuloalveolar glands that structurally resemble mucus secretory glands. Each gland is outerly covered by fibrous capsule and is made up of many glandular lobules which are held together by fibrous connective tissue and smooth muscle fibres.

The glandular epithelial cells vary in size and shape from columnar to low cuboidal. The cytoplasm of these epithelial cells are provided with mucoid droplets and acidophilic spindle-shaped bodies. The duct of the bulbourethral gland is lined by pseudostratified epithelium.

Function : The clear, mucus-like glandular secretion serves to lubricate the penile urethra during sexual intercourse.

Urethra

The urethra is a long muscular passage which communicates with the exterior of the body through a muscular structure, called **penis.** The male urethra differs functionally from the female urethra and is divided into two portions—pelvic portion and spongy portion. The pelvic portion extends from the neck of the urinary bladder to the penis and receives most of the ducts of accessory glands. The spongy portion remains embedded within the corpus spongiosum of the penis. The penis is the male copulatory organ which consists of **body** and a **glans.** There is fold of loose skin that attaches to the penis at the junction of the body and glans, known as **prepuce**. The glans is shorter than the body. It is cylindrical and ends in a rounded tip. The tip bears the **urethral orifice**.

Histology : The urethra is made up of strands of smooth muscle fibres and elastic fibres. The body of penis is composed of three highly erectile vascularised spongy tissue layers. Two dorsal layers are known as **corpora-cavernosa** and one ventral layer is called corpus spongiosum. The terminal part of the penis is called the glans which is formed only by the terminal end of the **corpus spongiosum**. The penis is enveloped by tunica albugenia. The **os-penis** is present on the dorsal surface of the glans.

Functions :

(i) Assists in transport of seminal fluid to the interior of the female genital tract.

(ii) Acts as a common passage both for the transfer of semen as well as urine.

IN FEMALES

In female the following accessory organs are seen to assist the functional activities of reproductive system.

Oviduct

Two narrow oviducts **(Fallopian tube)** are placed mainly on the dorso-lateral regions of the ovaries. This tubular structure is supported by broad ligament and is referred to as **uterine tube.** The oviduct is approximately 10 to 12 cm long and 1 mm in diameter. Each oviduct can be divided into four segments; such as **infundibulum, ampulla, fimbriae** and **isthmus.**

The terminal funnel-like triangular expansion of the cranial part of oviduct is known as **infundibulum** which is adjacent to ovary. The posterior longest segment of the infundibulum is known as ampulla and it is the site of fertilization. The infundibulum is provided with irregular ventral projections and these projections are called **fimbriae.** They extend from the mouth of the infundibulum toward the ovary. The **isthmus** is the narrow medial segment of the posterior part of the oviduct adjacent to the uterus [Fig 11.2].

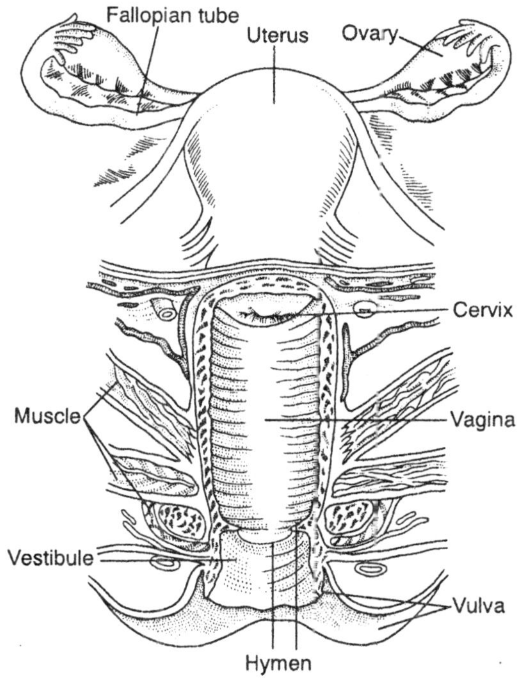

Fig. 11.2: The vagina is a tough muscular canal situated between the uterus and the vulva. Its corrugated structure is specifically designed to give it the amazing elasticity needed for the birth of a baby.

Histology : Histologically it is composed of three layers :

(i) **Serosa :** The serosa is the outermost layer of the oviduct and is composed of mesothelium and a thin layer of filbrous connective tissue.

(ii) **Muscularis layer :** This layer is organised into an inner, relatively thick circular layer and an outer, thinner longitudinal layer. The boundary between these layers is often indistinct.

(iii) **Mucosa layer :** The inner mucosa layer exhibits relatively thin longitudinal folds that project into the lumen of the oviduct throughout its length. These folds are most numerous and complex in the ampulla and become smaller in the isthmus. The mucosal lining is simple columnar epithelium and is composed of two kinds of cells—ciliated and non-ciliated epithelial cells.

Functions :

(i) After ovulation the oviduct helps to transport the ovum from the ovary to the uterus.

(ii) Provide the necessary environment for fertilization and initial development of the zygote to the morula stage.

Uterus

The uterus is the bicornuate 'y' shaped elongated organ. It is the largest organ of the female reproductive tract, extending between the oviducts cranially and vagina caudally. Anatomically the uterus consists of two **horns,** a **body** and a **cervix.** The two **horns** converge in the midline to form the **uterine body**. The body is the large upper portion of the uterus. The large anterior upper rounded portion of the body is known as **fundus.** The **cervix** is the lower, barrel-shaped part of the uterus separated from the body by the **isthmus.** The lumen of the cervix has a constricted opening or **os** at each end. The **internal os** communicates with the cavity of the uterus and the end which opens into the vagina, called **external os.**

Histology : Histologically the uterine wall is composed of three layers. From the lumen outward they are :

(i) **Endometrium :** The inner lining of the uterus is mucosal layer. It is made up of epithelium, spiral artery, uterine gland, etc. The thickness of this layer varies in different phase of reproductive cycle.

(ii) **Myometrium :** It is the thick muscular layer which is continuous with the muscle layer of the uterine tube and the vagina. The smooth muscle fibres extend into the ligaments connected to the uterus. This layer is richly supplied with blood capillaries and lymphatic vessels.

(iii) **Perimetrium :** It is the outer serous layer or visceral peritoneal covering of the uterus. The perimetrium layer consists of a mesothelium and a thin layer of loose connective tissue. Beneath the mesothelium, a layer of elastic tissue is usually prominent. This layers covers the entire posterior surface of the uterus but only a part of the anterior surface. The remaining part of the anterior surface is made up of fibrous connective tissue.

Both myometrium and endometrium undergo cyclic changes each month to prepare the uterine bed for nidation. If an embryo implants, the cycle stops, and both the layers undergo considerable development during pregnancy.

Vagina

It is a dorsoventrally flattend organ and internally many longitudinal ridges are present. In other words, it is a pink coloured fibromuscular tube extending from the cervix to the vestibule which is the area between the labia minora. In a virgin, the opening into the vagina may be surrounded by folds of mucous membrane called the **hymen,** extending into the vaginal lumen.

Histology : The vaginal wall consists of an inner mucosal layer, an intermediate muscular layer and an outer adventitial layer.

(i) **Mucosal layer :** The inner mucosal layer has numerous transverse folds and is lined with stratified squamous epithelium. Connective tissue papillae from the underlying lamina project into the epithelial layer.

This layer is devoid of any glands but the vaginal surface is lubricated by mucus from the cervix.

(ii) **Muscular layer** : This intermediate layer is organised into two indistinct, intermingling smooth muscle layers—an outer longitudinal layer and an inner circular layer. The outer layer is much thicker than the inner.

(iii) **Adventitial layer** : This layer is organised into an inner dense connective tissue layer and an outer loose connective tissue layer. The inner layer contains numerous elastic fibres and the outer layer is provided with numerous blood capillaries and lymphatic vessels and nerves.

Mammary gland

The mammary glands, or breasts, are a distinguishing feature of mammals. The mammary glands though accessory organs of reproduction are really specialised sweat glands in the subcutaneous tissues. The mammary gland in the functional state is a compound tubulo-alveolar gland. During embryonic development, growth and development of breast tissue occur in both sexes. Multiple glands develop along paired epidermal thickenings, called **mammary ridges (milk lines),** which extend from the developing axilla to the developing inguinal region. In humans, normally only one group of cells develop into a breast on each side. Each breast covers a nearly circular space anterior to pectoralis muscles from 2nd rib to the 6th rib and from the sternum into the axilla [Fig 11.3].

In males, the glands remain rudimentary. In females, the mammary glands undergo further development under hormonal influence. These glands are also influenced by changes in ovarian hormone levels during each menstrual cycle. The initiation of milk secretion is induced by prolactin secreted by the anterior pituitary. The ejection of the milk from the mammary gland is stimulated by oxytocin released from the neurophysis. With the change in the hormonal environment at menopause, the glandular component of the breast atrophies, and is replaced by fat and fibrous connective tissue.

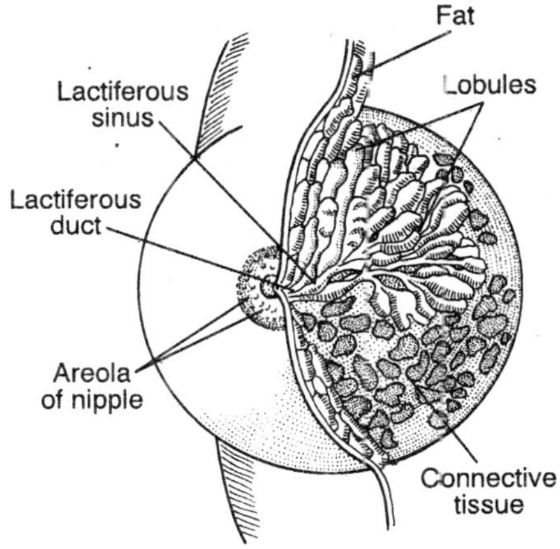

Fig. 11.3: Structure of the mammary gland showing its different structures.

Histology : Breast is a cutaneous structure. It develops as an evagination of the surface epithelium into the underlying connective tissue as solid columns of cells. Later on, the cell columns become hollowed out into ducts. These ducts branch out into terminal tubules which end in alveoli that secrete milk.

The alveoli remain modified muscle fibres, called myoepithelium. These are elongated and longitudinally striated cells. On each side the breast comprises of 15-20 lobes separated by connective tissue septa. In the lactating phase the number and size of alveoli increase and the secreting cells remain filled up with minute fat droplets. The secretion of this gland is discharged by rupture of the free ends of the cells, leaving the nucleus and basal lamina intact. At menopause the involution occurs, the gland atrophies, fatty tissue degenerates and only fibrous tissues persist. At puberty the structural components of the mammary glands are composed of glandular tissue. In functional state the mammary gland is a compound tubulo-alveolar gland. The larger ducts open at the nipple where a stratified squamous epithelium is continuous with two-layered columnar of the primary duct. The larger ducts (lactiferous ducts) are lined by an inner tall columnar layer and an outer cuboidal layer of epithelial cells. Smaller ducts have a single layer of colummar epithelial cells. The smallest ducts and alveoli contain irregularly depressed myoepithelial cells near the basement membrane. The basement membrane is enveloped by a loose stroma, especially about the smallest intralobular ducts and alveoli. The intralobular stroma contrasts with the interlobular stroma. Fatty lobules into which ducts project and in which lobules develop, contribute the looser intralobular stroma and more compact interlobular stroma.

Lactating breast produces milk containing unique proteins, casein, lactoglobulins, lactoalbumin, lactose and fats. Fats first appear in the secretory cells as small droplets. These fat droplets enlarge as they become more apically located and these droplets are always surrounded by smooth membranes. Fat is often observed in the epithelial cells of the smaller ducts and alveoli of nonlactating mammary gland [Fig 11.4].

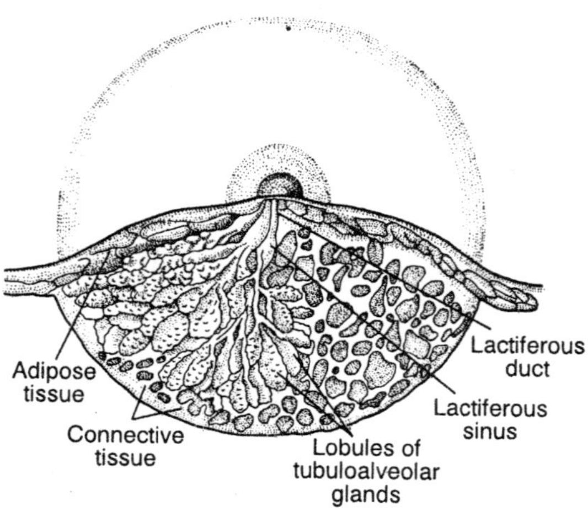

Fig. 11.4: Schematic drawing of the human breast as seen during lactation. The breast is composed largely of branched tubuloalveolar glands contained within an extensive connective tissue stroma and variable amounts of adipose tissue (Modified from Warwick R, Williams PI, eds. *Gray's Anatomy*. 35th ed. Edinburgh : Churchill Livingstone, 1973).

After parturition there will be irritation of secretory activity, and enlargement of breast takes place due to the accomulation of the secreting materials. The secretion released in the first few days after parturition is known as **colostrum.** This premilk is an alkaline, yellowish secretion with a higher protein, vitamin A, sodium, and chloride content and a lower lipid, carbohydrate, and potassium content than milk. It contains considerable amounts of antibodies. The antibodies in the colostrum are believed to be produced by the lymphocytes and plasma cells that infiltrate the loose connective tissue of the breast during its development and proliferation and are secreted across the glandular cells. As these wandering cells decrease in number after parturition, the production of colostrum stops, and lipid-rich milk is produced.

Hormonal regulation of breast development and lactation

In women, the initial growth and development of the breast at puberty occur under the influence of estrogens, and progesterone are produced by the maturing ovary. Estrogen causes the development of mammary ducts and progesterone stimulates the formation of lobules and alveoli. Optimum growth of breast also requires the presence of growth hormone and prolactin. Subsequent changes to this initial growth, slight changes in the morphology of glandular tissue take place during each ovarian cycle.

During pregnancy breasts develop further owing to the development of lobules and alveoli. This is caused by the simultaneous action of estrogen, progesterone, GH, adrenal corticoids and prolactin. At this time the corpus luteum and placenta continuously produce estrogens and progesterone. Estrogen present in the circulation stimulates proliferation of the lactiferous duct components, and progesterone stimulates the growth of alveoli. Immediately after birth, the sudden loss of estrogen and progesterone secretion from the placenta and corpus luteum

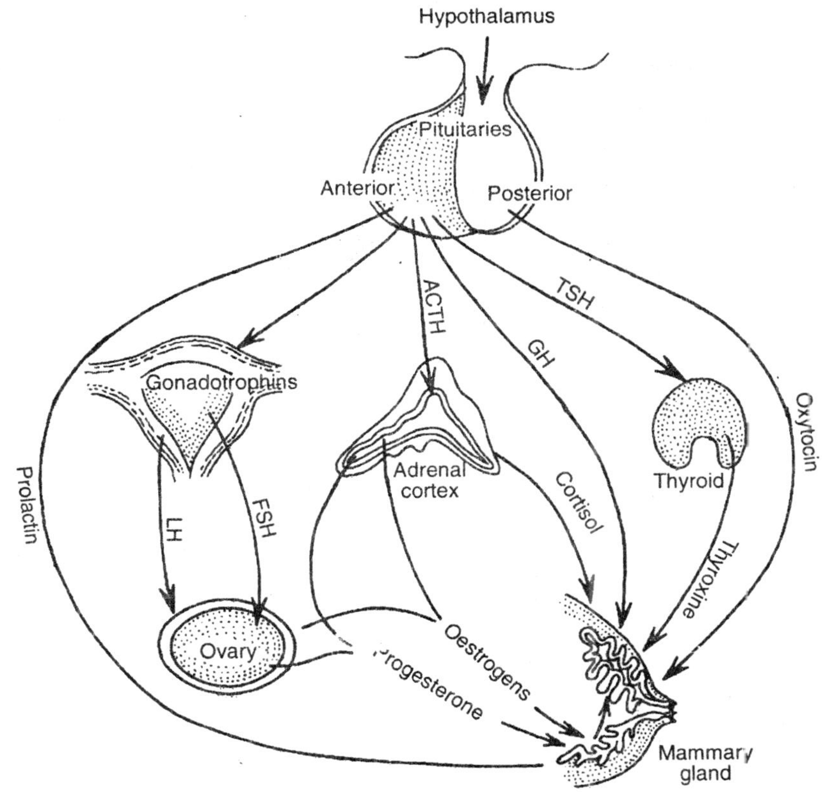

Fig. 11.5: The principal hormones that control the development and the function of the breast.

allows the prolactin to assume its lactogenic role. Production of milk also requires adequate secretion of growth hormone, adrenal glucocorticoids and parathyroid hormones.

During breast feeding the act of suckling initiates sensory impulses from receptors in the nipple to the hypothalamus. Now the impulses reduce the release of prolactin inhibiting factor and the prolactin is then released from the anterior pituitary. The sensory impulses also cause the release of oxytocin from the posterior pituitary. This oxytocin stimulates the myoepithelial cells that surround the base of the alveolar secretory cells and the base of the cells in the larger ducts, causing to contract and eject the milk from the alveoli and the lactiferous ducts [Fig 11.5].

The nipple is perforated at the tip by 15-20 minute openings of lactiferous ducts, each of which is an excretory duct from one lobules to the surface. The skin of the nipple extends outwards upon the surface of the breast for 1-2 cm to form a brown coloured **areola.** This areola contains numerous large sebaceous glands. These sebaceous glands secrete lipid material which protects and lubricates nipple during nursing of the infant.

- **Galactorrhoea** is a condition associated with excess breast milk production without child birth (excessive lactogenesis). It is mainly due to hypersecretion of pituitary PRL. This may be due to a pituitary adenoma (prolactinoma).

SECONDARY SEX CHARACTERS

Puberty is the final phase of the complex process of sexual maturation, a process by which an individual acquires reproductive competency. The dramatic developmental and behavioural changes in the male and female result from enhanced gonadal hormone secretion by the gonads. Dimorphic secondary sex characteristics are typical of all vertebrates.

A. Secondary sexual characters in male

The sexual characters in male are formed due to the influence of gonadal hormones that are liberated from the male gonad. These characters are characterised by morphological, physiological, sexological and psychological changes.

1. Morphological features :

(i) Development of muscles on the neck and shoulder region.

(ii) Less deposition of fat in the subcutaneous tissue.

(iii) The body structure becomes longer, muscular and stouter than females.

(iv) Rudimentany mammary glands are seen.

(v) Well-developed larynx and voice becomes deeper (masculine voice).

(vi) The hairs grow all over the body surface forming surface hairs and development of moustache and beard.

(vii) Growth of hairs within the nostrils known as nasal hairs.

(viii) Development of hairs on outer rim of the auricle of external ears which are known as auricular hairs.

2. Physiological features :

(i) Increased heart rate increases cardiac output and high blood pressure.

(ii) BMR increases and the respiratory rate becomes rapid.

(iii) RBC count increases.

(iv) The androgen and testosterone are secreted gradually.

(v) Increased muscle protein synthesis is found.

(vi) Accumulation of Ca^{++} increases in bones

3. Sexological features :

(i) The accessory sexual structures like epididymis, vas deferens, urethra, prostate, seminal vesicles, Cowper's glands are well developed.

4. Psychological features :

(i) Appearance of sexual desire towards opposite sex is noticed.

(ii) The male individuals become initiative, aggressiveness, idealism and interest in social problems.

B. Secondary sex characters in female

1. Morphological features :

(i) Disposition of hairs all over the body are fine and scarce.

(ii) More subcutaneous fat deposition all over the body specially in the neck, abdomen, pelvis and supraclavicular region.

(iii) The mammary gland is well developed along with huge deposition of subcutaneous fat in that area.

(iv) Body stature and height are comparatively lower than male individual.

(v) The larynx is less developed with high toned voice (feminine voice).

(vi) The pelvic region is broad and wide.

(vii) Narrow shoulders and broad hips.

(viii) There is no beard or moustache, hairs on the head are longer.

2. Physiological features :

(i) The heart rate, cardiac output and blood pressure are increased.

(ii) BMR is lowered.

(iii) RBC count is comparatively lesser than male.

(iv) Less Ca^{++} deposition in bones.

(v) Ovary matures, ovulation takes place and periodic menstruation occurs.

(vi) The female gonadal hormones like estrogen and progesterone are liberated in the blood from the ovary.

3. Psychological features :

(i) Highly developed emotivity and affections.

(ii) Maternal and family sentiments with practical outlook are observed.

4. Sexological features :

(i) The accessory sexual structures like Fallopian tube, vagina, uterus, vulva, clitoris and the glands in the mucosa of the female genital tract are developed.

(ii) Sexual desire towards the opposite sex is noticed.

Role of sex hormones on accessory sex organs

A. In males : The testis secretes masculinizing steroidal compounds (C_{19} steroids) grouped as **androgens** or male sex hormones into the blood stream. **Testosterone** is the chief androgen. Two other androgens secreted by the testis are **androstenedione** and **dehydroepiandrosterone.** They are secreted by the Leydig cells of testes. Small amounts of androgens may be secreted by adrenal cortex. This androgen promotes the growth as well as development, maintenance and functions of male accessory sex organs.

Androgens stimulate protein synthesis in the male accessory glands by direct stimulating effect on DNA and RNA polymerase by increasing the synthesis of mRNA in the nucleus and increased amino-acyl transferase at the ribosomal level. The protein synthesis induces the growth of muscles so that the male body becomes muscular and tough (a tough masculine body). Androgens also act on the prostate and seminal vesicles to secrete fructose which appears to function as nutrient to spermatozoa.

Testosterone causes development of the secondary sex characters of males, e.g., appearance of hairs on the face (moustache and beard), axilla and pubic region as well as on chest and back in some individuals, deepening of the pitch and voice, etc.

B. In females : Female sex hormones secreted by the ovary are mainly of two types—estrogens and progesterone. These are steroidal compounds. Estrogens are secreted from the maturing Graafian follicle whereas the progesterone is secreted from the corpus luteum. These two hormones are responsible for the development of pubertal changes in a girl. With the onset of secretion of these hormones from the ovary of a girl, she attains sexual maturity (adolescence). They facilitate the growth and development of accessory sex organs of females, e.g., fallopian tubes, uterus and vagina. The estrogen not only helps to increase the size of vagina but also accelerates to change the vaginal epithelium from cuboidal into stratified type. The estrogen also causes marked proliferation of endometrium during ovulatory phase and stimulates the growth of endometrial glands.

Estrogen and progesterone often act synergistically, viz., (i) progesterone can cause the premenstrual changes in the endometrium, only after the proliferative changes has been already done by estrogen. Progesterone alone will have no effect. (ii) Glandular development of breasts chiefly by proliferation of ducts, as seen during pregnancy, only occur by their combined action.

Both progesterone and estrogen also help in the appearance of secondary sex characters of females, e.g., softness of skin, development of breasts, axillary and pubic hairs, deposition of fat in the particular regions of the body such as thigh and hip, etc. so that the body structure becomes typically feminine. Estrogen maintains the sexual behaviour of females.

CHAPTER 12

Hormonal Disorders

Hormones secreted by the endocrine gland exert their influence on almost all physiological functions of the body. Hormones can alter the rate of a physiological process but cannot initiate it. Thus, their effects in the body are merely quantitative rather than qualitative. They regulate the growth and development of the body, integument and its derivatives, digestion, metabolism, and reproductive processes. It is often found that the action of one hormone is opposed by the action of another hormone and sometimes hormones act synergistically. The molecular mechanism by which the hormones produce their effects at their target cells is very complicated. For normal physiological activities of the body it is seen that a delicate balance is maintained in the level of various hormones and any disturbance in the levels of hormones secreted by hypo-or-hyper secretion of the endocrine glands owing to various reasons may cause several diseases. This is called endocrine or hormonal disorders.

DISORDERS OF PITUITARY HORMONES

Dysfunction of pituitary gland may cause hyposecretion or hypersecretion of one or more hormones. Under-secretion of pituitary gland may cause a result of destruction of normal glandular cells within the pituitary gland by an expanding tumour, disruption of hypothalamo-hypophyseal vascular connections or disease of hypothalamus. Tumours originating in a type of cell produce the signs of over-activity of not only those cells but also the signs of hyperactivity of adjacent cells due to irritation or symptoms of hypoactivity of the adjacent cells owing to degeneration caused by pressure.

Again, any disorder produced in adenohypophysis has adverse effects on other endocrine glands as this part produces trophic hormones which regulate the activities of all the other endocrine glands.

A. Hyper-activity or hypersecretion in young

(a) Gigantism : This disease is caused by hypersecretion of STH in young condition. This condition is rare and the excessive growth of normal pattern leads to extremely large individuals with normal bodily proportions. The growth period is prolonged due to delay in the closure of epiphyses. It is characterised by the following features.

1. Morphological features :

(i) Abnormal height in body which measures about 7 to 8 ft.

(ii) Unusual length of limbs and hands.

(iii) Well-built muscle.

(iv) Thick lips.

(v) Thickening of skin of eyelids and nose [Fig. 12.1].

2. Physiological features :

(i) Excessive sweating.

(ii) Increased BMR.

(iii) Glycosauria is noticed.

(iv) Less Ca^{++} in blood.

3. Psychological features :

(i) Individuals are normally intelligent.

4. Sexological features :

(i) The primary and secondary sex characters are ill developed.

(ii) Inhibition of sexual activity is noticed.

Effects of STH

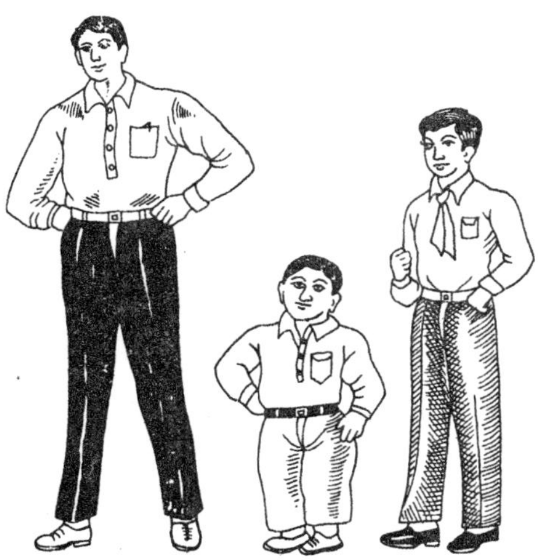

Fig. 12.1: Figure showing—A. Gigantism, B. Dwarfism and C. Normal human size.

• Hypersecretion of STH in adult

(b) Acromegaly : Tumors of somatotrophs of the adenohypophysis secrete large amounts of growth hormone, leading to **acromegaly** in adults. It is characterised by—

1. Morphological features :

(i) Enlargement of hands and feet.

(ii) The hands are broaded with thickening of the fingers.

(iii) Abnormal enlargement of facial bones.

(iv) Protrusion of the lower jaw together with enlargement of nasal bone and suborbital ridges.

(v) The subcutaneous tissues of the hands, feet, nose, lips and skin increase in amount and develop deep furrows.

(vi) Enlarged tongue is observed.

(vii) The visceral organs enlarge and the skin becomes thickened.

(viii) Generalised overgrowth of hairs all over the body surface [Fig. 12.2].

2. Physiological features :

(i) BMR is increased.

(ii) Increased secretion of sweat is noticed.

(iii) Hyperglycaemia is often observed.

(iv) The skeletal changes predispose to **osteoarthritis**.

3. Psychological features :

(i) Individual becomes not so intelligent.

(ii) May cause mental disturbances.

4. Sexological features :

(i) In both cases gonads become reduced in size.

(ii) The sexual functions in both may be decreased.

(iii) There is loss of libido effect in male.

(iv) Menstrual disturbances and ill developed mammary glands occur.

• Hypersecretion of antidiuretic hormone

(c) Oedema : In patients with hypersecretion of antidiuretic hormone, a high fluid intake may cause water intoxication. Such patient may develop **oedema** with low plasma osmolality and high blood pressure.

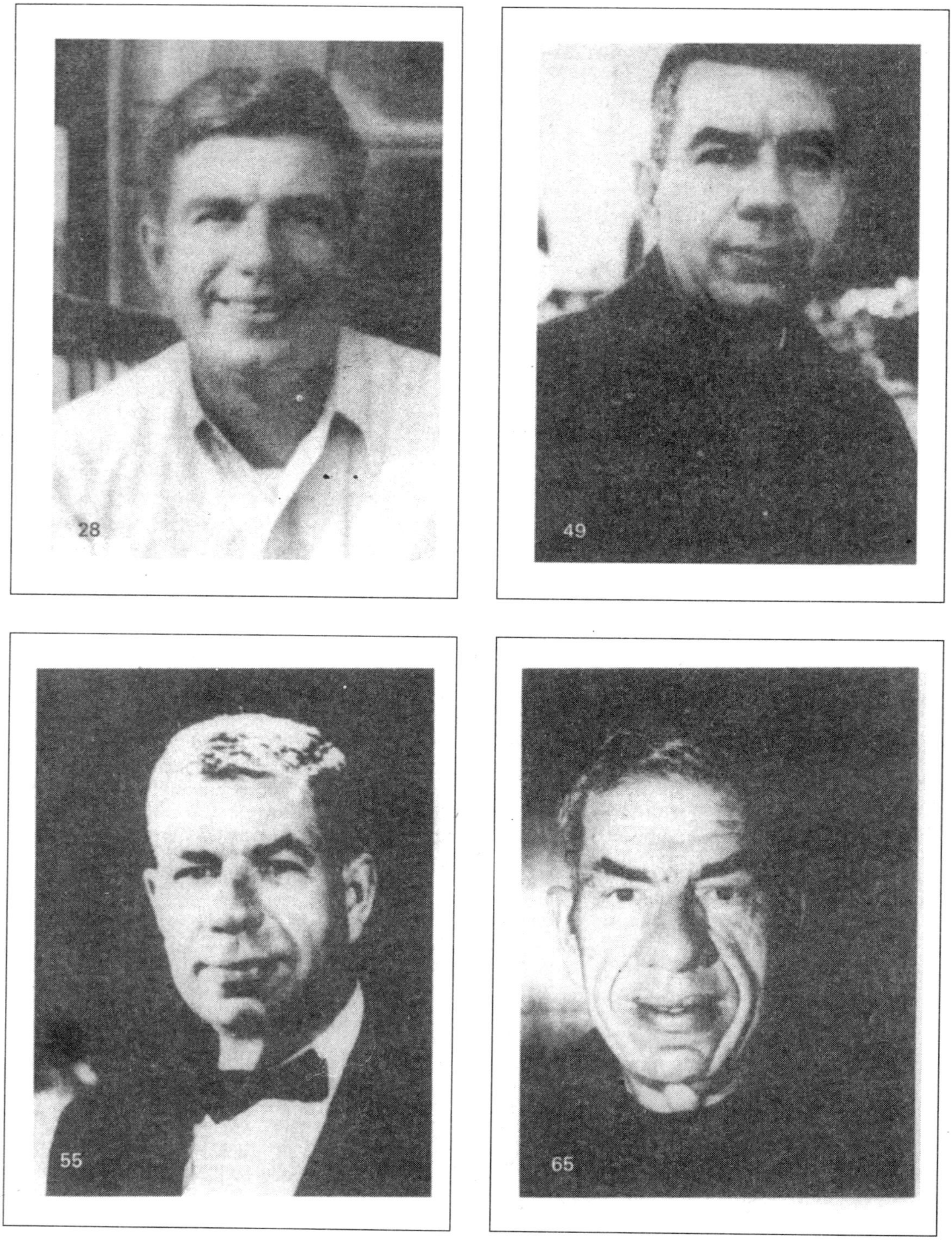

Fig. 12.2(i): Serial photographs of an acromegalic patient at the ages indicated. Note the gradual increase in size of the nose, lips, and skin folds.

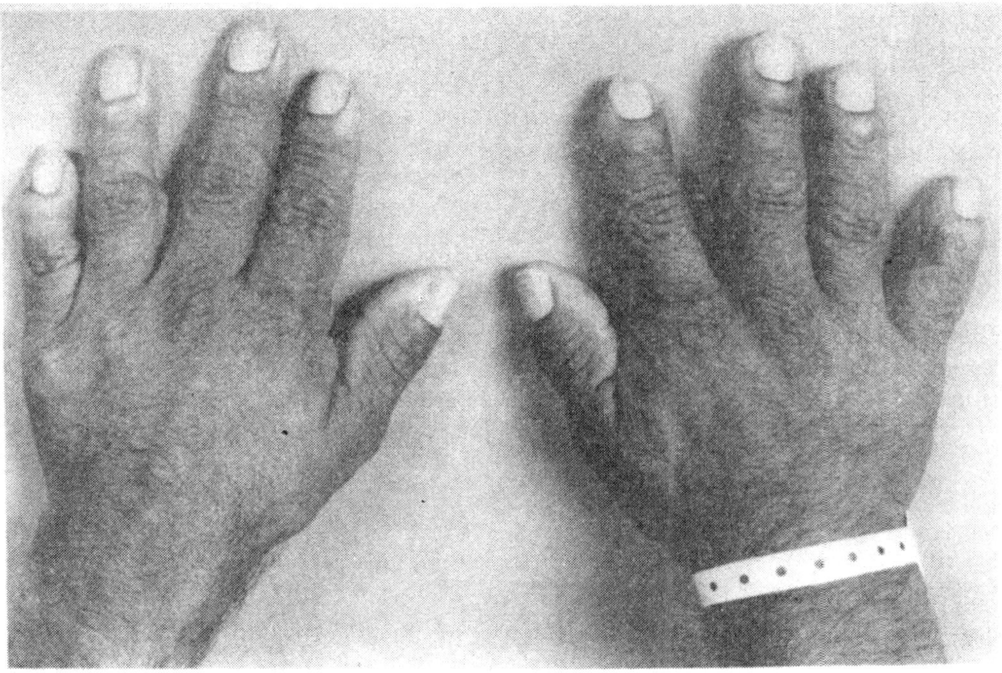

Fig. 12.2(ii): Markedly increased soft tissue, bulk and blunt fingers in a middle-aged man with acromegaly.

> **Note : Hypersecretion of STH** in adult is characterized by overgrowth of extremities. In this condition, unlike **gigantism,** the person does not become very tall because the long bones do not increase in length after attaining adulthood; but the flat bones of face, hand, feet, etc. continue to grow excessively and become disfigured. The visceral organs also enlarge and the skin becomes thickened. Due to the above changes the person assumes a gorilla like appearance.

B. Hyposecretion of growth hormone

Decreased secretion of STH is most commonly noticed in cases of pituitary insufficiency or hypopituitarism and its effects are difficult to separate from the associated failure of other pituitary hormones. In prepubertal life and in adult deficiency of STH produces profound impairment of growth.

• Hyposecretion of growth hormone in childhood or prepubertal life

(a) Dwarfism : It is caused due to decreased secretion of growth hormone in prepubertal life or childhood. It shows the following features :

1. Morphological features :

(i) Stunted growth and the adult reaches a maximum size of 3 feet.

(ii) Abnormal skeletal growth.

(iii) An adult pituitary dwarf resembles a normal child with large head.

(iv) Round face.

(v) Skin becomes smooth [Fig. 12.3].

2. Physiological features :

(i) BMR is low.

(ii) The ossification and dentation remain normal.

(iii) Adiposity may be seen.

(iv) Hypoglycaemia is observed.

(v) Accumulation of nitrogen product is increased.

(vi) The growth is impaired.

3. Psychological features :

(i) Intelligence is normal in proportion to age.

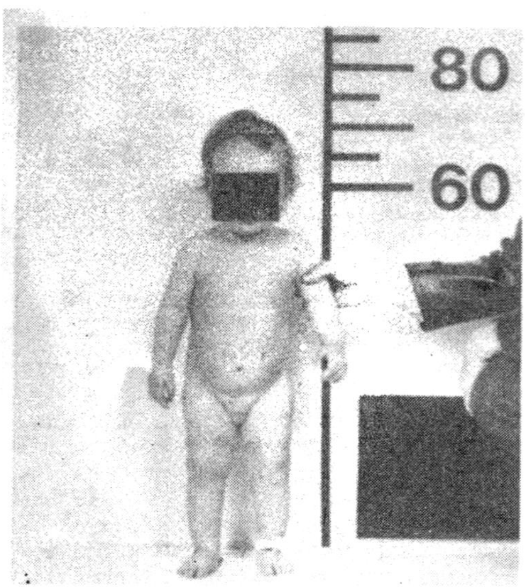

Fig. 12.3: A 12-month old boy with congenital hypopituitarism. At 12 months, length was 66.5 cm (–2 SD) and weight was 8.5 kg (–3 SD). The penis was less than 1.5 cm long, and both testes were descended (each 1 cm in diameter).

4. Sexological features :

(i) Underdeveloped gonads.

(ii) Secondary sex characters do not develop.

(iii) The sexual functions are undeveloped.

Kinds of Dwarfism : It is caused by hypoactivity of the acidophil cells of the pituitary gland in the young. There are four types of dwarfism.

(i) **Lorain-Levy type of dwarfism (Infantilism) :** Here the plasma IgF-I level is reduced and the plasma growth hormone-binding protein concentration is also reduced indicating genetic defects in the extracellular portion of the growth hormone receptor. The growth of the individual is stunted and the adult reaches a maximum size of 3 feet. Sex organs and secondary sex characters do not grow. Intelligence level is normal in proportion to age and the metabolism also becomes normal.

(ii) **Brissaud type dwarfism (Fat boy of Dickens) :** Same as Lorain-Levy type dwarfism plus excessive deposition of fat in the body. They have round and chubby face. However, they are lethargic and sleepy. Secondary sexual characters such as moustaches and beard do not grow and growth of hair over the body is also scarce.

(iii) **Pigmy type dwarfism :** It is characterised by short stature which can result from abnormalities in GH metabolism other than deficient secretion and thus, GH levels are normal. Their small stature is due to other factors, either a slightly abnormal and less efficient GH molecule or a failure of peripheral response to GH or deficient somatomedin secretion.

• Hyposecretion of STH in case of adult

(b) Acromicria : Hyposecretion of STH in case of adults (who have already attained normal height) results in a condition, called **acromicria,** and it is caused by hypoactivity of the acidophil cells in the adult and it is characterised by the following features. It is the **antithesis of acromegaly**.

1. Morphological features :

(i) Abnormal small facial features.

(ii) Bones of face, hands and feet are small.

(iii) Loss of hairs.

(iv) The skin becomes wrinkle and dry.

(v) Adiposity is also observed.

2. Physiological features :

(i) BMR is reduced.

(ii) Polyuria condition is found.
(iii) Less Ca^{++} level in blood.

3. Psychological features :

(i) Idiotic behaviour is noted.
(ii) Mentally backward condition.

4. Sexological features :

(i) Loss of sexual function.
(ii) Gonads are reduced in size.

• Hyposecretion of Vasopressin/ADH

(c) Diabetes incipidus : Deficiency of antidiuretic hormone (ADH) due to defects in hypothalamus or posterior pituitary (neurohypophysis) leads to a pathological condition, called **diabetes insipidus.** In this condition the urine becomes insipid (or tasteless) hence, it is so named. The symptoms are :

(i) Passage of a large volume of dilute urine **(diuresis)**.
(ii) Drinking of a large amount of water owing to excessive thirst **(polydypsia)** to compensate the loss of water through urine.
(iii) The urine of polydypsea patient has a low specific gravity because it becomes diluted.
(iv) The frequency of excretion of a large amount of diluted urine is increased **(polyuria)**.
(v) Electrolyte disorder (**hypokalemia**) is noticed.
(vi) Physical and mental retardation.
(vii) Dilation of urinary bladder is found.

Hyposecretion of oxytocin :

(i) In deficiency of oxytocin—the parturition, or delivery of the body is delayed and becomes difficult.
(ii) There is difficulty in breast feeding due to defect in milk ejection from the mammary gland (breast).
(iii) Milk formation in the mammary glands is not impaired.

DISORDERS OF THE HORMONES OF THYROID

A. Hyposecretion or malfunction of thyroid gland

Malfunction or less secretion from the thyroid gland produces **cretinism** in infancy or childhood and **myxoedema** in adults.

(a) **Cretinism** : It is the condition in children due to severe thyroid deficiency. Hyposecretion of pituitary TSH may cause hypoactivity of thyroid gland. Congenital lack of thyroid gland also induces in development of cretinism. Symptoms do not appear till after six months, because enough hormone is present in mother's milk. The most characteristic features are as follows [Fig. 12.4] :

1. Morphological features :

(i) Linear growth is severely retarded.
(ii) Stunted skeletal growth.
(iii) Short club-like fingers.
(iv) Rough, thick, dry and wrinkled skin.
(v) Hairs scanty.
(vi) Bloated idiotic-look face.
(vii) Thick parted lips and large protruding tongue.
(viii) Saliva dribbling.
(ix) Broad nose with depressed bridge.
(x) Pot bellied abdomen, umbilicus often protruding.
(xi) Muscular weakness.
(xii) Deformed bones and teeth.

2. Physiological features :

(i) Appetite is reduced. Motility of the gastrointestinal tract is reduced and there is often constipation.
(ii) BMR is lowered.
(iii) Low body temperature.
(iv) Irregularly deposit of fat specially above the clavicles.
(v) Low blood sugar is noticed.
(vi) Low RBC count is found.

(vii) High serum cholesterol.

(viii) Resistance is lowered and susceptible to cold, toxins and inter-current infection.

(ix) Less creatine excretion is observed.

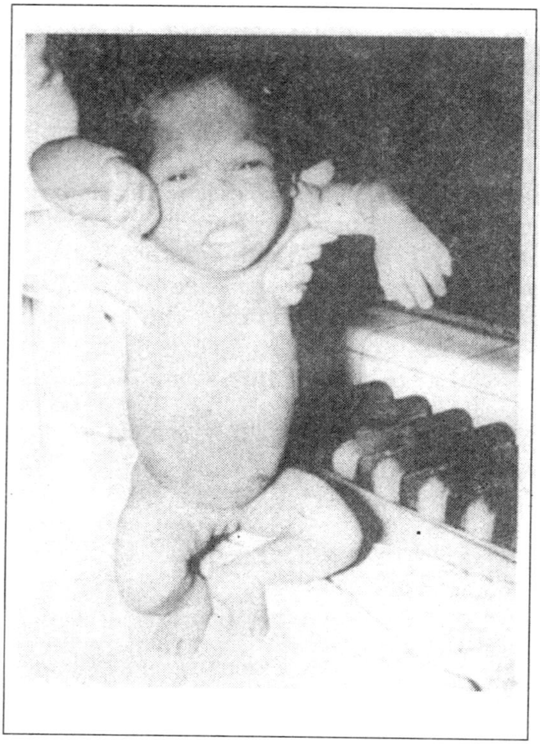

Fig. 12.4: A 9-month old infant with hypothyroidism (cretinism). Note the puffy face, protuberant abdomen, umbilical hernia, and muscle weakness (infant cannot sit up unassisted).

3. Psychological features :

(i) Various degress of idiocy and mental growth are seen.

(ii) Cretins are often deaf and dumb.

(iii) Intelligence level is severly subnormal.

4. Sexological features :

(i) Ill-developed sex glands and sex organs.

(ii) Retarded secondary sex characters are observed.

(b) **Myxoedema or Gull's disease**

Hypothyroidism in the adult is referred to as myxoedema. It is caused by the hypoactivity of thyroid gland or also hyposecretion of pituitary TSH. This disease generally occurs more in adult female than adult male owing to decrease or absence of thyroid hormone. This condition [Fig. 12.5] is characterised by following features—

1. Morphological features :

(i) Skin colour becomes yellow due to deposition of mucinous protein in the cutaneous tissues.

(ii) Swollen, puffy, pale and oedematous face and thus exhibits mongoloid appearance.

(iii) Cheeks look like parchment.

(iv) Swelling in the neck region.

(v) Loss of hairs from the axillae, pubis, head and eyebrows.

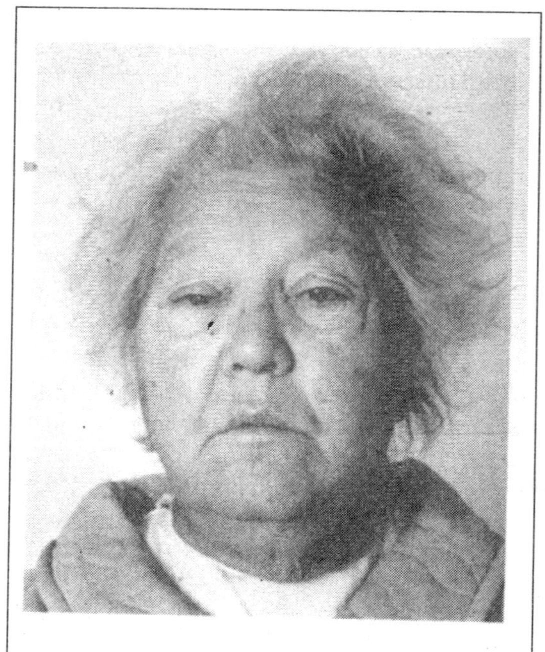

Fig. 12.5: Hypothyroidism in adult (myxoedema). Note puffy face, puffy eyes, frowsy hair, and dull and apathetic appearance.

(vi) Fat deposition over the body is irregular.
(vii) Swelling of the tongue and larynx.

2. Physiological features :

(i) Low BMR.
(ii) Respiratory rate is reduced.
(iii) Cholesterol level is very high.
(iv) Decreased heart rate.
(v) Patients are anaemic and plasma albumin level is high.
(vi) Glucose level in blood is reduced.
(vii) Reduced heart rate and cardiac output.
(viii) Body weight increases and appetite is reduced.
(ix) Nitrogen excretion is reduced.

3. Psychological features :

(i) Mental faculties are reduced.
(ii) The patient suffers from loss of memory.
(iii) Reflexes are very slow.
(iv) The patient is lethargic, dull, apathetic and sleepy.
(v) Inability to tolerate cold.

4. Sexological features :

(i) Sexual functions are degenerated.
(ii) Loss of libido and failure of fertility.
(iii) Impotency in male and amenorrhoea in female are observed.
(iv) Reproductive glands, organs and secondary sexual characters are all degenerated.

Arteriosclerosis

Lack of thyroid hormone increases the quantity of blood cholesterol because of altered fat and cholesterol metabolism and diminished liver excretion of cholesterol in the bile. The increase in blood cholesterol is usually associated with increased artherosclerosis and arteriosclerosis. Therefore, many hypothyroid patients, particularly those with myxoedema, develop arteriosclerosis, which in turn results in peripheral vascular disease, deafness, and often-extreme coronary sclerosis with consequent early death (**Guyton** and **Hall** 2000).

B. Hypersecretion of thyroid gland

The condition of excessive secretion and action of thyroid gland is known as **hyperthyroidism** or **thyrotoxicosis** which is always associated with **goitre.** This disease is caused by hypersecretion of thyroid hormones. Hypersecretion of pituitary TSH or thyrotoxicosis may help in the development of hyperactivity of thyroid gland and it secretes excess T_3 and T_4. However, the most common type of hyperthyroidism is the **Grave's disease** or **Exopthalmic goitre** in which goitre is associated with protrusion of the eyes. Grave's disease (named after **R. J. Graves**, 1797-1853, an Irish physician, who discovered it) is an autoimmune disease due to over production of a thyroid stimulating immunoglobulin by the B-lymphocytes, i.e., this disease may be mediated by an immunoglobulin known as long acting thyroid stimulator (LATS). LATS binds to TSH receptors and activates thyroid cell functions even in absence of circulating TSH.

(a) **Grave's disease or Exopthalmic goitre :**

1. Morphological features :

(i) Enlargement of thyroid gland occur.
(ii) Decreased body weight.
(iii) Soft, moist and flashed skin.
(iv) Protrusion of eyeball with less twinkling of eyelids.
(v) Hands are usually warm and moist.
(vi) Muscles become easily fatigued.
(vii) Hairs are fine and friable [Fig. 12.6 and 12.7].

2. Physiological features :

(i) Decrease of body weight.
(ii) Increase in heart rate.

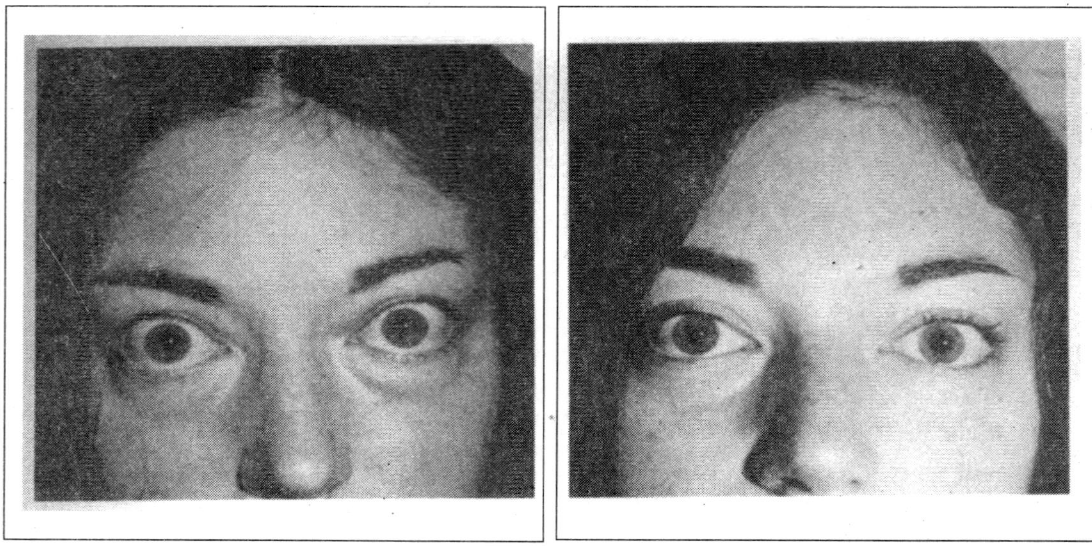

Fig. 12.6(i): Patient with mild ophthalmopathy of Graves disease. **Left :** Before radioactive iodine therapy. Note white sclera visible above and below the iris as well as mild periorbital oedema. **Right :** After radioactive iodine therapy. Marked improvement is noted.

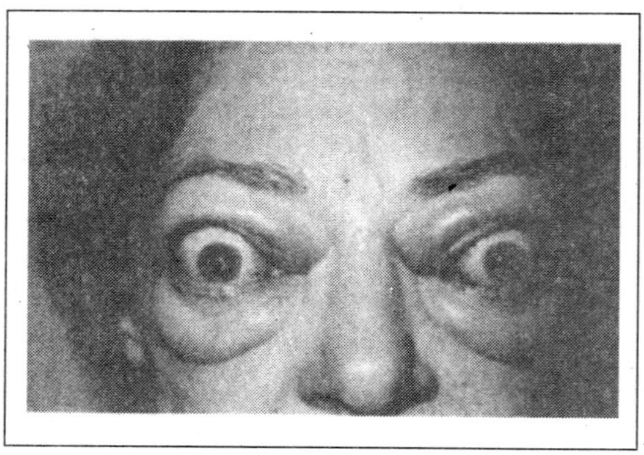

Fig. 12.6(ii): Severe ophthalmopathy of Graves' disease. Note marked periorbital oedema, injection of corneal blood vessels, and proptosis.

(iii) Increase in body temperature and BMR.

(iv) Increase in sweating and tolerance to heat.

(v) Due to excessive catabolism weight loss is noted.

(vi) Increased appetite.

(vii) Goitre may also occur due to tumor in pituitary or thyroid gland.

(viii) Osteoporosis occurs due to loss of calcium and phosphorus from bones.

(ix) Exhibits hyperglycaemia and glycosuria is diminished.

(x) Cholesterol content and increased iodine contents in the blood are observed.

(xi) There will be increased vitamin need, specially vitamins A, B, and C.

(xii) Skin becomes soft and moist due to sweating.

(xiii) Blood pressure is increased.

3. Psychological features :

(i) Individual becomes emotional and slightly restless.

(ii) There will be acute nervousness and irritability.

(iii) Individual becomes nervous and sleepless.

4. Sexological features :

(i) Alteration of libido effect is seen.

(ii) There will be impotency in male and amenorrhoea in female.

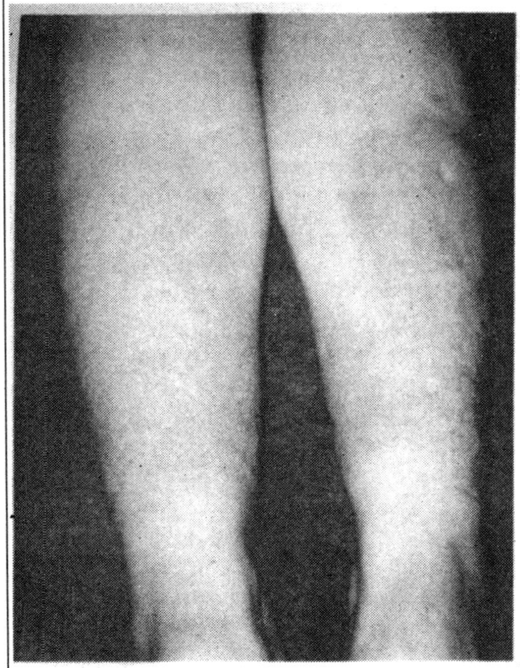

Fig. 12.7: Dermopathy of Graves' disease. Marked thickening of the skin is noted, usually over the pre-tibial area. Thickening will occasionally extend downward over the ankle and the dorsal aspect of the foot but almost never above the knee.

(iii) The menorrhagia may occur in female and finally there may be complete stoppage of menstruation.

• **Goitre :** Goitre means swelling of the neck owing to enlargement of thyroid gland. This is a non-inflammatory and non-neoplastic enlargement of thyroid gland. The overgrowth of the gland may be associated with hypothyroidism (low level of T_3 and T_4 in blood), as well as hyperthyroidism (high level of T_3 and T_4). Hypothyroidism takes place mainly in dietary deficiency of iodine. This is also called **endemic goitre** which was formerly more common in hilly areas where the food and drinking water lacked iodine. Nowadays this is rare because of the use of iodised common salt. Goitre with hyperthyroidism occurs most commonly in Grave's disease. Goitre can be divided into following types :

1. **Simple goitre :** In this type of goitre the gland becomes enlarged to produce normal level of hormones due to deficiency of iodine. Simple type of goiter can be differentiated into three kinds.

   (i) **Colloid goitre** is an endemic and benign goitre. This kind of goitre is prevalent in areas where the drinking water is deficient in iodine. There is no hypertrophy or hyperplasia. So in order to produce normal levels of the hormone the gland becomes hypertrophied. The alveoli are distended with colloid lined by cubical or flattened epithelial cells. Use of iodised salt reduces the incidence of this disease.

   (ii) **Diffuse parenchymatous goitre :** In this disease the alveoli are not distended with colloid-like goitre. The cells lining the alveoli are of columnar type. These columnar epithelial cells linining the follicles hypertrophy multiply in number due to which the lumen of the follicles become obliterated.

   (iii) **Nodular goitre** : This kind of disease is characterised by nodular swelling in some part of the thyroid gland.

2. **Toxic goitre :** When swelling or enlargement of the thyroid gland results in excessive secretion of thyroid hormones, this condition is called **toxic goitre.** The follicular epithelial cells are hypertrophied and hyperplastic. Toxicosis does not mean excessive secretion but toxic symptoms are developed owing to hyperthyroidism. Grave's disease is always associated with toxic goitre.

3. **Hokkaido goitre :** While deficiency of iodine may cause endemic goitre or endemic cretinism, a very high concen-

tration may also result hypothyroidism by inhibiting iodine organification—the **Wolff-Chaikoff effect.** e.g., during the synthesis of thyroid hormones, inorganic iron is taken up from the blood and converted into organic form by reacting with the amino acid tyrosine. High concentration of iodine inhibits organification of iodine and causes hypothyroidism. This may also be named as a **Hokkaido goitre** because in Hokkaido the Japanese people consume large amounts of sea-weeds having 10 to 20 mg of iodine per day or more causing a good number of goitre with hypothyroidism but no cretinism. High content of iodine may also interfere with release of T_4 and T_3 from the thyroid gland and causes hypothyroidism.

4. **Exopthalmic goitre :** Due to excessive secretion of thyroxine, the thyroid gland becomes enlarged, i.e., hypertrophy and hyperplasia. This type of goitre is associated with protrusion of the eyeball with a 'starling' look—less twinkling of the eyelids. It is caused due to deposition of fat in retro-ocular region. The other important features are—increased heart rate, BMR and body temperature; sweating and intolerance to heat, body weight decreased and fat stores depleted, tremor, anxiety, mental instability and restlessness.

5. **Endemic goitre :** The term goitre means a greatly enlarged thyroid gland. It has been shown that about 50 milligrams of iodine are required each year for the formation of adequate quantities of thyroid hormone. In certain areas of the world, notably in the Swiss Alps, the Andes, the Great Lakes region of the United States and certain parts of the Western and Eastern Himalays, India, insufficient iodine is present in the soil, for the foodstuffs to contain even this minute quantity. Therefore, in the days before iodized table salt, many people who lived in these areas, developed extremely large thyroid glands, called **endemic goitre.** The mechanism for development of large endemic goitre is the following (**Guyton** and **Hall** 2000) : lack of iodine prevents production of both thyroxine and triiodothyronine. As a result, no hormone is available to inhibit production of TSH by the anterior pituitary, which causes the pituitary to secrete excessively large quantities of TSH. The TSH then stimulates the thyroid cells to secrete tremendous amounts of thyroglobulin colloid into the follicles, and the gland grows larger and larger. But because of lack of iodine, thyroxine and triiodothyronine production does not occur in the thyroglobulin molecule and therefore, does not cause the normal suppression of TSH production by the anterior pituitary. The Follicles become tremendous in size, and thus, the thyroid gland may increase to 10 to 20 times normal size (**Guyton** and **Hall** 2000).

HYPOTHYROIDISM

Reduced production of thyroid hormones is referred to as **hypothyroidism.** It produces two kinds of disorders. In infants and young the disease is called **Cretinism** and in adults reduced activity of the thyroid gland causes a disorder, known as **Myxoedema.**

Causes :

(i) Deficiency of iodine in diet.

(ii) Defective thyroglobin formation and secretion.

(iii) Radioactive iodine therapy or X-ray therapy causes hypothyroidism.

(iv) Genetic defects can also lead to synthesis of abnormal hormones resulting in defects in iodine trapping or organification.

(v) Intake of goitrogenic substances can also lead to hypothyroidism.

(vi) Failure in the conversion of T_3 and T_4 in the peripheral tissue is also responsible for hypothyroidism.

(vii) Thyroid activity can also be reduced by antithyroid drugs as well as autoimmune disease.

(viii) Pituitary adenoma, pituitary ablation or pituitary destruction are also the causes of reduced production of thyroid hormones.

(ix) Damage of hypothalamo-hypophyseal system is another factor for hypothyroidism.

HYPERTHYROIDISM

Abnormally high thyroid secretion is called **hyperthyroidism or thyrotoxicosis** which is caused due to primary thyroid over-activity. Enlargement of the thyroid associated with hyperfunction produces a wide range of symptoms. Grave's disease and Plummer's disease are the common disorders in which goitre is associated with thyrotoxicosis and exopthalmia. Practically thyrotoxicosis results when tissues are exposed to over secretion of thyroid hormones.

Causes :

(i) The thyroid gland is diffusedly enlarged and there is protrusion of the eyeball owing to swelling of the extraocular muscles and connective tissue within the rigid bony walls of the orbit.

(ii) Grave's disease is an autoimmune disease in which circulating antibodies formed against TSH which activates the TSH-receptor, making the gland hyperactive. These antibodies are known as TSH-R (stim) Ab which may bind to TSH-receptors on thyroid follicle membrane and thus stimulating the secretion of T_3 and T_4.

(iii) Hyperactivity of the thyroid is due to the presence of another factor with a much more protracted thyroid stimulating action. This substance is known as Long Acting Thyroid Stimulator (LATS). LATS is one of a group of IgG immunoglobulins.

(iv) Lesions on thyroid gland are responsible for hypersecretion of T_3 and T_4 even under low TSH.

Thyrotoxicosis : It results when tissues are exposed to abnormally high thyroid hormone secretion. Hyperplastic growth of the thyroid gland can lead to severe thyrotoxicosis In **thyrotoxicosis,** due to mental stimulation, the patient becomes very nervous, irritable and restless. Grave's disease and plummer's disease are notable examples.

• **Hashimoto's disease :** It is another disorder which is caused due to damage or destruction and hypofunction of thyroid gland. This disease is characterised by the following clinical symptoms—exaggeration of normal lobular pattern, infiltration of lymphocytes, destruction of epithelial cells, degeneration of follicular basement membrane, etc. By the observation of high titre of thyroid auto-antibodies in the serum the diagnosis of Hashimoto's disease is confirmed.

• Euthyroid sick syndrome

Many non-thyroid conditions can alter thyroid function. Even though, the person is actually euthyroid, he/she will appear to be hypothyroid. For example, fasting, anorexia nervosa, malnutrition and unrelated diabetes mellitus are all metabolic disturbances that bring about marked decreases in circulating T_3 and increase in rT_3. Thyroid hormones also are altered in a variety of liver and renal disease as a consequence of numerous infections and following myocardial infections. Some conditions may alter levels of T_4, TSH, T_3 and/or rT_3. These alterations in thyroid parameters by peripheral disorders constitute the so-called *euthyroid sick syndrome,* reflecting normal responses of the euthyroid person to the generalized disease state (**Guyton** and

Major physiological manifestations of hyper—and hypothyroidism

Hypothyroidism	Hyperthyroidism
(i) Decreased secretion of thyroid hormone is noticed.	(i) Excess secretion of thyroid hormone is observed.
(ii) Blood levels of T_3 and T_4 are low but that of TSH is high.	(ii) Blood levels of T_3 and T_4 are high and that of TSH is low.
(iii) Basal metabolic rate (BMR) becomes low.	(iii) Elevated BMR.
(iv) Perspiration becomes slow.	(iv) Perspiration becomes high.
(v) Low body temperature.	(v) High body temperature.
(vi) Cold intolerance.	(vi) Heat intolerance.
(vii) Decreased appetite.	(vii) Increased appetite.
(viii) Weight gain.	(viii) Weight loss.
(ix) Coarse, dry palm as well as skin, subdermal thickening.	(ix) Warm, moist palms.
(x) Impaired intestinal glucose absorption.	(x) Enhanced intestinal glucose absorption.
(xi) Lethargy, depression, Sleepiness, tiredness.	(xi) Nervousness, anxiety, restlessness, insomnia.
(xii) Enlargement of thyroid is not associated with protrusion of eyeballs.	(xii) Enlargement of thyroid is associated with protrusion of eyeballs.
(xiii) Decreased cardiac output and low pulse rate.	(xiii) Increased cardiac output and high pulse rate.
(xiv) Low blood cholesterol level is noticed.	(xiv) High blood cholesterol level is seen.

Hall 2000).

• Thyroid storm

Thyroid storm is an acute, life-threatening, thyroid hormone induced hyper-metabolic state in patients, thyrotoxicosis. Thyroid storm may be the initial presentation of thyrotoxicosis in undiagonised children. Common clinical presentation includes fever, trachaecardia, neurologic abnormalities and hypertension followed by hypotension and shock. Because thyroid storm is invariably fatal if left untreated, rapid diagonosis and aggressive treatment are critical. Fortunately, this condition is extremely rare in children.

Causes : Besides surgery, thyroid storm is triggered by radioactive iodine therapy, uncontrolled diabetes, emotional stress, abrupt withdrawl of anti-thyroid medication, excessive palpation of thyroid gland in hyperthyroid patients, thyroid hormone overdose, pulmonary thromboembolism, toxemia of pregnancy, labour, trauma, acute infection, severe drug reaction or myocardial infection. Radioiodine causes a sharp rise of stimulating TSH receptor, antibodies are released during the first few weeks after radioiodine ablation. Thyroid storm generally occurs in this period, although one patient has developed thyroid storm 5 weeks post ablation.

Diagnosis/Treatment : Thyroid storm is diagnosed on the basis of symptoms. Although laboratory tests indicate thyrotoxicosis (by elevated thyroid hormone levels) there is nothing to distinguish thyroid storm from ordinary hypothyroidism.

- **Idiopathic nontoxic colloid goitre**

Enlarged thyroid glands similar to those of endemic colloid goitre also frequently occur in people who do not have iodine deficiency. These goitrous glands may secrete normal quantities of thyroid hormones, but more frequently, the secretion of hormone is depressed, as in endemic colloid goitre. The exact cause of the enlarged thyroid gland in patients with idiopathic colloid goitre is not known (**Guyton** and **Hall** 2000). However most of these patients show signs of **mild thyroiditis**.

Cause : Therefore, it has been suggested that the thyroiditis might cause slight hypothyroidism, which then leads to increased TSH secretion and progressive growth of the noninflamed portions of the gland. This could explain, why these glands usually are nodular, with some portions of the gland growing, while other portions are being destroyed by thyroiditis (**Guyton** and **Hall** 2000). In some persons with colloid goitre, the thyroid gland has an abnormality of the enzyme system, required for formation of the thyroid hormones.

Abnormalities (according to Guyton and Hall, 2000) :

(i) Deficient iodine trapping mechanism, in which iodine is not pumped adequately into the thyroid cells.

(ii) Deficient peroxidase system, in which the inorganic iodides are not oxidized to the active form, i.e. organic iodine state.

(iii) Deficient coupling of iodinated tyrosines in the thyroglobulin molecule, so that the final thyroid hormones cannot be formed.

(iv) Deficiency of the deiodinase enzyme, which prevents recovery of iodine from the iodinated tyrosines that are not coupled to form the thyroid hormones (this is about two thirds of the iodine), thus, leading to iodine deficiency.

(v) Finally, some foods contain goitrogenic substances that have a propylthiouracil type of antithyroid activity, thus, also leading to TSH stimulated enlargement of the thyroid gland.

DISORDERS OF THE PARATHYROID HORMONE

A. Hypoparathyroidism or hyposecretion of PTH :

(a) Tetany : Accidental damage to the parathyroids or their blood vessels during thyroid surgery or hypoactivity of parathyroid glands, i.e., deficiency of PTH leads to a condition known as **tetany;** it is a nervous condition caused by hypothyroidism and characterised by intermittent or continuous tonic muscular contractions of the extremities. The sign and symptoms are as due to fall of calcium (from 10 mg to 6 mg/100 ml) and rise of phosphate in the blood, caused by hypoparathyroidism. Tetany is produced in animals by the removal of the parathyroid glands two or three days after the operation or hypoparathyroidism. It is severe in young persons than older persons and also more severe in pregnant condition [Fig. 12.8]. The features are as follows :

1. Morphological features :

(i) **Carpopedal spasm** or **Trousseau's sign**—slight pressure on the limbs may elicit the elbow and wrist flexed and fingers flexed at the metacarpophalangeal joints but extended at the interphalangeal joints. Thumb in the palm and finger-tips are drawn together.

(ii) Pedal spasm is the dorsiflexion of the ankle joint and planter flexion of the toes.

(iii) There will be deficient development of hairs and nails. The hairs fall and the nails are easily broken.

(iv) Cutaneous disturbances such as erosion and ulcerations are sometimes observed.

(v) Dental lesions take place; defects in enamel formation and growth of root occur.

(vi) Convulsions are the most serious complications.

2. Physiological features :

(i) Increase in body temperature.

(ii) Respiration becomes rapid and noisy owing to respiratory muscular spasms.

(iii) The calcium and phosphate levels of urine become increased.

(iv) Osteoporosis and osteomalacia are found.

(v) Blood coagulation becomes slower and defective.

(vi) Heart rate is increased.

(vii) Reduced intestinal uptake of Ca^{++}.

(viii) Muscle twitches due to neuromuscular hyper-irritability.

(ix) Spasm of respiratory muscles and glottis leading to asphyxia.

(x) Blood calcium level is lowered which results in neuromuscular hyperexcitability.

3. Psychological features :

(i) Mental retardation occurs.

(ii) Shows anxiety, irritability and depression.

> • **Causes of Tetany :** (i) Lowered ionic calcium in blood and tissue fluid is the immediate cause.
>
> (ii) Fall of calcium increases the neuroexcitory factors, viz, Na, K, etc. and causes tetany.
>
> Total calcium has no relation with tetany. But lowering of total calcium owing to diminished plasma protein does not affect tetany. This reveals that calcium which remains bound with protein is not physiologically active.

B. Hypersecretion of PTH

(a) Osteitis fibrosa cystica : Hyperparathyroidism (a high blood level of PTH) occurs due to parathyroid tumors or diffuse

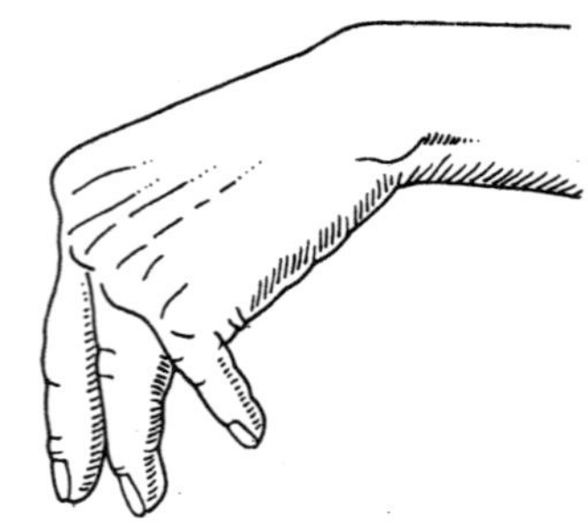

Fig. 12.8: Position of hand in hypocalcaemic tetany (Trousseau's sign).

hyperplasia of the parathyroid glands. Oversecretion of parathormone results in abnormally high blood calcium levels associated with lowered blood phosphate levels. In this condition the bones become rarefied, weak and fragile. Then it is known as **osteitis fibrosa cystica** in which the damaged bone tissue is replaced by cavities filled with fibrous tissue. The characteristic features of this disease are :

1. Anatomical features :

(i) General weakness in the body.

(ii) Bones become rarefied, weak and fragile.

(iii) Loss of muscular tone.

(iv) Renal disorders owing to the formation of cysts and stones in the kidney.

(v) Retention of phosphate depresses serum calcium levels and reduced synthesis of Vit D_3 by the kidney impairs intestinal calcium absorption.

2. Physiological features :

(i) Demineralisation of bones of varying degrees of severity is often observed.

(ii) Loss of appetite.

(iii) Nausea, vomiting, increased thirst, etc. are the general symptoms.

(iv) Mental retardation occurs.

(v) Polyurea due to the damage of the renal tubules inhibiting the reabsorption of water and there is increased secretion of calcium in the urine.

(vi) Urine calcium level is increased.

In man **primary hyperparathyroidism** is usually the result of the presence of a **benign tumor (adenoma)** of one or more of the parathyroid glands. **Secondary hyperparathyroidism** often results from a peripheral defect of parathormone action. It is a frequent consequence of chronic renal failure.

DISORDERS OF PANCREATIC HORMONES

Insulin and **glucagon,** the chief hormones of pancreas, regulate the metabolism of carbohydrate, protein and fat. These two hormones are functionally opposite to each other. Glucagon is a **catabolic hormone,** i.e., it stimulates catabolism of those foods, thereby depleting the reserve food stores of the body, and insulin is essentially an **anabolic hormone** because it helps to increase the storage of food in the body.

• **Hypofunction of insulin : Diabetes mellitus.** Due to less secretion or lack of insulin, the stored liver glycogen breaks down (glycogenolysis) into glucose due to the action of glucagon. In absence of insulin, the glucose cannot enter the cell or cell cannot oxidise the glucose properly. Thus, the amount of glucose in the blood increases. This is called **hyperglycaemia.** When the amount of glucose in the blood exceeds the renal threshold value (180 mg/100 ml blood), glucose appears in the urine. Presence of glucose in the urine is known as **glycosuria.** These conditions (i.e., hyperglycaemia with glycosuria) are collectively known as **diabetes mellitus.** The severity is dependent on the extent of the deficiency in insulin release. Diabetes mellitus was first described about 1500 B.C in Egypt. **Mellitus,** the Latin word for honey, characterises the high sugar content of the urine of diabetics. The word **diabetes,** derived from the Greek word **diabaincin** for 'siphon', refers to the copious excretion of water that characterises the disease. For centuries the disease was known as the "pissing evil" in England, indicating the large volume of urine passed by people suffering from diabetes.

• **Who discovered insulin?**

Banting and **Best** (1922) discovered insulin.

Symptoms of diabetes mellitus :

(i) The urine becomes sweet and its specific gravity is raised due to the presence of sugar in it.

(ii) Increased thirst.

(iii) Increased appetite (Polyphagia).

(iv) A feeling of fatigue, weakness and hunger.

(v) Extreme anxiety and irritability.

(vi) Tremors develop and fine movements are not possible.

(vii) Blurring of eyesight is noticed.

(viii) Vasomotor disturbances, such as flushing or palor, perspiration and chilliness.

(ix) Unexpected weight loss is observed.

(x) Vulval itching occurs in woman.

(xi) Frequent voiding of urine (Polyuria).

(xii) Hyperglycaemia may be associated with cardiovascular and other complications.

Types of diabetes mellitus : It can be distinguished into two types :

1. Insulin dependent diabetes mellitus (IDDM) or type-I : In patients with insulin dependent diabetes mellitus there is a marked decrease in the number of insulin-containing β-cells.

2. Non-insulin dependent diabetes mellitus (NIDDM) or type-II : It is the more common form of diabetes.

• **Insulin dependent diabetes mellitus (IDDM) or type-I :** The pathogenesis may result from the development of islet cell-surface antibodies. It is caused by marked deficiency of insulin or marked decrease in number of β-cells of pancreas. It has been found that cytotoxic autoantibodies to β-cells lead to β cell destruction. The causes responsible for the development of cytotoxic antibodies are not known. Autoantibodies play a role in the pathogenesis of several other endocrine-based disease states.

IDDM is a juvenile-onset diabetes which develops in youth within ten to fourteen years. The symptoms begin rather abruptly and the control of the disease almost always requires insulin replacement therapy. There is evidence that juvenile–onset diabetes may also be caused by a virus but initiation may require more than a single virus infection. The symptoms may only be manifested when sufficient damage has been caused by a number of infections such as mumps and rubella.

Clinical symptoms :

(i) Hyperglycaemia : It is a condition in which blood sugar level increases above the normal level, i.e. above 120 mg per 100 ml. When the blood sugar level exceeds the renal threshold value, i.e., 180 mg per 100 ml of blood, then sugar appears in the urine. Continuous hyperglycaemia condition occurs when peripheral tissues do not utilize glucose and the liver releases excess of glucose. Hyperfunction of anterior pituitary, adrenal cortex, etc. causes hyperglycaemia.

(ii) Glycosuria : This is a condition when the glucose level exceeds 180 mg glucose per 100 ml of blood above the normal blood glucose level, i.e., 60-100 mg glucose per 100 ml of blood. At this time the renal tubules fail to reabsorb the entire quantity of glucose filtered. Consequently some glucose that remains unabsorbed is excreted along with the urine and, therefore, sugar appears in the urine.

(iii) Protein catabolism : Hyposecretion of insulin stimulates pronounced protein catabolism in skeletal muscle and the amino acids produced provide further substrate for gluconeogenesis in the liver. The conversion of proteins through amino acids into glucose, which cannot be metabolised and excreted in the urine, leads to wasting of muscles and loss of weight in the diabetic patient.

(iv) Ketogenesis : Hyposecretion of insulin may cause synthesis of ketone bodies. The increased breakdown of fats leads to high levels of free fatty acids in the plasma which further inhibit the uptake of glucose by skeletal muscle and are metabolised to ketone bodies such as acetone, β-hydroxybutyric acid and aceto-acetic acid in the liver. The accumulation of these strong acids in the plasma leads to severe **metabolic acidosis.**

• **Non-insulin dependent diabetes mellitus (Previously called adult (maturity) onset diabetes or type-II :** This type is the more common form of diabetes and is usually found in middle aged to elderly adults. The majority of people who suffer from **maturity onset diabetes** have above normal levels of insulin, but their tissues do not respond to the hormone. This condition is called **insulin resistance** which may be caused by a number of factors. The resistance to insulin can be divided into three types : (i) pre-receptor, (ii) receptor and (iii) post-receptor resistance. This and other observations strongly support the notion of abnormal glucose recognition by the pancreatic islet as a fundamental defect in NIDDM.

(i) **Pre-receptor resistance :** This may be due to : (a) antibodies against insulin; (b) mutant insulin structures like defect in primary structure of insulin β-chain at one or more positions; (c) familial-hyperpro insulinemia and the mutation occurs at cleavage site of A or B chain.

(ii) **Receptor resistance :** This may occur due to :

Type A : (a) Decrease in number of insulin receptor on target cell and/or decrease in affinity of the receptor to the hormone. (b) Point mutation in insulin receptor gene prevents processing of the receptor precursor. (c) Impaired expression of receptor tyrosine kinase activity. (d) Point mutation blocks insertion of mature receptor into the plasma membrane of the target cell.

Type B : Receptor blocked by circulatory antibodies to the receptor.

(iii) **Post-receptor resistance :** This is owing to the following :

(a) Decreased capacity of β-cells to compensate for the underlying insulin resistance by increased secretion of insulin.

(b) Possible under expression (down regulation) of β-cell glucose transporters.

(c) Autoantibodies to the GLUT-2 glucose transporter of β-cells.

(d) Mutation of the glucokinase gene may prevent uptake and metabolism of glucose necessary for the mechanism of insulin secretion.

Symptoms of NIDDM : There are about 10 million people with diabetes mellitus in the limited states. Among these 80% of the people have NIDDM. The symptoms of polyuria (frequency of urine), polydispia (increased thirst), blurred vision, paresthesia and fatigues are manifestations of hyperglycaemia. The vast majority of NIDDM have normal levels of insulin but their tissues do not respond to the hormone. However most individuals of type II show obesity and chronic skin infections. It has been revealed that upper body obesity is strongly associated with hyperlipidemia, hypertension and NIDDM, whereas lower-body obsesity is usually not.

• **Abnormal characteristics of diabetes :** Hyperglycaemia, glycosuria, ketosis, acidosis, diabetic coma (unconsciousness), polyuria, weight loss in spite of polyphagia (condition of increased appetite) and polydipsia (condition of increased thirst) are the abnormal characteristics.

Diabetes mellitus : Disease produced by deficiency of secretion or action of insulin. It may be of two types insulin dependent diabetes mellitus (IDDM in which insulin secretion is low) and non-insulin dependent diabetes mellitus (NIDDM in which there is a tissue insensitivity to insulin).

DISORDERS OF ADRENAL CORTICAL HORMONES

Deficiency of corticoid hormones owing to hypofunction of adrenal cortex causes to a clinical condition, called **Addison's disease** whereas hypersecretion of these hormones produces **Cushing's disease.** An excessive production of aldosterone leads to a disease, called **Conn's disease.** Secretion of excess sex hormone (androgen) from the adrenal cortex leads to a disease, called **virilism.**

Hypofunction of adrenal cortex

• **(a) Addison's disease :** Deficiency of corticoid (corticosteroid) hormones owing to hypofunction of adrenal cortex causes a clinical condition, called **Addison's disease.** The disease may be of primary origin and

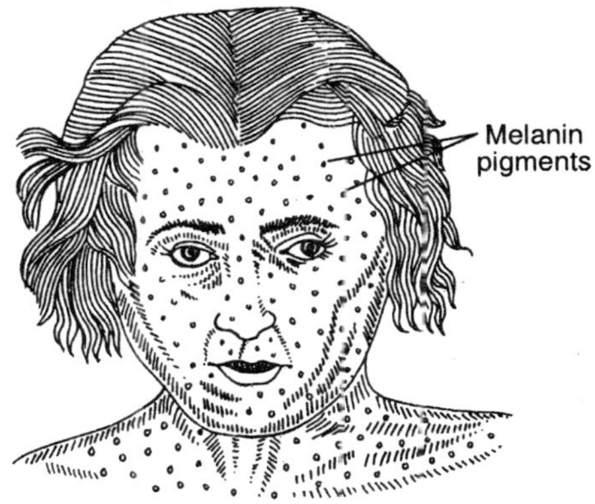

Fig. 12.9: Addison's disease.

involves total destruction of the glands. Frequently it may be due to bilateral tububercular destruction or due to tubercular infection. **Thomas Addison** (1855) first described this disease [Fig. 12.9]. It is characterised by the following features :

1. **Morphological features :**
   - (i) There is increased pigmentation or bronzing of the skin (specially the exposed areas of the skin) due to melanin synthesis.
   - (ii) Muscular weakness and easy fatiguability is due to loss of sodium

Distinguish between Diabetes mellitus and Diabetes insipidus

Subject	Diabetes mellitus	Diabetes insipidus
1. Cause	(i) It is caused by the deficiency of secretion of insulin.	(i) It is caused by the deficiency of secretion of ADH.
2. Symptoms	(i) Hyperglycaemia occurs, i.e., blood sugar level is high.	(i) Hyperglycaemia does not occur.
	(ii) Glycosuria occurs, i.e., sugar is excreted through urine.	(ii) Glycosuria does not occur.
	(iii) Polyuria occurs, i.e., large volume of urine is excreted but the specific gravity of urine is high i.e., diuresis does not occur.	(iii) Here also a large volume of urine is excreted having low specific gravity, i.e., diuresis occurs.
	(iv) Polydipsia (excessive thirst) and polyphagia (excessive hunger) are noticed.	(iv) Polydipsia takes place but polyphagia is not found.

chloride and defective power of glycogen formation.

(iii) Oedema occurs owing to loss of water from the capillaries.

2. Physiological features :

(i) Loss of appetite.

(ii) Fall of blood pressure.

(iii) BMR is reduced.

(iv) Reduction of fluid and blood volume.

(v) Persons show subnormal body temperature (i.e., below 96 °F).

(vi) Blood glucose level is low and persons suffer from weight loss.

(vii) Disturbances in ionic balance.

(viii) Gastro-intestinal disturbances and vomiting occur.

(ix) Renal insufficiency is due to glomerular filtration causing low urine volume and nitrogen retention.

3. Psychological features :

(i) Patients show restlessness.

(ii) Lack of mental concentration and insomnia.

(iii) Diminished mental process.

(iv) Shows slowness of thought.

(v) Sluggish movement is noticed.

4. Sexological features :

(i) Depression of sexual activity.

(ii) Both primary and secondary sexual characters are ill developed.

B. Hypersecretion of adrenal cortex

Overactivity of adrenal glands causes following syndromes :

(a) **Cushing's syndrome :** It is a disease characterised by a collection of symptoms caused due to excessive secretion of **glucocorticoids.** This disease was first described by **Cushing** in 1932. Primary Cushing's syndrome is due to adrenocortical tumors or adrenal hyperplasia. Pituitary tumors causing excess secretion of ACTH may be the reason of this syndrome (secondary origin). The clinical features are as following :

1. Morphological features :

(i) Excessive hair growth (**hirsutism**).

(ii) Increased deposition of fat on the trunk (but not on the limbs), face (rounded or moon-face), characteristic pad of fat at the back of the neck (a buffalo hump) and abdomen.

(iii) Osteoporosis due to bone decalcification and loss of protein matrix.

(iv) The skin is thin with purplish striations.

(v) Wound healing is slow and poor.

(vi) Fish-like mouth.

(vii) Minor injuries cause bruises.

(viii) Asthenia and wasting of muscles of the limbs.

(ix) Central obesity occurs.

2. Physiological features :

(i) The hyperglycaemia is caused due to the stimulation of neo-glucogenesis and inhibition of oxidation of glucose in tissue.

(ii) Glucose intolerance.

(iii) Eosinopenia, lymphocytopenia and plycythaemia are observed.

(iv) Retention of sodium and diminution of potassium level in the plasma.

(v) There will be rise of blood volume, increased cardiac output and rise of blood pressure.

(vi) Polyurea and polydipsia are noticed due to loss of large volume of water.

3. Psychological features :

(i) There will be mental derangement which will cause diminished mental process.

(ii) Hypertension occurs.

4. Sexological features :

(i) In females masculinisation with development of male secondary sex characters such as growth of beard, moustaches, musculature, etc.

(ii) In male impotency with atrophy of testes occurs.

(iii) Underdeveloped mammary glands in female.

(iv) In females amenorrhoea, sterility, etc aslo occur.

(b) **Conn's syndrome :** An excessive production of **aldosterone/mineralo corticoids**- commonly due to a tumor of zona glomerulosa tissue of the adrenal cortex is termed **Conn's disease** or **primary aldosteronism. W. J. Conn** described this disease in 1955. It is characterised by the following features.

1. Morphological/anatomical features :

(i) Muscular weakness is developed due to the depletion of potassium.

(ii) Muscle cramp occurs.

(iii) Cirrhosis of liver with ascites (hydroperitoneum) is found.

(iv) Bone becomes fragile.

2. Physiological features :

(i) Renal distal tubular excretion of potassium and hydrogen ions in exchange of reabsorbed sodium are observed.

(ii) Loss of hydrogen ions may lead to metabolic alkalosis.

(iii) Congestion may cause cardiac failure.

(iv) Hypernatremia is usually associated with water retention.

(v) Prolonged potassium depletion damages the kidneys resulting in polyuria.

3. Psychological features :

(i) Severe hypertension.

(ii) Mental disturbance is also noticed.

(c) **Adrenogenital syndrome :** It is a disease characterised by a collection of symptoms due to increased secretion of cortico-sexual hormones by the hyperactivity of zona-reticularis of adrenal cortex. The main characteristic of the syndrome is the overproduction of adrenal androgens. It is associated with tumors of the adrenal cortex. Adrenogenital syndrome occurs both in male and female and shows sex-reversal. This syndrome may be congenital in childhood or may acquire in adult stage.

(d) **Adrenal virilism or masculinity** : Hyper-secretion of male hormones or androgens from the adrenal cortex of **adult females** leads to **virilism** which is characterised by the following features.

(i) Growth of beard and moustaches.
(ii) The voice becomes husky and male-like.
(iii) The pubic hairs grow in male pattern.
(iv) Clitoris enlarges to look like penis.
(v) Uterus and ovaries degenerate.
(vi) Menstruation stops.
(vii) Sterility develops.
(viii) Mammary glands reduce in size.

(e) **Adrenal feminization** : Excessive secretion of female sex hormone from the adrenal cortex of **adult male** produces the signs of **feminization** which is characterised by the following features :

(i) Appearance of feminine voice.
(ii) Development of breast occurs.
(iii) Atrophy of testis is noticed.
(iv) Loss of sex desire and impotency develops.
(v) Scanty body hairs.
(vi) Penis reduces in size.

> **Note : Congenital adrenogenital syndrome** : Excessive formation of sex hormones in childhood of both females and males leads to precocious development of sexual characters.
>
> **1. In male children :** Early puberty sets in resulting in the development of secondary sexual characters.
>
> (i) Precocious growth of sex and body—producing the so, called 'Pocket Hercules' or 'Infant Hercules'.
> (ii) Early development of testes.
>
> **2. In female children :**
>
> (i) Menstruation starts early in life.
> (ii) Breasts develop fully in size.
> (iii) Growth of haris on the pubis and axillae.

DISORDERS OF ADRENAL MEDULLARY HORMONES

A. Hyperfunction of adrenal medulla : Phaeochromocytoma : It is a catecholamine-producing tumor that arises from chromaffin cells most commonly in the adrenal medulla. The common clinical manifestations are :

(i) Severe hypertension—excessive effects of epinephrine or norepinephrine.
(ii) Increased secretion of catecholamines occurs due to the presence of tumor.
(iii) Blood pressure is associated with headache, angina pectoris or blanching of the face.
(iv) Facial flushing or sweating, rapid palpitations, fever, and sometimes hypotension.
(v) High BMR.
(vi) High O_2 consumption.
(vii) There may also be nervousness or anxiety, diabetes mellitus and various types of emotional disturbances.
(viii) Myocarditis is sometimes observed.

B. Hypofunction of adrenal medullary hormone

Hypofunction of adrenal medullary hormone is very rare. Hyposecretion of epinephrine is responsible for the disturbance of autonomic nervous system. So the person shows orthostatic hypotension and hypoglycaemia.

DISORDERS OF SEX HORMONES

The human reproductive system is very much complicated. Because of the complexity of the reproductive system, it is no surprise that there are many events that can account for abnormalities in sexual development. Most of the defects have a genetic basis and they may result from a failure of steroid hormone biosynthesis or a failure of their action on target tissues.

A. In male

(i) Male pseudohermaphroditism : It is due to be chromosomal abnormalities, mutant genes, or defective gonadogenesis. In some cases male pseudohermaphroditism may be due to a defect in LH receptors of foetal Leydig cells of testis. Actually male pseudohermaphroditism can be developed by hyposecretion of testosterone and testosterone secretion may be owing to defect in synthesis of androgen receptors. A number of inborn errors of androgen production can also result in this type of syndrome.

A male pseudohermaphrodite is one whose gonads are exclusively testes but whose genital ducts or external genital organs or both-exhibit a female phenotype or that of an incompletely differentiated male.

(ii) Gynecomastia : In this condition growth of the mammary gland tissue of the male may be common during the neonatal period and the enlargement of the mammary gland is generally attributed to maternal hormones reaching the foetus during gestation. Prepubertal gynecomastia may result from a peripheral conversion of androgens produced by the testes and adrenals to estrogens. Adolescent gynecomastia may be associated with hyposecretion of testosterone/estradiol ratio. In adult males the slow increase in the prevalence of this syndrome is accentuated over the age of 45, may also be accounted for by the age-related increase of testosterone/estrogen levels. The clinical report revealed that a 70 yr old man developed gynecomastia. The etiology of the breast enlargement could not be immediately determined.

(iii) Pubarche/premature adrenarche : Pubarche refers to the isolated development of sexual hairs at an early age owing to increased levels of adrenal androgens. It is believed that adrenal androgens rather than testosterone (which can be converted to DHT) are responsible for early growth of sexual hairs.

(iv) Male climacteric phase : Inhibition of Leydig cell function and fall of androgen level may produce this disease. Although androgen therapy may not improve sexual function, muscle activities may be restored, thus counteracting the negative nitrogen balance that is a sequel of androgen deficiency.

(v) Germinal cell aplasia : Elevated FSH levels may produce this symptom. Here the seminiferous tubule is thickly populated by Sertoli cell. This disease may originate from congenital absence of germ cells.

(vi) Testicular atrophy : Increased estrogen secretion by an adrenal tumor may inhibit pituitary-hypothalamic activities, resulting in inhibition of pituitary gonadotropin secretion, which finally leads to testicular atrophy. This kind of syndrome is also called **'Feminizing Adrenocortical Carcinoma'**.

(vii) Hypogonadism : Defects in the normal development of secondary sexual characters at puberty may result from failure of pituitary gonadotropin secretion, defects at the level of the gonads or at the level of hypothalamus [Fig. 12.10].

It is two types—

(a) **Primary hypogonadism** : It occurs owing to the failure in the production of gonadal steroids in any one of a number of cases or to some defect in the hypothalamus resulting in a failure to secrete GnRH or due to Leydig cell deficiency.

(b) **Secondary hypogonadism** : It results from a defect in pituitary gonadotropin secretion and hypothalamic hypogonadism (defect in GnRH secretion).

The clinical features are : (i) Impotence. (ii) Inhibition in the production of germ cells (iii) Loss of libido effect (iv) Reduced androgen secretion and prostate involution.

(viii) Hypergonadism : It involves overproduction of pituitary gonadotropic secretion and it may be of two kinds—

(a) **Primary hypergonadism** : It may derive from tumors that secrete excess androgens. Feminizing tumors of gonadal or adrenal origin secrete

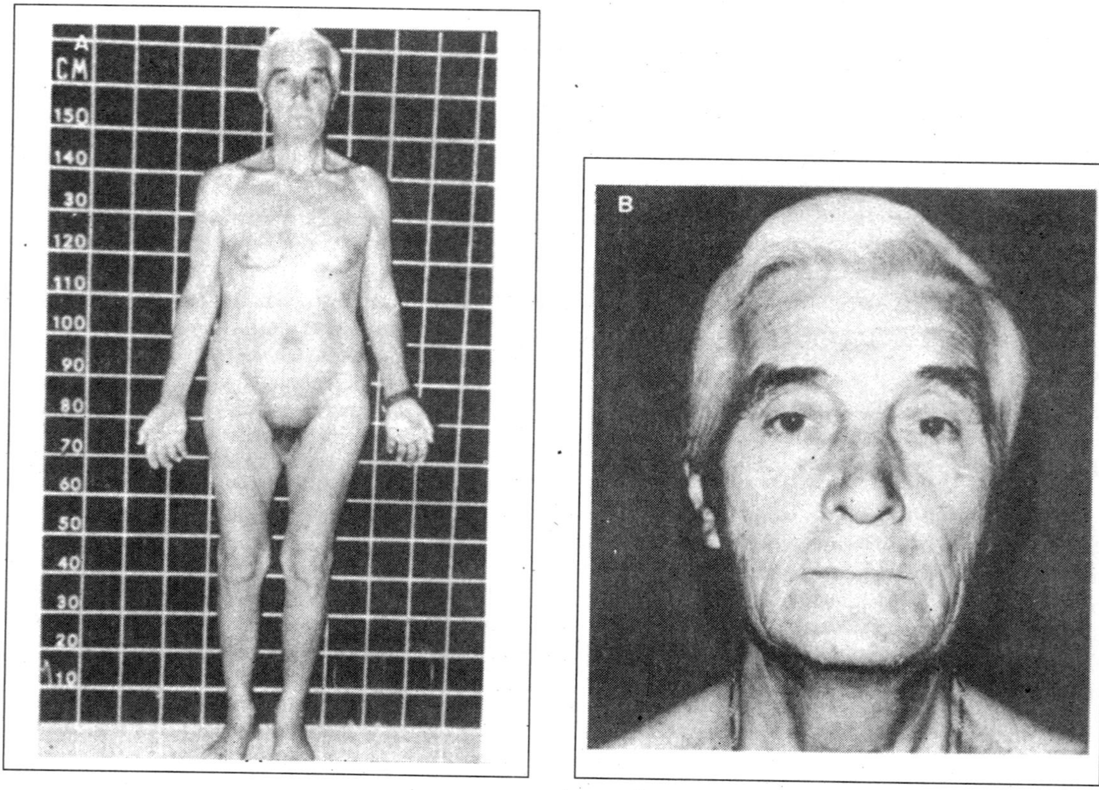

Fig. 12.10: A. Hypogonadal habitus. Note absence of body and facial hair as well as feminine body distribution. B. Hypogonadal facies. Note absence of facial hair and fine wrinkles around the corners of the eyes and lips.

estrogens have also been documented in the male.

(b) **Secondary hypergonadism :** It involves overproduction of pituitary gonadotropic hormones. Gonadal dysfunction in hyper prolactinemia is now widely recognised.

• **Pseudohermaphroditism :** Individual possessing testis but in the presence of external and internal genitalia with a female phenotype are called male pseudohermaphroditism. Gonadal cells do not match genital phenotype.

Pathophysiology :

1. Androgen insensitivity syndrome.
2. 5-α reductase deficiency.
3. Testosterone biosynthesis defect.
4. Anti Mullerian Hormone defect.
5. Impaired androgenization.

(ix) Testicular feminization : It is a X-linked recessive disorder with incomplete virilization.

Pathophysiology :

1. Insensitive to androgen.
2. AMH is not perfect.
3. Testes descends to the level of inguinal ring.
4. A short vagina forms the urogenital sinus.
5. At birth children with female sex because of the loss of androgen activity is noticed.

(x) Benign prostatic hyperplasia : Prostatic hyperplasia is a common occurence in aging men. The hyperplasia of the gland is due to accumulation of dihydrotestosterone (DHT). This hormone acts as a mediator to enhance the intracellular binding of the androgen and the process is accelerated by estrogen. Here the estrogen acts as 'androgen receptor' of the gland. It has been shown that these androgen receptors allow for androgen mediated growth even in the face of declining androgen production in advanced age. So both gynaecomastia and prostate hyperplasia may relate to the declining ratio of androgens to estrogens, which is common in the aging process of men.

B. In females

(i) Amenorrhoea : In human female the term amenorrhoea designates a relatively common disturbance, characterised by an absence of the monthly menstrual flow. The disease relates to a hyposecretion of estrogen and a failure, therefore, in the monthly proliferative growth of the endometrium resulting in an absence of monthly sloughing of the uterine lining. It is of two types—

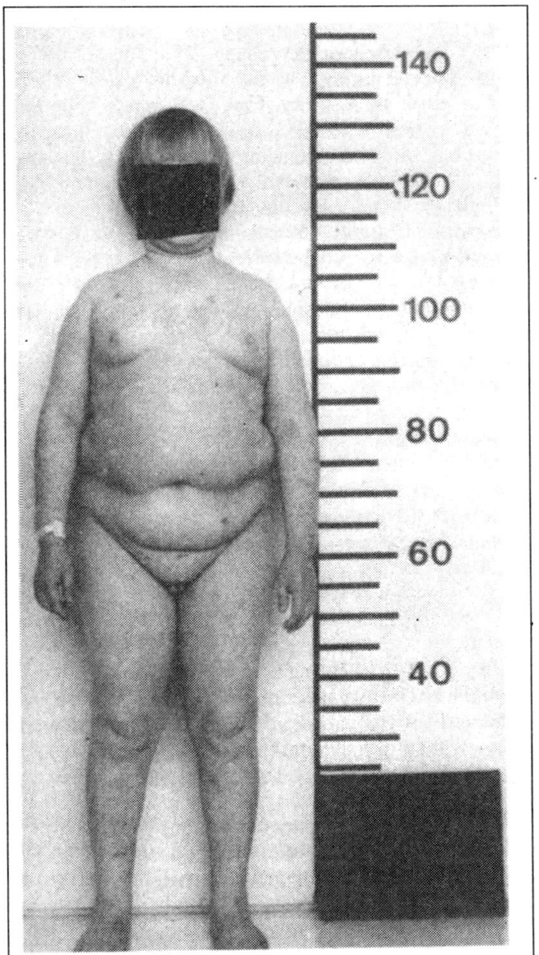

Fig. 12.11: Twenty year old male with congenital deficiency of GH, GnRH, TSH, and ACTH.

(a) **Primary amenorrhoea :** The failure of the menses to be initiated at puberty is referred to as **primary amenorrhoea.**

It is due to failure of gonadal maturation or more specifically to a defect in estrogen biosynthesis. So primary amenorrhoea is the condition when menstrual bleeding has never occured.

(b) **Secondary amenorrhoea :** Cessation of the cycle in women with previously normal periods is known as **secondary amenorrhoea,** i.e., sudden failure of menses after regular menstrual flow in pubertal condition.

If during regular periods, the flow is scanty, it is called **oligomenorrhoea** and, if profuse, it is termed as **dysmenorrhea.** Pregnancy and menopause are, of course, examples of normal physiological bases for failure to resume the menses. Failure of pituitary gonadotropin release or hyperprolactinemia are defects that result in amenorrhoea.

(ii) Hirsutism : This is defined as the presence of hairs in women on areas of the body where hairs usually are not present like men. Hairs are mainly located on the face, chest, areola of the breasts or the abdomen above the pubic symphysis. The etiology of hirsutism is mainly due to increased androgen production by the ovary and/or the adrenal gland. The presence of excess unbound androgen leads to the development of hirsutism and this is only one manifestation of hyperandrogenic conditions. The degree of this condition does not correlate with the degree of androgen production or the circulating levels of serum testosterone. The severity of hirsutism depends

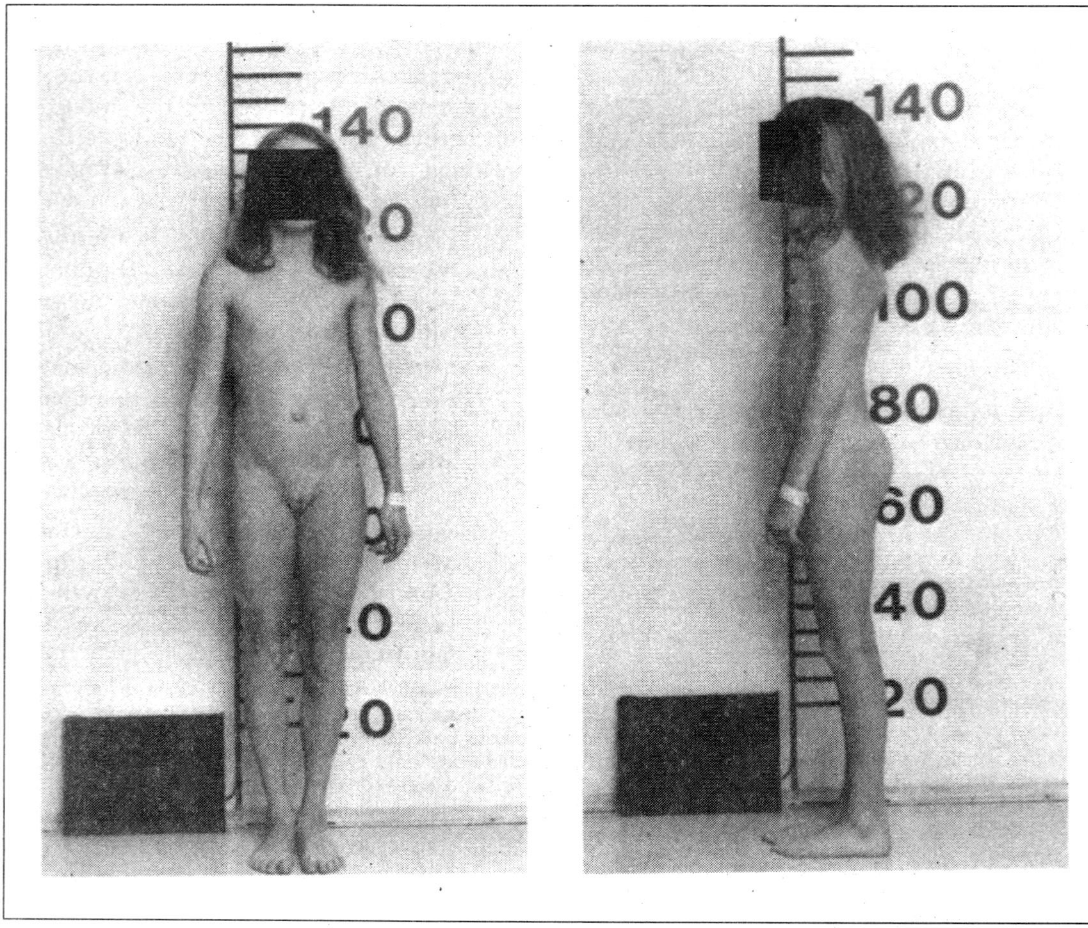

Fig. 12.12: Girl 13 4/12 years old with constitutional delay in growth and puberty. History revealed a normal growth rate but short stature at all ages. Physical examination revealed a height of 138 cm (–4.5 SD) and a weight of 28.6 kg (–3 SD). The patient had early stage 2-breast development, with 1 cm of glandular tissue on the right breast and 2 cm on the left breast. The vaginal mucosa was dulled, and there was no pubic hair.

on the availability and metabolism of testosterone by the integument. The integument of hirsute women is highly sensitive as compared with nonhirsute women. The peripheral effects of androgen, in addition to hirsutism, are to induce sebaceous glands to secrete sebum. This leads to oily skin.

Again, the effect of excess androgen secretion on the hypothalamic-pituitary gonadal system depends on the sensitivity of that system to androgen. Thus, some women may be hirsute by having regular menstrual cycles

(iii) Virilization : The females will be converted into male due to the increased secretion of male sex hormone (androgen) from zona reticularis of adrenal cortex. The general appearance, face, masculine voice, muscular body, reduced breast size, loss of female body are the main features. Beard and moustache grow and there will be growth of hairs all over the body surface. Menstruation stops, ovaries and uterus degenerate and clitoris enlarges. It is actually the combination of hirsutism and masuculinization.

(iv) Polycystic ovary : Hyposecretion of ovarian estrogen and hypersecretion of ovarian androgen are the major abnormal hormonal features of the polycystic ovarian syndrome. The women with this disease show infrequent ovulation or not at all. Excessive adrenal androgen secretion converts androstenedione to estrone (E_2). This elevated estrone may be inhibitory to pituitary FSH secretion but stimulatory to LH secretion, thus causing to failure of follicular development and ovulation.

(v) Hypogonadism : It is due to the failure in the production of normal gonadal steroids and this hyposecretion of female steroid hormones may cause this syndrome. Result is the development of amenorrhoea and polycystic ovary, failure of ovulation, etc.

(vi) Hypergonadism : Hypergonadism in female may derive from tumors of ovary that secrete excess estrogen and to a secondary defect (hypergonadotropic hypergonadism) involving overproduction of pituitary gonadotropic hormones. The clinical features are anovulatory bleeding in premenopausal women, irregular bleedng after menopause, precocious puberty in children, etc.

Female pseudohermaphroditism

Sex steroidal hormone imbalance in female foetus results **female pseudohermaphroditism.** Female pseudohermaphrodites possess ovaries but the external genitalia and gonoducts are like that of male. The male type of external genitalia are developed owing to excessive secretion of androgens. Female pseudohermaphroditism causes congenital adrenal hyperplasia resulting in failure of cortisol production.

(vii) Feminizing adrenocortical carcinoma : Excessive estrogen secretion by an adrenal tumor may inhibit pituitary-hypothalamic activities, resulting in hyposecretion of pituitary gonadotropin which causes testicular atrophy.

(viii) Premenstrual syndrome (PMS) : It is defined as the cyclic recurrence, in the luteal phase of the menstrual cycle, of a combination of distressing physical, psychological or behavioural changes of sufficient severity to result in deterioration of interpersonal relationships and/or interference with normal activities. This syndrome is one of the most common disorders of the reproductive aged woman. PMS occurs due to disorders of both the levels of reproductive hormones including estradiol, progesterone, FSH, LH, and ovarian and adrenal androgens. Nevertheless, no clear correlation has been recorded between gonadal steriod levels and the so called PMS or other menstrual cycle-related behaviours.

(ix) Galactorrhoea [Hyperprolactinemia] : It describes the secretion of breast milk in states unassociated with nursing. It can result from hyperprolactinemia.

Excess milk production is found due to hypersecretion of prolactin (PRL). Not only does hyperprolactinaemia lead to galactorrhoea but amenorrhoea and anovulation are complicating sequelae of excessive prolactin secretion in mother. Breast engorgement owing to excessive lactogenesis results from excessive prolactin secretion from a pituitary adenoma. The probable cause of prolactinoma is unknown but a failure of hypothalamic release of prolactin inhibiting factor causes to lactotroph hyperplasia, and eventually adenoma formation is occurred. The onset of excess milk production in mother may date to normal postpartum lactation that fails to be discontinued.

Casuse :

1. Pituitary adenoma.
2. Hypothyroidism.
3. Interference with dopamine action.

(x) Endometriosis : It is a common disorder characterised by the presence of tissue resembling endometrium outside of its normal position lining the uterus. The glands and stroma of endometriosis are usually responsive to gonadal hormones and the biochemical changes induce ectopic endometrium within the uterine cavity.

DISORDERS OF GASTRO-INTESTINAL HORMONES

There are two well-documented examples of direct involvement by gastrointestinal (GI) hormone in abnormal clinical conditions. Most endocrine tumors of the GI system originate in the pancreatic islets and these tumors secrete hormones that are originated there (e.g., insulin and glucagon); these tumors may also secrete vasoactive intestinal peptide (VIP) or gastrin. This VIP stimulates intestinal water secretion, and tumors consisting of VIP secreting cells are responsible for **pancreatic cholera** or the **water diarrhoea syndrome.** Patients with the **Zollinger-Ellison syndrome** have high circulating gastrin levels of tumor origin.

• **(a) Gastrointestinal syndrome**

(i) **Watery diarrhoea syndrome or Pancreatic cholera :** This disorder is formed due to the development of tumors in the pancreas. Although these pancreatic tumors secrete hormones that are normally produced there, these tumors may also secrete VIP or gastrin. The VIP secreting cells stimulate intestinal water secretion. It is known as **pancreatic cholera or water diarrhoea syndrome** (or **syndrome of profuse watery diarrhoea).**

(ii) **Zollinger-Ellison syndrome :** Patients with Zollinger-Ellison syndrome have high circulating gastrin levels of pancreatic-tumor origin. In this disorder, excessive secretion of gastrin may cause overproduction of gastric acid and the result is severe duodenal ulcer formation. It is also called **gastrinoma.** Two different types of the Zollinger-Ellison syndrome may exist, type I—due to a hyperplasia of the antral G cells and type II—due to gastrinoma of the pancreatic islets.

• **(b) Achalasia :** In this disorder, regulation of the lower oesophageal sphincter, which is important in preventing the reflux of gastric contents, may be regulated by one or more gastrointestinal hormones. Gastrin and motilin control the contractions of the lower oesophageal sphincter, while VIP is particularly potent as an inhibitor of lower oesophageal tone. In this disorder food accumulates in the oesophagus and the gastroesophageal junction fails to relax preventine food from passing leading to obstruction of the passage of food into the stomach. This condition is known as **Achalasia.** The smooth muscle of this junction is hypersensitive to normal circulating levels of gastrin, which could account for the prolonged contraction, characteristic of this disorder. Hyposecretion of these hormones may cause this disorder.

DISORDERS OF CALCIUM METABOLISM

(a) **Osteoporosis :** Osteoporosis is a malformation of bone matrix due to negative protein balance and is generally found in postmenopausal women and elderly people owing to diminution of sex hormone. Excessive secretion of adrenal cortical hormone also causes this disease due to excessive protein catabolism. Osteoporosis is characterised by decalcification and loss of bone matrix from the skeleton, resulting in shrinkage, distortion and increased brittleness of the bones. It is of two types :

(i) **Postmenopausal osteoporosis or type I :** The pathogenesis that occurs after menopause is related to a decrease in gonadal steroids and is characterised by vertebral crush, fracture of the forearm just above the wrist and hip.

(ii) **Senile osteoporosis or type II :** In elderly people with osteoporosis, there is not only reduced 1, 25 $(OH)_2P_3$ secretion, but also PTH plasma levels are diminished. It is mainly a consequence of decreased ability to absorb sufficient dietary calcium. It is believed that vitamin D deficiency is a real risk.

(b) **Osteomalacia :** This disorder is characterised by a failure of normal mineralization of bone in the adult. It is a form of adult ricket. The undermineralization of cartilage and bone (i.e.. undermineralization is due to decreased PTH levels) results in retardation of growth and in development of characteristic skeletal deformities.

It is classified as vit D-responsive or vit D-resistant. The vit D-responsive disorder may be due to a deficiency in dietary intake of vit D precursors, inadequate exposure to sunlight or intestinal malabsorption of Ca^{++}. Whereas the vit D-resistant disorders may be due to acquired renal-tubular phosphate wasting, defective collagen matrix formation and specific hereditary defects in the metabolic transformation of vit D.

This disorder occurs in women during pregnancy and lactation when a large amount of calcium is depleted from the pregnant woman (mother).

(c) **Paget's disease :** This focal disorder is characterised by the presence of excessive numbers of both osteoclasts and osteoblasts which leads to structurally weakened bone tissue. Paget's disease is fairly common in England and certain Northern European countries. Although this disorder is believed to be transmitted by a simple autosomal dominant gene, the etiology remains elusive. Osteoclasts from the bone of this patient may be enlarged and contain large numbers of nuclei. Virus like inclusions have been seen in the nuclei of some patient's osteoclasts. Certain individuals may be born with the genetic such ceptibility to osteoclastic invasion by c virus organism.

Chapter 13

Insect Endocrine Glands : Secretion and Function

In some invertebrates there are some specialised nerve cells which act like endocrine organs. Chemical substances produced in these cells are carried by blood to various tissues to regulate their functions. Their nerve cells are called **neurosecretory cells** and their secretory products are known as **neurosecretions** or **neurohormone.** The neurosecretory cells are modified neurons, and the neurohormones act as the link between the nervous and endocrine systems.

In insects, endocrine gland and neurosecretory cells have combined to form the neuroendocrine system. Neurosecretory cells are numerous in insects and there are two kinds of neurosecretory cells; **type-A** which stain with para-aldehyde fuchsin and **type B** which do not. The neurosecretory cells are provided with electron dense granules and these cells can exhibit bluish colour from the reflected light owing to the light scattering effect of colloidal sized particles.

ENDOCRINE GLANDS IN INSECTS

Corpus cardiacum is one of the neuroendocrine gland of insects which originates from the nervous system and is seen behind the brain in close association with the dorsal aorta. It receives axons from the neurosecretory cells in the brain and serves as a storage and release site for its secretions. That's why it is recognised as **neurohaemal organ.** There are four kinds of cellular elements, such as— (i) the bulbous endings of neurosecretory axons whose perikarya are found within the dorsum of the brain, (ii) the perikarya of neurosecretory cells that send axons into nerves which supply various peripheral organs, (iii) intrinsic corpus cardiacum cells and (iv) glia-like cells. The cells of corpora cardiaca are capable of producing secretions and they also act as storage release centres. **Brain hormone (BH)** is secreted by the neurosecretory cells of the brain which serves to activate corpora cardiaca. **Prothoracicotropic hormones (PTTH)** are secreted by the corpora cardiaca which in turn stimulate the prothoracic glands. **Prothoracic gland hormone (PGH)** is secreted by the prothoracic gland. Chemically it is **ecdysone.** This hormone is known to trigger moulting as it acts on the tissues to promote all of the changes characterising a moult.

Corpus allatum

These are endocrine organs of epithelial origin in insects. Here aggregation of ectodermal cells, proliferated from the surface epithelium in the vicinity of the mouth parts, are present in the posterior margin of the brain. These ectodermal cells are fused to form a gland, the **corpus allatum.** In *Peri-*

planeta sp the corpora allata are commonly paired and laterally placed or these epidermal cells are fused to form a single structure in *Rhodinus* sp. In the butterfly (*Pieris* sp), few large cells with polymorphic nuclei persist in corpus allatum. The corpus allatum of bug (*Pentatoma rufipes*) comprises of almost syncytial mass of small cells with cell boundaries barely distinguishable. A nearly columnar epithelium surronding the embryonic lumen is noticed in adult phasmid (*Bacillus rossii*).

The corpus allatum secretes a hormone, called **juvenile hormone (JH)**, to keep the larval cells active. This hormone regulates morphogenesis and so promotes metamorphosis, that is, development of the larva into adult through pupal stage. The absence of the JH causes the death of larval cells and they are used as nutrients for the growing imaginal buds [Fig 13.1].

glands depending upon final location. The tissue of the prothoracic glands exhibit cyclic secretory activity, reaching a maximum between moults. The gland becomes rudimentary in adults.

The ecdysial glands produce a hormone, called ecdysone, which brings about moulting and development of imaginal discs and reproductive organs.

• Regulation of Hormones on Metamorphosis

It may be defined as a post-embryonic extension of the developmental potential and involves dramatic changes in habit, habitat, morphology, physiology and behaviour of the larva so that it is transformed into the adult having entirely different habitat and structure. Insect metamorphosis is a special form of moulting, i.e., it consists of differential destruction of certain tissues,

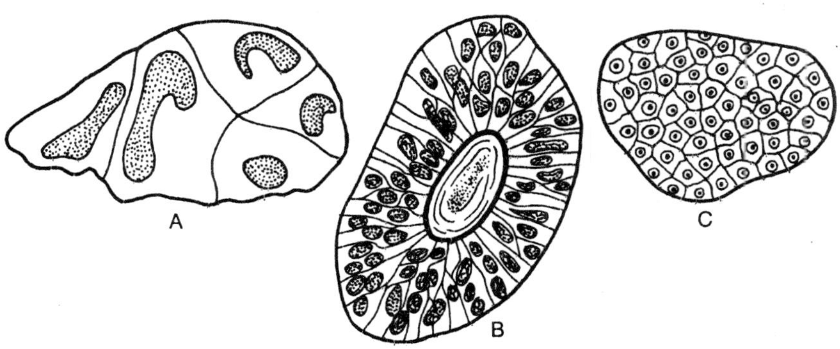

Fig. 13.1: Histological structure of corpora allata of different insects : A. *Pieris brassicae*, few large cells with polymorphic nuclei, B. *Pentatoma rufipes*, an almost syncytial mass of small cells, and C. *Bacillus rossii*, a nearly columnar epithelium surrounding the embryonic lumen.

Thoracic gland or ecdysial gland

The prothoracic glands are a pair of small glands in the first thoracic segment. This gland is observed in immature insect with the exception of Apterygote. They are also known as prothoracic glands. These glands comprise of irregular masses of tissue which are intimately associated with tracheae. These tissue are ectodermal in origin. These glands are also recognised as peritracheal or ventral

accompanied by an increase in growth and differentiation of tissues. Usually moulting comprises mainly the casting off an old cuticle and the acquisition of a new one. This change of cuticle is essential for growth and morphogenesis.

During the period of post-embryonic growth (after hatching) an insect undergoes a series of ecdyses or cast off its integument; by this process it attains its maximum size.

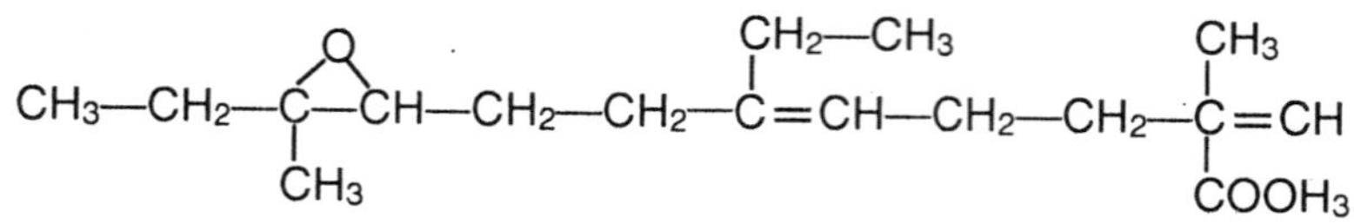

A

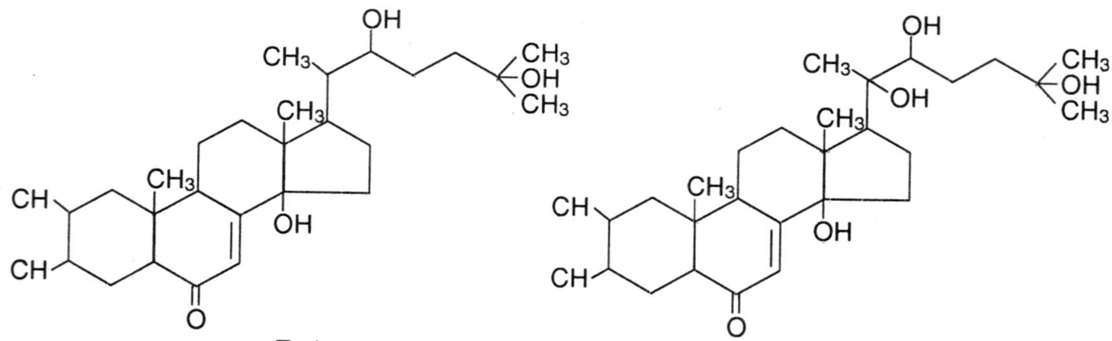

α-Ecdysone B β-Ecdysone

Fig. 13.2: A. Structure of Juvenile hormone of the moth *H. cecropia*, B. Structures of ecdysones.

The interval or stage between the two moults or ecdyses is known as a **stadium;** and the form attained by an insect in any stadium between two ecdyses or moults is termed as **instar.** When it emerges from an egg it is in its first instar, at the end of this stadium it undergoes an ecdysis or moulting and assumes the second instar and so on. The final instar is the adult or **imago.** The changes of an insect undergo to become an imago are collectively called metamorphosis. This special form of moulting or metamorphosis is under the control of different hormones.

Types of metamorphosis

Insects exhibit the following kinds of metamorphosis.

(i) **Epimorphosis or ametabolic metamorphosis** : During metamorphosis the wingless insects (apterygotes) undergo very minor changes in form, as the immature instars differ from the adult only in size and development of gonads and external genitalia. Those insects are termed as **ametabolous insects** and undergo **ametabolous development.** This type of development is considered to be primitive, for the insect goes through moults without changing its appearance, merely getting bigger. Such insects are said to undergo **epimorphosis,** i.e., the change from young to adult is negligible. The stages are **egg, juvenile** and **adult.** Example—silver-fish, springtail [Fig 13.3].

> **Note :** Schmidt-Neilsen, 1983 has argued that the term ametabolous is less desirable because it mixes with a Latin ending, so he preferred the term ametabolic.

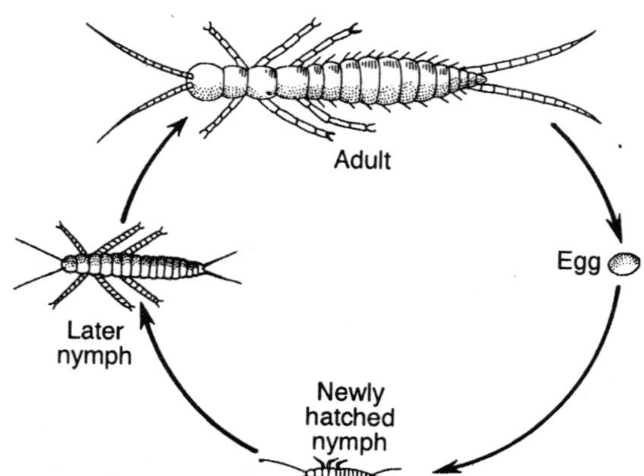

Fig. 13.3: *Lepisma* (silver fish); stages of the life history exhibiting no metamorphosis (ametabolic metamorphosis).

(ii) **Gradual metamorphosis or incomplete metamorphosis or hemimetabolic metamorphosis** : The winged insects or exopterygotes undergo a **gradual** or **incomplete metamorphosis** and is referred to as **hemimetabolous development** where the immature instars, commonly known as nymphs, resemble the adults in many respects including the presence of compound eyes but they lack functional wings, gonads and external genitalia. The wings of nymphs develop externally as bud-like outgrowths in the early instars and increase in size as the animal grows by successive moults and

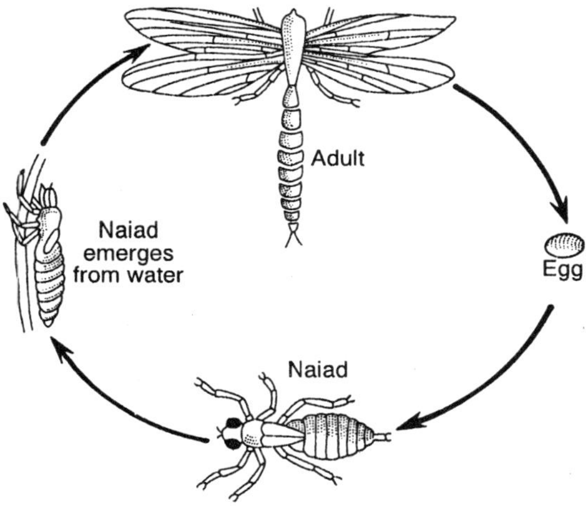

Fig. 13.4: Dragon-fly (Odonata) stages of life history exhibiting hemimetabolic metamorphosis or to say incomplete metamorphosis.

becomes winged adult. The aquatic naiads (nymphs) have tracheal gills or other modifications for aquatic life. The stages are **egg**, **nymph** and **adult**. This type of metamorphosis includes the grasshoppers, cockroaches, mantids, dragon-fly etc [Fig 13.4].

(iii) **Complete metamorphosis or holometabolic metamorphosis** : The endopterygota (ants, bees, butterflies, moths, flies, etc) undergo a **complete metamorphosis** and this developmental process is referred to as **holometabolous development.** Complete metamorphosis separates the physiological process of growth (larva) from those of **differentiation** (pupa) and **reproduction** (adult). Each stage acts efficiently without competition with the other stages, for the larvae often live in entirely different environments or surroundings and eat different foods. In endopterygota, the immature instars are recognised as larvae, which are quite dissimilar to the adults and are adapted to different environmental situations. The larvae lack compound eyes but usually have mandibulate mouth parts or chewing mouth parts. They may or may not have thoracic or abdominal legs. In these insects, the changes in the transformation from the last instar larva to the adult are compressed into a single intervening instar surrounded by a

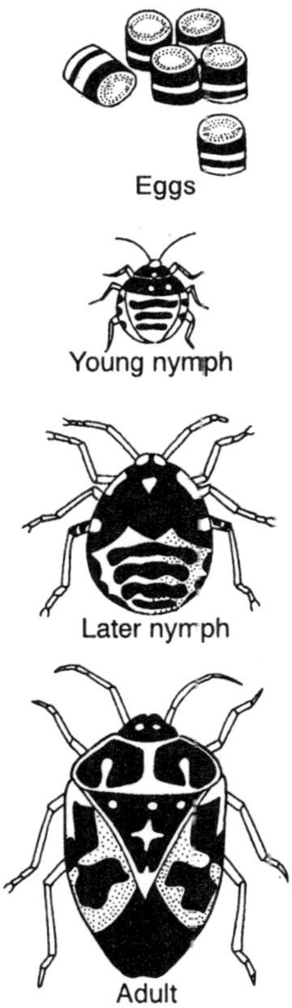

Fig. 13.5: Beetles; stages of the life history exhibiting paurometabolous metamorphosis.

'case' or 'cocoon', called **pupa.** In most cases the larval instars resemble one another except for a few minor morphological details and in size. However, some holometabolic insects pass through one or more larval instars that are completely different from the others (e.g., some members of Diptera, Coleoptera). This is known as **hypermetamorphosis.** The stages of endopterygota are **egg, larva,** and **adult.** The adults do not undergo further moulting [Fig 13.6 and 13.7].

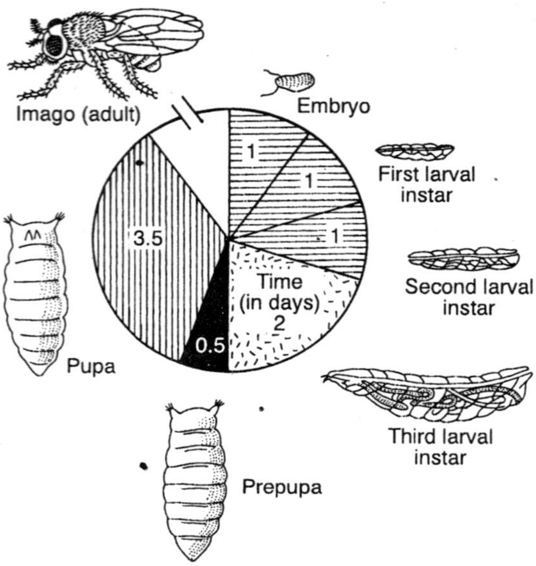

Fig. 13.6: Life cycle of *Drosophila,* a holometabolous insect. It includes following developmental stages : the embryo, three larval instars, prepupa, pupa and adult. The number represents the duration of each stage in days.

(iv) **Paurometabolous metamorphosis or development :** In beetles, Cockroaches, grasshoppers etc the newly hatched form or larval form is terrestrial, similar to the adult. It resembles the adult in external body form but lacks wing rudiments and external genitalia. Here the development is gradual metamorphosis. The special adult characters (i.e., wings and external genital organs) appear gradually or only in the last moult. Except for gonads and the flight muscles, the internal structures do not undergo much change [Fig 13.5].

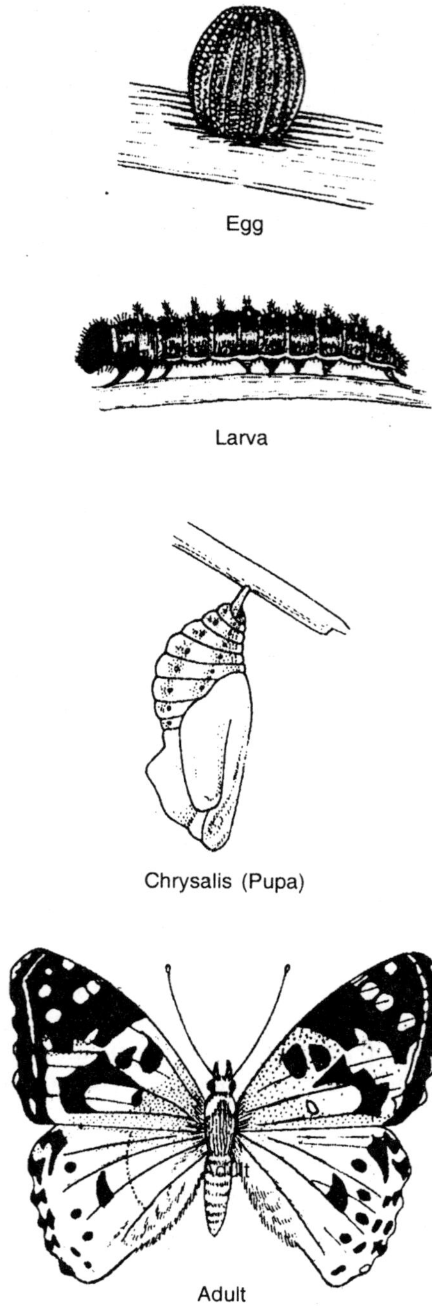

Fig. 13.7: Butterfly. Stages of life history exhibiting holometabolic (complete) metamorphosis.

ENDOCRINE OR HORMONAL REGULATION IN INSECT METAMORPHOSIS

The sequence of events of moulting cycles and metamorphosis of insects have been found under precise hormonal control. In brief, certain stimuli associated with the state of nourishment cause the neurosecretory cells of the brain to discharge the "brain hormone" (BH), which is carried by neurosecretary cell axons to the corpora cardiaca (insect endocrine glands), from where it is released into the blood.

> **Note :**
>
> **Hormones required :** Brain hormone (BH) or prothoracicotropic hormone (PTTH), Ecdysome, Juvenile hormone (JH).
>
> **Tissues involved :** Lateral neurosecretory cells of the brain, corpus cardiacum, corpus allatum, prothoracic gland.

Role of BH in insect metamorphosis : This hormone then stimulates the thoracic glands (or their equivalent) to produce a hormone which causes the epithelial cells to begin the processes which lead to moulting. At the same time at all moults except the last, the corpora allata (insect endocrine glands which are located near brain) secrete a hormone which ensures the development of another larval instar. During the last moult, the corpora allata are inactive and the adult is produced.

These hormones are named according to their functions. The brain hormone because of its effect upon the thoracic gland is called **ecdysone** or **moulting hormone** or MH because it initiates moulting or ecdysis; and that form the corpora allata is called **juvenile hormone** (JH) because it ensures the retention of juvenile characters. These insect hormones have following role in the insect moulting and metamorphosis.

Juvenile hormone and its involvement in insect moulting and metamorphosis

The juvenile hormone controls the growth, moulting and onset of metamorphosis of insects. In the insect, whose life cycle consists of 4 larval moults, a larval-pupal moult and a pupal-adult moult; it has been observed that in every case the developing system, having been diverted to some degree during embryonic development, moves towards expression of the adult organization. The hormonal controls operate to determine when the major event occurs, to what extent development can be temporarily arrested and how long juvenile state may be prolonged. For example, in the presence of the ecdysone or prothoracic gland hormone (PGH), juvenile hormone (JH) promotes larval development or maintains the status quo and so prevents metamorphosis. The presence of JH in an immature insect, whether larva or pupa, ensures that when the immature insect moults, it remains its larval or pupal characters and does not differentiate into an adult. In other words, withdrawl of JH initiates metamorphosis. Conversely, implantation of the JH secretion gland from a 2nd stage larva to a 4th stage larva maintains the larval state, in effect inhibiting metamorphosis so that larval growth continues and a giant larva is produced.

During the early larval instars, both JH and ecdysone (i.e., MH) are formed prior to moult. It is known that JH interacts with ecdysone to stimulate larval maturation during each stage of development. The concentration of JH evidently decreases toward the end of a larval instar allowing the ecdysone to cause ecdysis.

Accordingly, if the corpora allata are removed in the last larval stage of honeybee or the giant **cecropia,** a silk moth, for instance, instead of a normal pupa appearing a monstrous form, intermediate between a pupa and an adult, is developed. However, if these glands are surgically removed during one of the earlier stages, the larvae undergo precocious pupation at the very next stage and eventually develop into midget sized adult insects. The larval form is developed in the presence of a high JH concentration, the pupa in the presence of a very low JH concentration and the adult when the JH is completely absent.

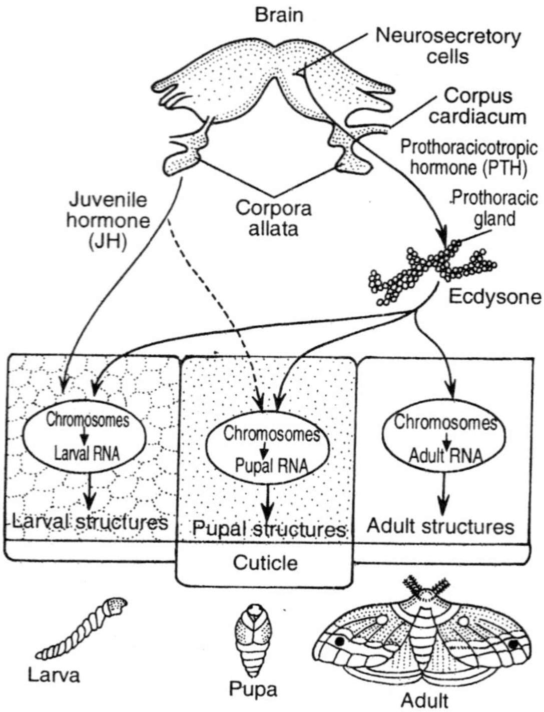

Fig. 13.8: Hormonal control of metamorphosis in the silk moth, *Cecropia*.

In both holometabolous and hemimetabolous insects, two separate and distinct peaks of ecdysone are noticed during the last immature instar. The first one is low and in absence of JH, the epidermal cells are reprogrammed from larval to pupal commitment in holometabolous insects and from nymphal to adult stage in hemimetabolous insects. The second ecdysone or MH peak being high, causes moulting in association with JH. At this phase the presence of JH prevents the imaginal discs from developing into adult structures during the pupal stage. Finally, the next peak of ecdysone or MH in the absence of JH causes adult development.

Ecdysone and Juvenile Hormone (JH) involvement

Ecdysone : Ecdysone is a steroid moulting hormone (MH) secreted from prothoracic gland or ecdysial gland of immature insects, with the exception of the Apterygotes. The ecdysial glands consist of irregular masses of tissue of ectodermal origin that are usually intimately associated with trachea. Depending upon its final location, these glands are also referred to as peritracheal or ventral glands. The cells of these glands exhibit cyclic secretory activity, reaching a maximum between moults and the ecdysial glands undergo atrophy in the adults.

It has been shown that the neurosecretory cells of brain of insects produce a prothoracic gland-stimulating factor (polypeptide) known as **brain hormone (BH)** or **prothoracicotrophin** that evokes the synthesis of ecdysone. It acts on the cells to promote growth and differentiations leading to maturation of the young. Two types of ecdysones can be synthesised by insects—α-ecdysone and β-ecdysone [Fig 13.2]. The latter steroid differs from α-ecdysone only by having a hydroxyl group at position 20.

Endocrine control of ecdysone on growth and metamorphosis in insects : Upon emergence from the egg, the immature insects gradually increase in size to reach adults through some mechanism, called moulting or ecdysis. Under the impact of ecdysone, at each moult the old cuticle is loosened and thrown off, the specialised epidermal cells are reabsorbed or discarded, and the ordinary epidermal cells which have been stimulated to grow and divide, give rise to new cuticle and the two new groups of specialised cells. The ecdysone functions directly upon those cells that are in a state of dormancy. Within few hours, the nucleolus is enlarged, RNA begins to accumulate in the cytoplasm and mitochondria enlarge and multiply by subdivision. By the time, the old cuticle is thrown off, the renewed epidermal growth has been virtually completed with locally expanded regions folded compactly while awaiting release from cuticular confinement. It has been shown that the muscles of the larva in *Rhodnius sp* dedifferentiate between moults and redifferentiate muscle fibres shortly before the next moult occur. To a degree the organism is renewed on occasion and at each time the volume of the growing animal doubles.

• **Juvenile hormone :** It is another hormone of insect secreted from **corpora allata.** It opposes metamorphosis and thus, prolongs the larval or the pupal stage of development. This hormone ensures the retention of juvenile characters.

Chemically this hormone (JH) is methyl 10 epoxy-7-ethyl-3, 11-dimethyl-2, 6-tridecadienoate in moth, *Hyalophora cecropia*. It is likely that considerable species variability may be found in chemistry of this hormone since the corpora allata vary in functional appearance.

Endocrine control of juvenile hormone (JH) and its role in insect moulting and metamorphosis : The juvenile hormone controls the growth, moulting and onset of metamorphosis of insects. Practically the corpora allata secrete juvenile hormone, which promote larval development and inhibit development of adult characteristics. It has been described to have **'status quo'** effect, which implies that it is more of an inhibitory substance than an active growth factor (**Williams**). In the insect, whose life cycle consists of four larval moults, a larval-pupal moult and a pupal-adult moult and in every case the developing system, having been diverted to some degree during embryonic development, moves toward expression of the adult organisation.

During the early larval instars, both MH and JH are formed prior to ecdysis. In fact JH interacts with MH to induce larval maturation in every stage of development. The concentration of JH decreases toward the end of a larval instar, allowing the ecdysone to cause moulting

The presence of JH in an immature insect, whether larva or pupa, ensures that when the immature insect undergoes moulting it retains larval or pupal characters and does not differentiate into an adult. In other words, withdrawl of JH initiates metamorphosis.

• Other hormones related to metamorphosis

Ecdysis triggering hormone (ETH) : It is the twenty six amino acid peptide hormone which is synthesised by the epitracheal glands that are housed segmentally in larvae, pupae and adults of *Manduca sexta*. This hormone may act upstream from the eclosion hormone in a series of cascade events leading to moulting i.e., it also plays an important role in ecdysis (**Zitnan et al**, 1996).

Eclosion hormone (EH) : It is one kind of hormone among insects which induces many aspects of pupal-adult ecdysis including the behaviour associated with ecdysis and subsequent degeneration of abdominal intersegmental muscles. This hormone is released from the brain by a circadian clock and declining ecdysteroid titers. It has been shown that, if the EH titer is artificially kept high the secretion of this hormone and its activity are inhibited.

Bursicon or Tanning hormone (BH or TH) : Bursicon is a hormone which is said to stimulate tanning and sclerotisation of the cuticle following moulting. It is commonly found in the neurohaemal organs associated with the ventral chain ganglia.

• Role of hormones in reproduction of insects

There are several hormones in insects which are suggested to influence the different phases of reproduction. These are—

(i) **Spermatogenesis :** Ecdysone regulates the permeability of the testes walls to induce the differentiating process of spermatocytes in insects. JH is shown to have some inhibitory effects on spermatogenesis.

(ii) **Oogenesis :** Oogenesis is a very much complicated phenomenon and it varies in different insects. In general, the hormones from corpus allatum assist in maturation of the egg. Again some substances like farnesol and farnesyl methyl ether can mimic the effects of corpora allata hormones and have a gonadotropic action. The secretions of the median neuro-secretory cells of brain stimulate corpus allatum and protein syntheis (required for the synthesis of yolk material). In addition to that ecdysone has been found to be incorporated in the regulation of oogenesis in female mosquitoes. Following a blood meal, lateral neurosecretory cells of the brain in mosquitoes secrete a hormone for the development of egg, which in turn, induces the ovary to release ecdysone. This ecdysone triggers the synthesis of egg yolk and the JH released by corpus allatum activates fat bodies and ovaries.

(iii) **Fertilization/Reproduction** : Both nervous and endocrine systems act accordingly to make reproduction success. The major centres are the neurosecretory cells of the brain and major events are the release of JH by corpora allata and either ecdysone secretion by ecdysial gland in immature insects or ecdysone biosynthesis by the ovary in adult insects. Now the hormones act either independently or together in association with nervous system to make reproduction success.

• Hormonal regulation of general body function

(i) **Nutrition** : The movement of alimentary canal in some insects that complement the action of digestive enzymes and absorption of food is said to be controlled partly by the neurosecretory cells. In cockroaches, **proctolin** (a neurohormone) regulates the peristaltic movements of the hindgut. In Diptera, the secretion of saliva is under the control of **5-hydroxytryptamine (5-HT)**, a neurohormone.

(ii) **Circulation** : Eclosion hormone (EH) is released from the brain and is suggested to control the heart beat. This hormone influences cardioacceleration which lasts only for 75 minutes of the eclosion period.

(iii) **Excretion** : It is reported that **antidiuretic hormones** are released by pars intercerebralis of brain, corpus cardiacum ventral chain ganglia and subesophageal ganglia in insects. These hormones regulate the production of excretion. In cockroaches, proctolin is responsible for motility of the hindgut which also acts as a neuromodulator to assist in the excretion process. Again, in *Locusta*, an antidiuretic hormone and a chloride transport-stimulating hormone (CTSH) have been shown to regulate both ion and water balance.

(iv) **Metabolism** : The hormones released by corpus cardiacum inhibit the oxidation of glucose in many insects. **MNCH** (median neurosecretory cell hormone) suppresses glycogen synthesis in mosquitoes. Again the DH (diapause hormone) is suggested to stimulate glycogen synthesis at the time of diapause stage.

The hormonal regulation of protein metabolism in insects has not been studied in detail. It is assumed that some hormones may directly or indirectly influence the metabolism of amino acids in general.

Lipid remain stored in the fat body in most insects. Many hormones are known to stimulate lipid content of haemolymph. The **AKH (adipokinetic hormone)** secreted from corpus cardiacum has considerable adipokinetic activity. But in cockroaches, AKH has no adipokinetic effect. In *Locusta*, storage of lobe of corpus cardiacum produces a hypoliparmic factor that opposes the action of AKH.

• Hormonal control of behaviour

Hormones play a very important role and they either act as **modifiers** or as **releasers** of behaviour, such as, ecdysis triggering hormone (ETH) and eclosion hormone (EH) in the moth, *Autheraea*, act both as releasers in triggering the pre-eclosion behaviour and as modifiers in turning on adult behaviour.

(i) **Migration** : Migration takes place often in some insects on the basis of endocrine variations correlated with environmental effects like crowding, short-day length and deficiency of food. In 'aphid groups' crowding results in the production of winged forms instead of wingless forms. This migratory behaviour depends on a particular balance between ecdysone and JH in the haemolymph. This is associated with the activity of corpus allatum.

(ii) **Dormancy** : It has been seen that insect development and general activity may undergo two kinds of suppression or dormancy in response to the changes in abiotic environment. Insects may undergo retardation of metabolism and development in adverse environmental conditions, when conditions are no longer adverse, both functions resume immediately. This kind of dormancy is known as **quiescence**. Again the development as well as growth does not necessarily resume immediately with the return of favourable conditions. This kind of dormancy is referred to as **diapause.**

Diapause is regulated by hormones. For example, the secretion of hormones from the subesophageal ganglia of the moths like *Bombyx* and **Phalaenoides,** induce diapause in the embryos. The arrest of development in the larval and pupal diapause has classically been attributed to an arrest of PTTH secretion. It is to be noted that biological clock directly controls PTTH release by a mechanism housed entirely within the brain while in other species the PTTH release may be arrested by high levels of JH. Indeed, high titers of JH levels at larval diapause lead to the invocation of JH in regulation of PTTH secretion in non-diapausing moults.

Acronyms Used in This Text

ABP—Androgen binding protein
AC—Adenylate cyclase
ACH—Acetylcholine
ACHR—Acetylcholine receptor
ADH—Antidiuretic hormone; Vasopressin
APCs—Antigen presenting cells
ANF—Atrial natriuretic factor
ANP—Atrial natriuretic peptide
AKH—Adipo kinetic hormone
BH—Brain hormone
CaM—Calmodulin
cAMP—Cyclic adenosine monophosphate
CAT—Chloramphenical acetyl transferase
CBG—Corticosteroid binding globulin; Transcortin
CBP—Calcium binding protein
CCK—Cholecystokinin
CCK—PZ—Cholecystokinin pancreozymin
CG—Chorionic gonadotropin
CGMP—Guanosine 3′, 5′—cyclic monophosphate
CGRH—Calcitonin gene-related hormone
CLIP—Corticotropin like intermediate lobe peptide
CMP—Cytidine monophosphate
COC—Cumulus oocyte complex
COMT—Catechol-o-methyl transferase
CPK—Creatine phosphokinase
CRE—cAMP response element
CRE β—cAMP response element binding protein
CRH—Corticotropin-releasing hormone
CT—Computed tomography/Calcitonin
CTSH—Chloride transport stimulating hormone
DAG—Diacylglycerol
DBH—Dopamine-β-hydroxylase

DH—Diapause hormone
DHEA—Dehydroepiandrosterone
DHT—Dihydrotestosterone
DIT—Diiodotyrosine
DOC—Dioxycorticosterone
DOPA—Dihydroxyphenylalanine
EDRF—Endothelium-derived relaxing factor
EDT—Ethylene diamine tetra acetate
EGF—Epidermal growth factor
EH—Eclosion hormone
ELISA—Enzyme-linked immunosorbent assay
EPO—Erythropoietin
ERC—Estrogen receptor complex
ERK—Extracellular regulated kinase
ETH—Ecdysis triggering hormone
FFA—Free fatty acid
FGF—Fibroblast growth factor
GABA—γ-aminobutyric acid
GAP—GTPasactivating protein/GnRH associated peptide
GDP—Guanosine di-phosphate
GH—Growth hormone
GI—Gastrointestinal
GRH—Growth releasing hormone
GPCR—G-protein coupled receptor
GTP—Guanosine triphosphate
GM-CSF—Granulocyte-macrophage colony stimulating factor
GnRH—Gonadotropin releasing hormone
GSBG—Gonadal steroid binding globulin
HCG—Human chorionic gonadotropin
HCS—Human chorionic somatomammotropin
HETE—Hydroxy-eicosa-tetraenoic acid
HIOMT—Hydroxy-indole-o-methyl transferase
HRC—Hormone receptor complex
HRE—Hormone response/regulatory element
5-HT—5-Hydroxy tryptamine
HSP—Heat shock protein
HTH—Homeostatic thymic hormone
IDDM—Insulin dependent diabetes mellitus .

IGF—Insulin-like growth factor

$InsP_3$—Inositol 1, 4, 5-triphosphate

IH—Inhibitory hormone

IP_3—Inositol triphosphate

IF—Inntibitory factor

IRS—Insulin receptor substance/substrate

ITP—Inosine triphosphate

JH—Juvenile hormone

JAK—Janus kinase

LATS—Long acting thyroid stimulator

LCAT—Lecithin cholesterol acyl-transferase

LDL—Low-density lipoprotein

LH—Luteinizing hormone

LSH—Lymphocyte stimulating hormone

LTH—Luteotropic hormone

MAO—Monoamine oxidase

MAPK—Mitogen-activated protein kinase

MEN—Multiple endocrine neoplasia

MEK—Mitogen effective kinase

MH—Moulting hormone

MIT—Mono-iodo-tyrosine

MIH—Mono-iodo-histidine

MNCH—Median neurosecretory cell hormone

MRH—Melanocyte releasing hormone

MRHIH—Melanocyte releasing hormone inhibiting hormone

MSH—Melanocyte stimulating hormone

NE—Norepinephrine

NLS—Nuclear location sequence

NIDDM—Non-insulin dependent diabetes mellitus

NO—Nitric oxide

OHSD—Hydoxy-steroid dehydrogenase

OMI—Oocyte maturation-inhibitor

OPKTs—Ovulation predictor kits

PAP—Prostate acid phosphatase

PALS—Periarterial lymphatic sheath

PCOs—Polycystic ovaries

PDGF—Platelet derived growth factor

PEPCK—Phosphoenol pyruvate carboxy-kinase

PGE—Prostaglandin E
PGF—Prostaglandin F
PGH—Prothoracic gland hormone
PIF—Prolactin-release-inhibiting factor
PIH—Prolactin-release-inhibitory hormone
PKA—Protein Kinase A
PKC—Protein kinase C
PLA—Phospholipase A
PLC—Phospholipase C
PM—Plasma membrane
PMS—Premenstrual syndrome
PNMT—Phenylethanolamine-N-methyl transferase
POMC—Pro-opio-melano-cortin
PP—Pancreatic polypeptide
PRH—Prolactin releasing hormone
PRIH—Prolactin releasing inhibiting hormone
PRL—Prolactin
PSA—Prostate specific antigen
PTH—Parathyroid hormone
PTTH—Pro-thoracico-tropic hormone
RAS—Renin-angiotensin system
RFLP—Restriction fragment length polymorphism
RTK—Receptor tyrosine kinase
RYRs—Ryanodine receptors
SHBG—Sex hormone binding globulin
SST—Somatostatin acute regulatory protein
STAT—Signal transduction activator of transcription
STH—Somatotropic hormone
TBG—Thyroxine binding globulin
TCT—Thyrocalcitonin
TBPA—Thyroxine binding pre-albumin; transthyretin
TEBG—Testosterone estrogen binding globulin
TH—Tanning hormone
TRC—Testosterone receptor complex
TRH—Thyrotropin releasing hormone
TSH—Thyroid stimulating hormone
TXA_2—Thromboxane A_2
VIP—Vasoactive intestinal polypeptide; Gastrin
VMA—Vanil mandelic acid

References

1. Histology: Ross and Reith
2. Histology: R. O. Greep
3. A Text Book of Histology: Bloom and Fawcett
4. Bailey's Text Book of Histology: W. M. Copenhavea, D. E. Kelly and R. L. Wood
5. A Text Book of Animal Histology: A. K. Berry
6. Simplified Course in Chordate Embryology and Histology: U. K. Agarwal and Usha Gupta
7. An Atlas of Histology: Freeman & Bracegirdle
8. Endocrinology: Mac E. Hadley
9. Endocrinology (Vol 1, 2 & 3): L. J. Degroot
10. Endocrinology: Ross. W. Hawker
11. Text Book of Endocrinology: Gorman & Wilson
12. A Text Book of Endocrinology: Robert H. Williams
13. Mammalian Endocrinology: A. K. Boral
14. General Endocrinology: Turner & Bagnara
15. Comparative vertebrate Endocrinology: P. J. Bentley
16. A Text Book of Comparative Endocrinology: Gorbman
17. Vertebrate Endocrinology: Norris and Bern
18. Endocrinology and Reproductive Biology: K. V. Shastry
19. Harper's Review of Biochemistry: D. W. Martin, P. A. Mayes and V. W. Rodwell
20. Fundamentals of Biochemistry: A. C. Deb
21. Biochemistry: D. Das
22. Biochemistry: U. Satyanaryan
23. Biochemistry: Lehninger
24. Human Physiology (Vol I & II): C. C. Chatterjee
25. Animal Physiology: Prosser & Brown
26. Animal Physiology: Mohan. P. Arora
27. Introduction to General Zoology (Vol II): Chaki, Kundu & Sarkar
28. Atlas of Anatomy: Trevor Weston

Index

DIFFERENT TYPES OF EPITHELIAL TISSUE

Different Types of Epithelial Tissue

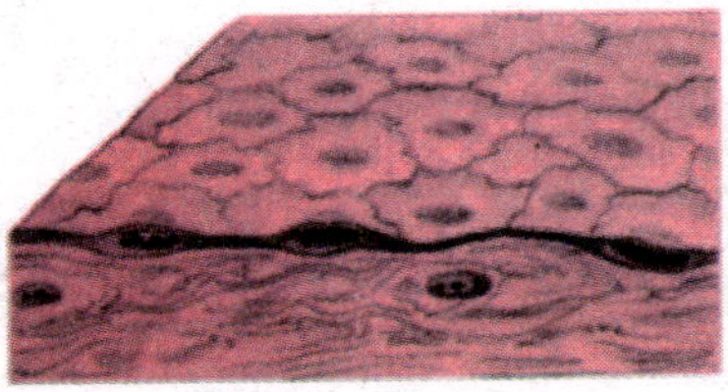

Simple squamous

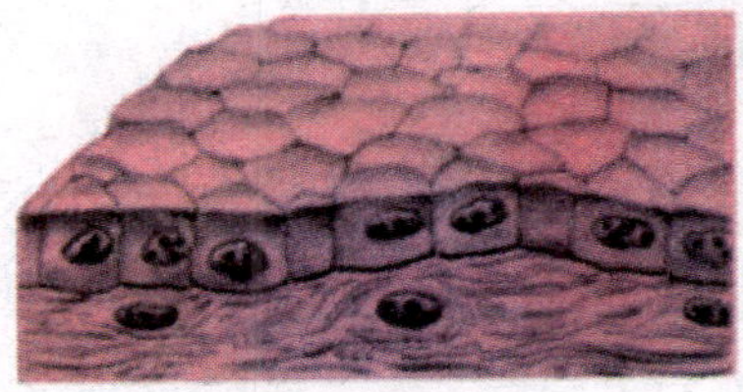

Simple cuboidal

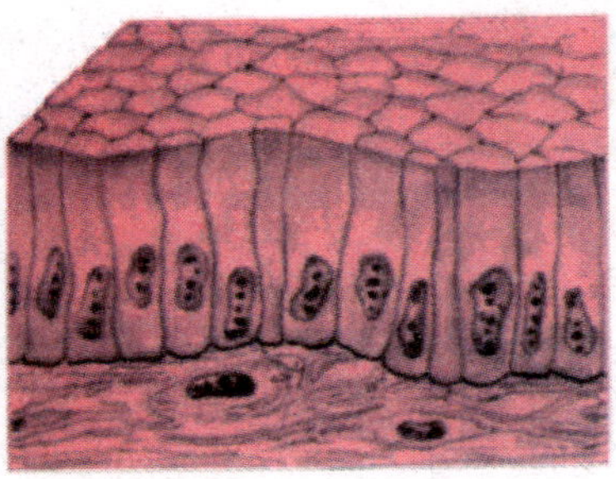

Simple columnar

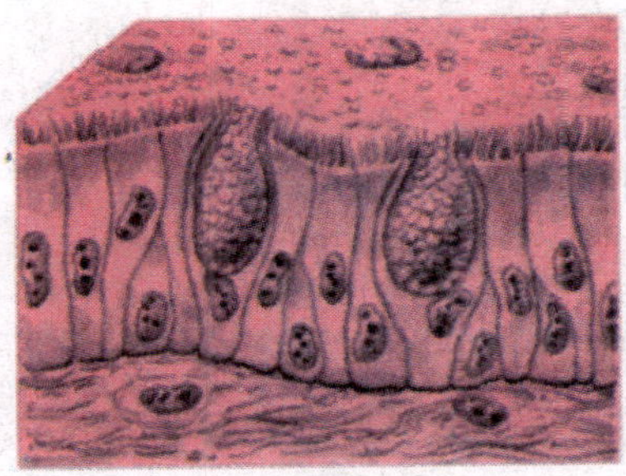

Pseudostratified columnar ciliated

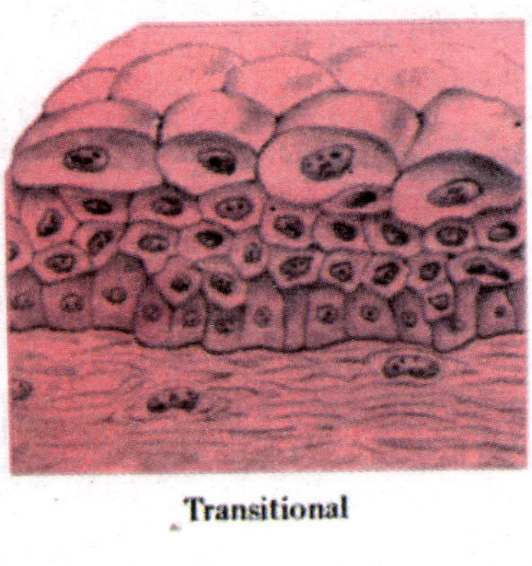

Transitional

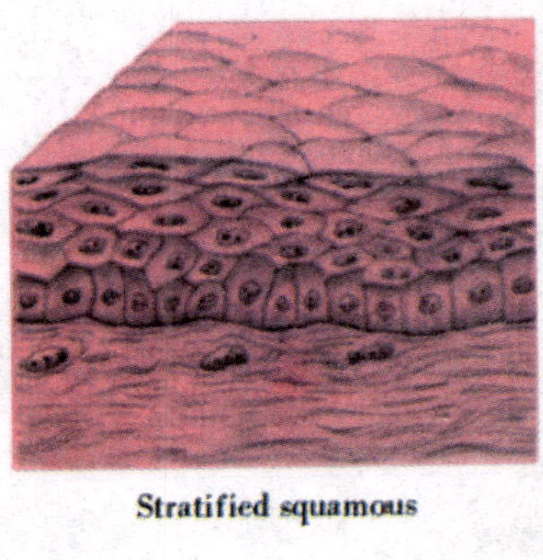

Stratified squamous

Diagrams illustrating the three-dimensional arrangements of cells in different types of epithelia and their descriptive nomenclature. (A. W. Ham and D. H. Cormack, 1979)

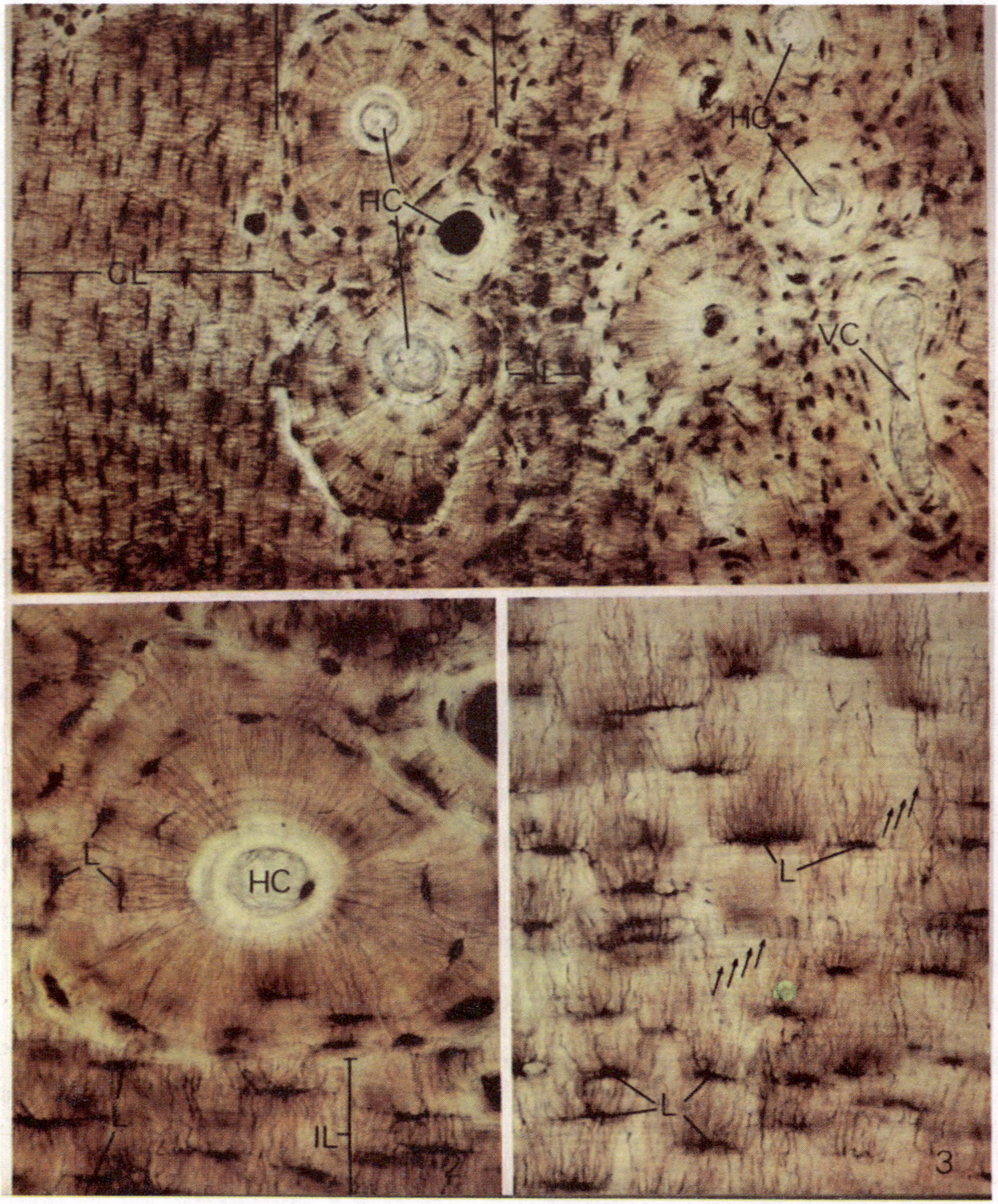

Photographs of Osseous Tissue.

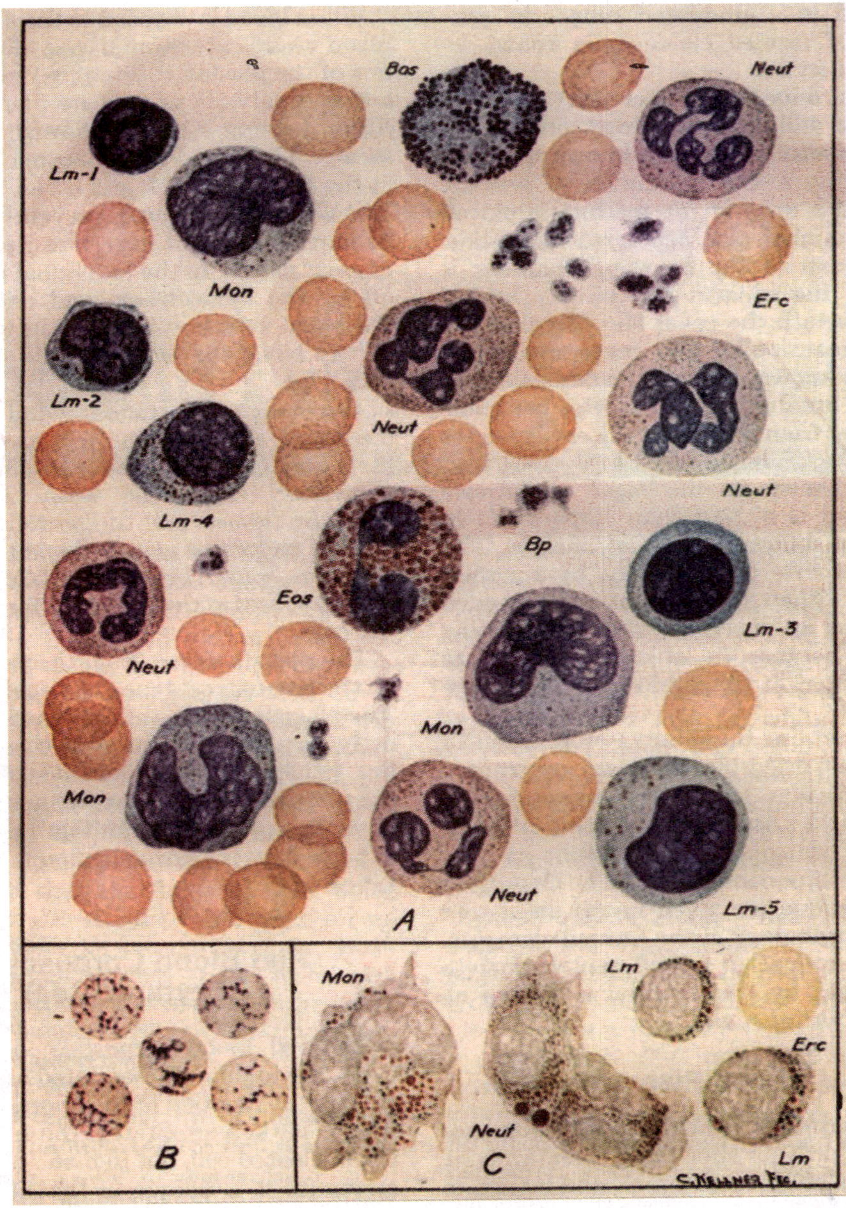

A. Cells from normal human blood. Wright's stain. *Bas*, basophilic leukocyte; *Bp*, aggregations of blood platelets; *Eos*, eosinophilic leukocyte; *Erc*, erythrocytes; *Lm-1 to 5*, lymphocytes; *1 to 3* are small and medium sizes and *4 and 5* are the less numerous larger forms; *Mon*, monocytes; *Neut*, neutrophilic leukocytes. ***B***. Reticulocytes from normal human blood stained with dilute cresyl blue. ***C***. Blood cells as seen after about 20 min of staining with neutral red and Janus green B in a supravital preparation. *Erc*, erythrocyte; *Lm*, small lymphocytes with bluish green mitochondria and a few neutral red granules; *Mon*, monocyte with mitochondria and numerous neutral red granules and vacuoles of varying size; *Neut*, neutrophilic leukocytes with staining of the neutrophilic granules and the formation of a few large vacuoles, which frequently appear after 15 to 20 min of staining. All figures ∞ 1550.

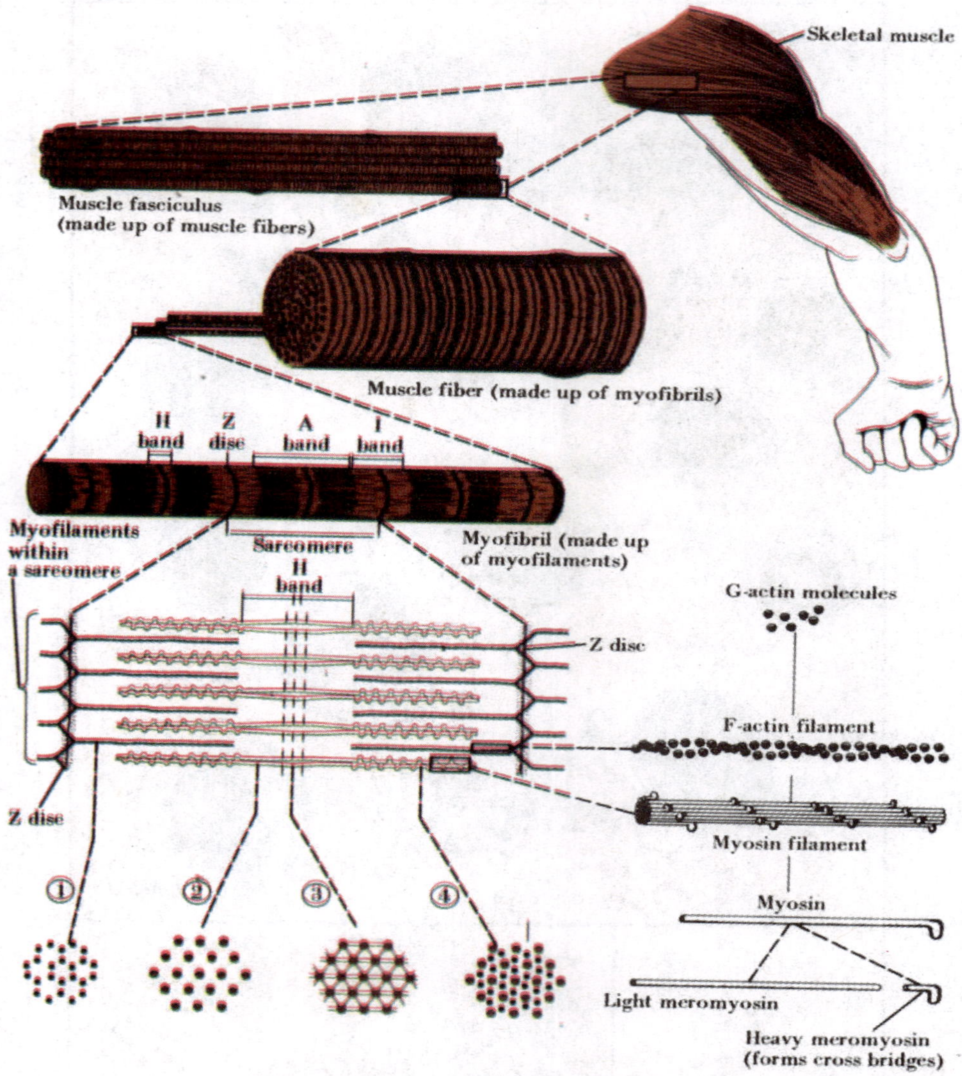

Organization of a skeletal muscle. A skeletal muscle consists of bundles of muscle fibers called fasciculi. In turn, each fasciculus consists of a bundle of elongate muscle fibers (cells). Within the muscle cell are longitudinal units, the myofibrils, which in turn are made up of myofilaments of two types: myosin (thick) filaments and actin (thin) filaments. The myofilaments are organized in a specific manner which impart to the myofibril, and in turn to the fiber, a cross-striated appearance. The functionally significant repeating unit of the myofibril is the sarcomere; it extends from one Z disc to the next Z disc. The A band marks the extent of the myosin filaments. Actin filaments extend from the Z band into the region of the A band, where they interdigitate with the myosin filaments as shown in the illustration. Items 1 to 4 show cross sections through different regions of the sarcomere: **(1)** through actin filaments of the I band; **(2)** through myosin filaments of the H band; **(3)** through the center of the A band where adjacent myofilaments are linked to form the M line; and **(4)** where actin and myosin filaments interdigitate in the A band, each myosin filament is within the center of a hexagonal array of actin filaments. Actin filaments can be broken down into globular actin molecules. Myosin filaments consist of myosin molecules; each one can be further broken down to a light and heavy meromyosin. (W. Bloom and D. W. Fawcett, 1975)

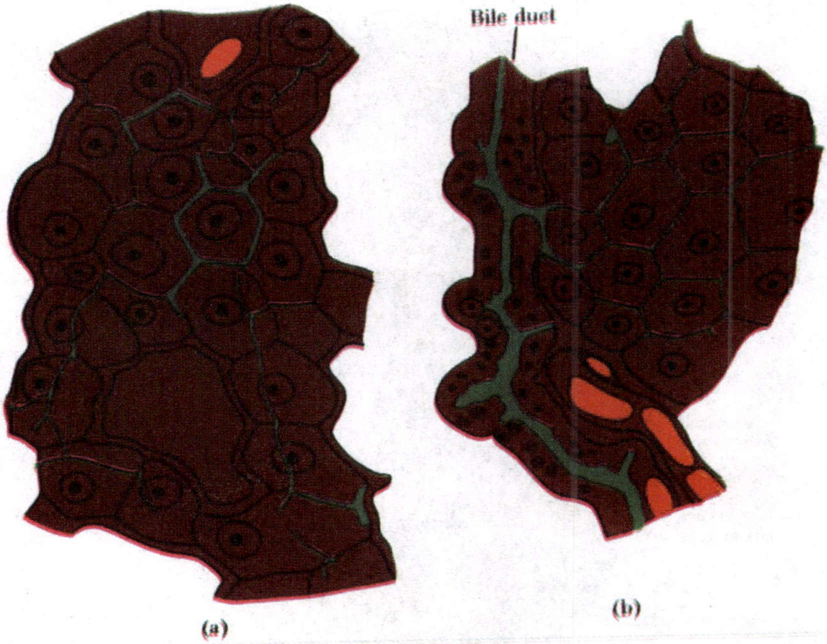

(a) Network of bile canaliculi demonstrated by intravenous injection of indigo carmine. Some bile canaliculi are clearly seen to form a band (green) about the hepatocyte. Thinner threads of dye show bile canaliculi just out of the main focal plane. (Special preparation fixed in potassium chloride formol; frozen section mounted in glycerine). **(b)** Bile canaliculi draining into duct. (Same type of preparation as in a) (H. Elias, 1949)

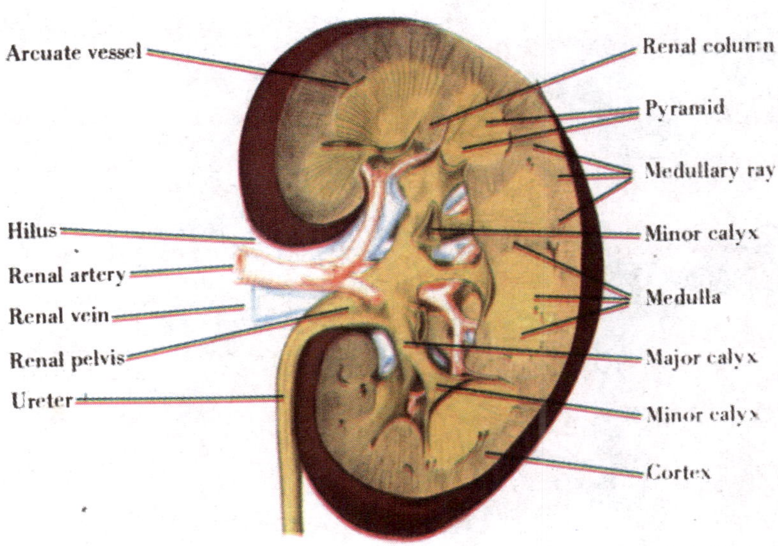

Diagram of a kidney seen from behind. Part of the kidney has been removed to show the internal structure. (Braus, 1924)

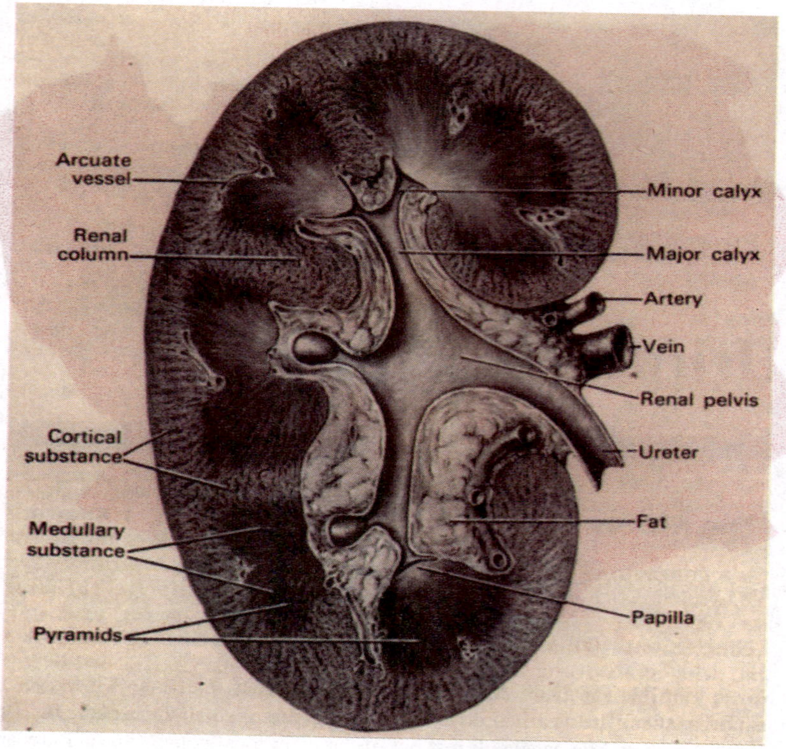

Longitudinal section of a human kidney. Natural size.

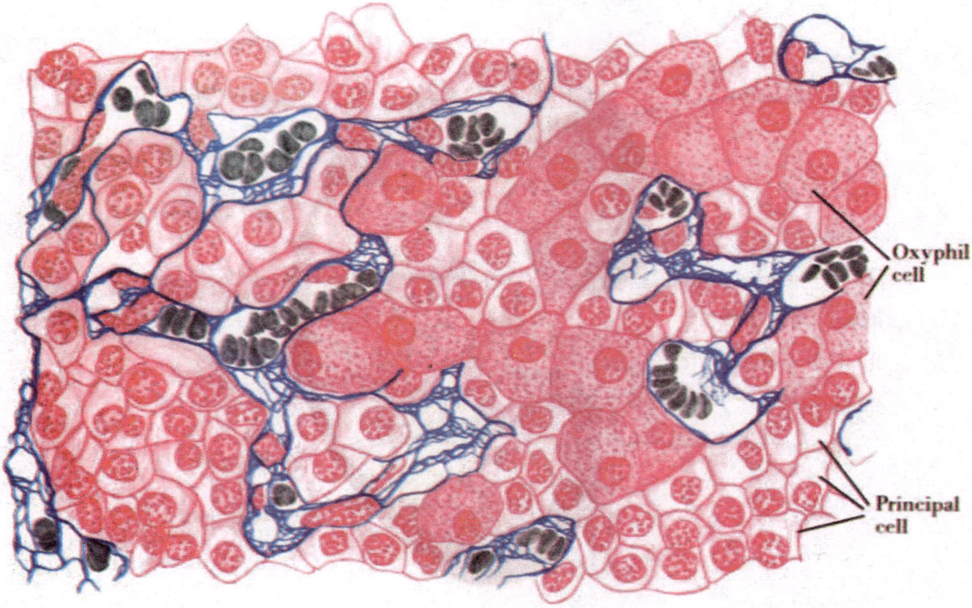

Drawing of cells within the human parathyroid gland. Principal cells are small and often vacuolated. The oxyphilic cells are much larger and contain fine granules. (W. Bloom and D. W. Fawcett, 1975)

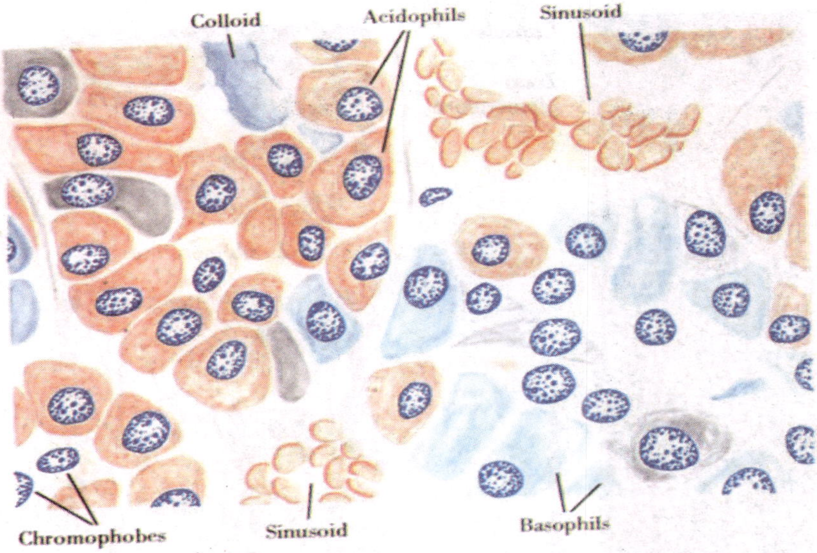

Drawing of cells within the human adenohypophysis. The drawing is of a histological section stained with aldehyde fuchsin-fast green-orange G. Acidophils appear orange; basophils, blue. Chromophobes appear lightly stained. The cords of cells are surrounded by a thin layer of connective tissue and sinusoids. (After Bailey, 1978)

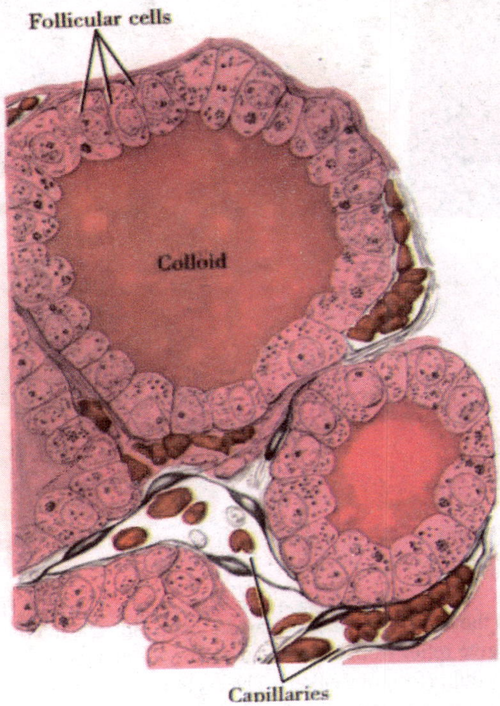

Drawing of a section through follicles of a human thyroid gland. Follicles consist of a single layer of epithelial cells surrounding a central mass of colloidal material. (After R. R. Bensley)

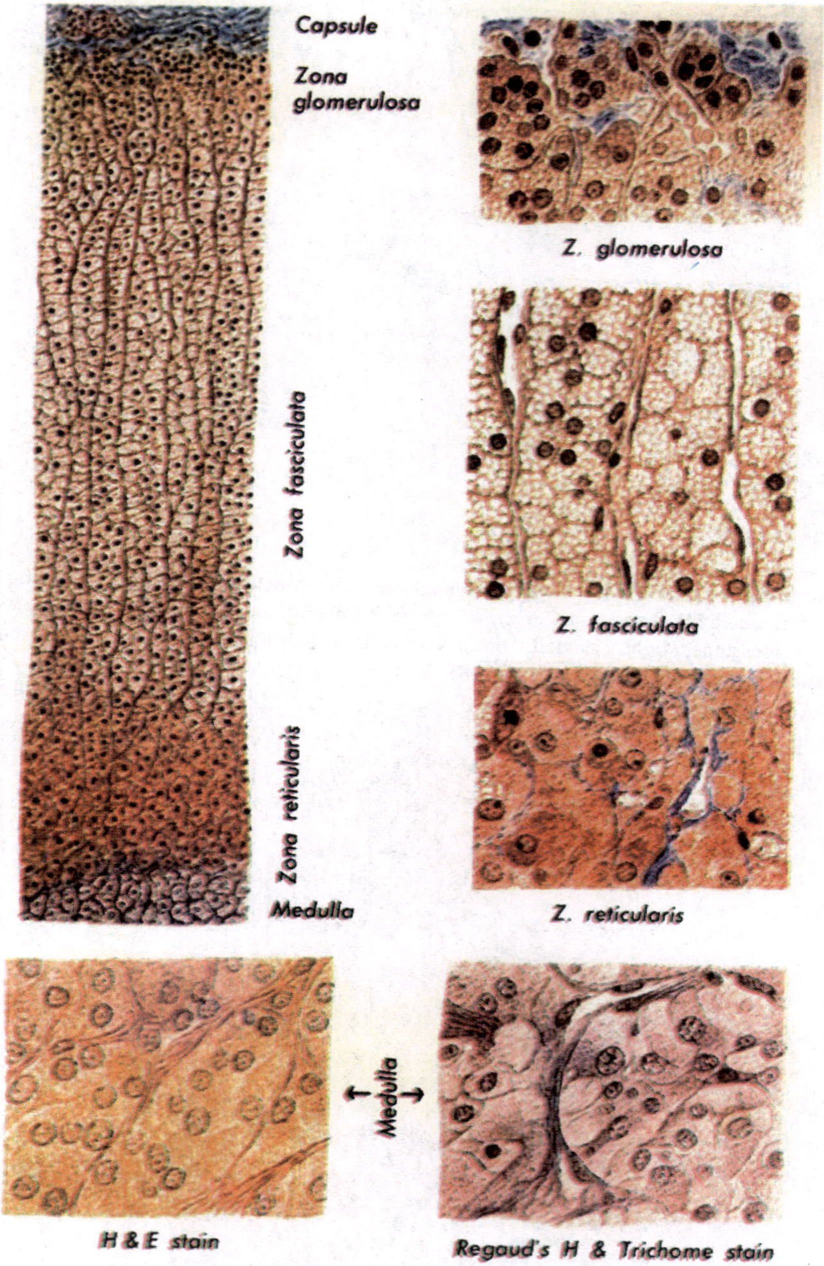

Sections through the right adrenal of a man 35 years old. The adrenal was removed in an attempt to give relief from a testicular tumor with metastases. The tissue was fixed in Helly's fluid (formol Zenker). The section used for all of the drawings, except the *lower left one*, was stained with Regaud's hematoxylin and Masson's trichrome. The low power (*upper left*) is ∞ 205; the others, ∞ 535.

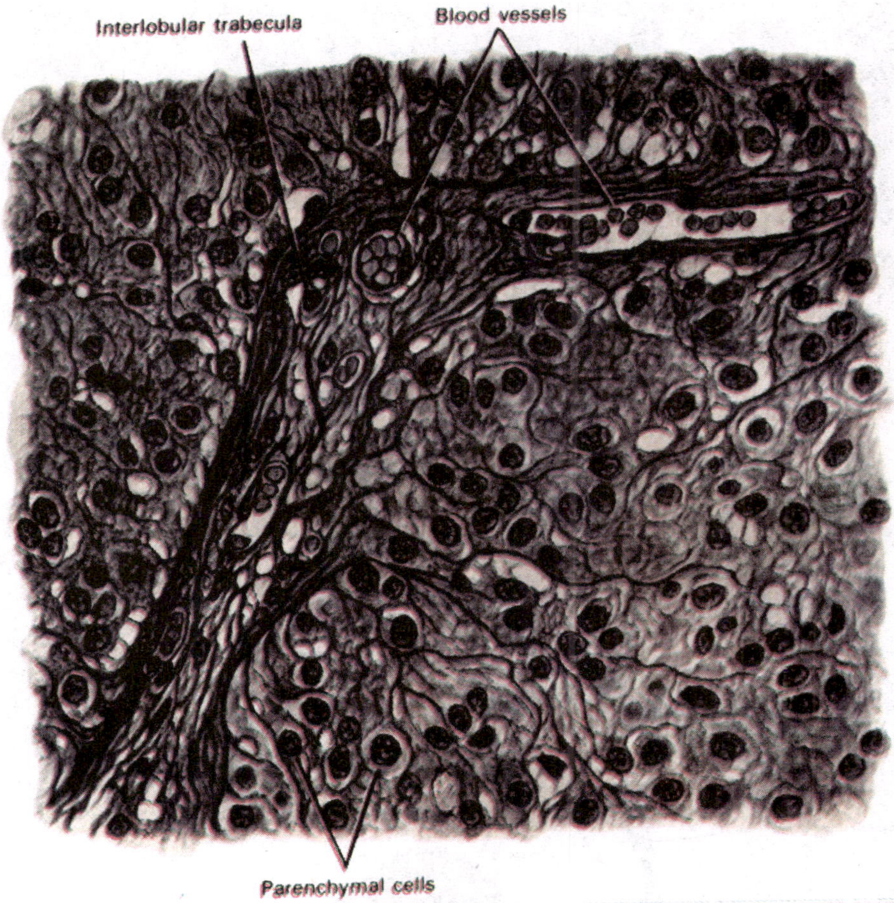

Section through the pineal gland of a woman 37 years of age. Hematoxylin-eosin. ∞ 535.

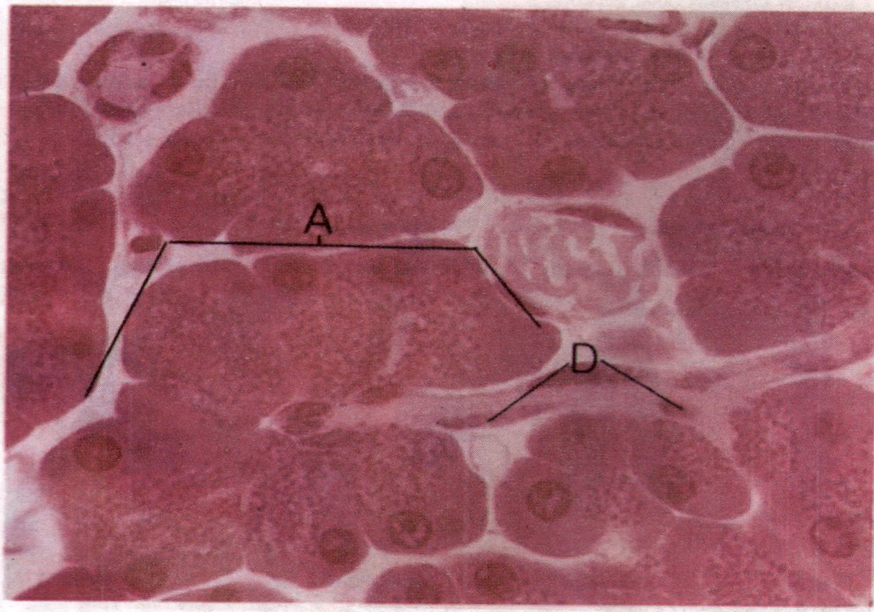

Photomicrograph of pancreatic acinus (A) with its duct (D). The small round objects within the acinar cells represent the stored secretory precursor material.

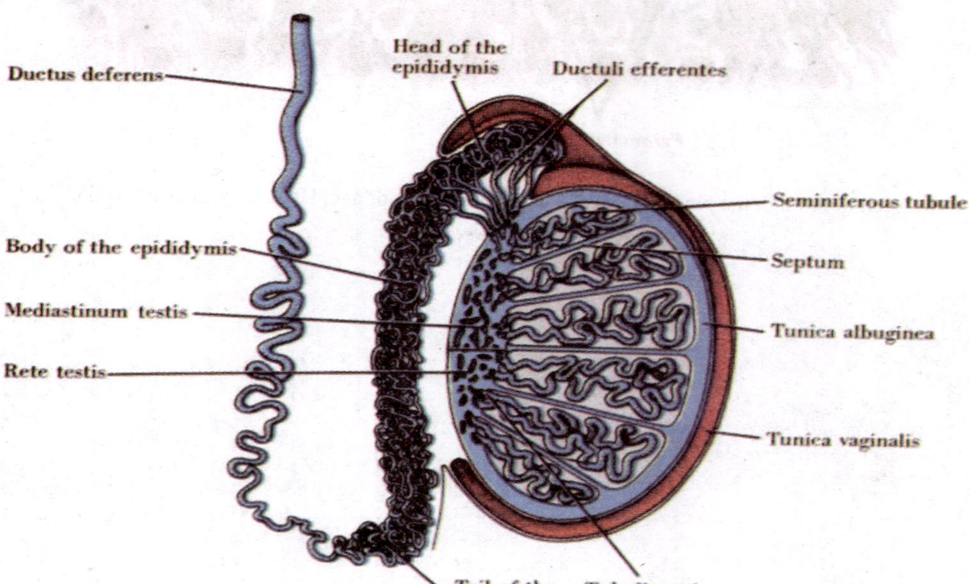

Schematic diagram of a longitudinal section through the human testis. The genital duct system, which includes the tubuli recti, rete testis, ductuli efferentes, ductus epididymidis, and ductus deferens, is also shown. (Modified from M. Dym, 1977)

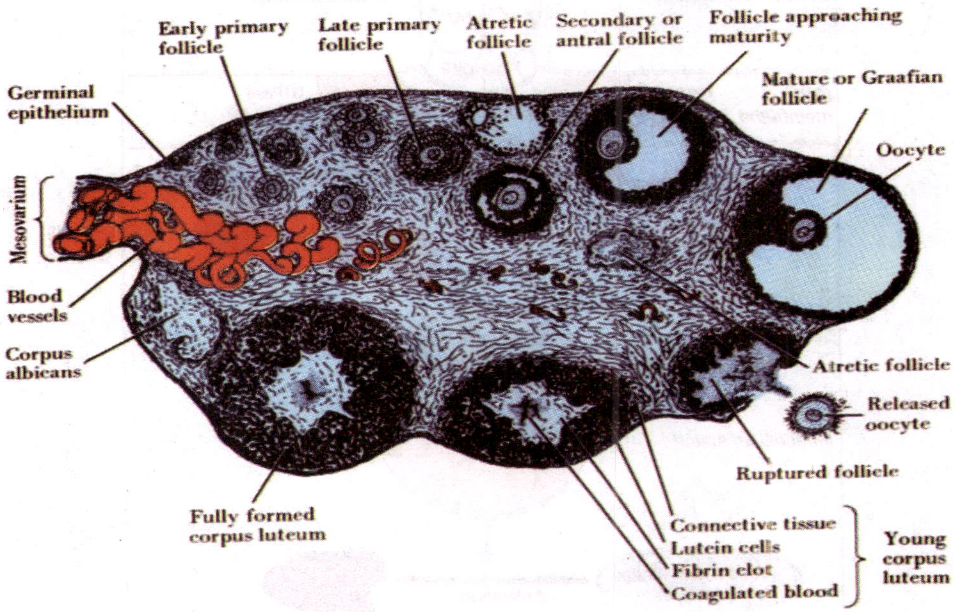

Schematic drawing of a section through the ovary. Highly coiled blood vessels are present in the hilum and medullary regions. (After C. E. Corliss)

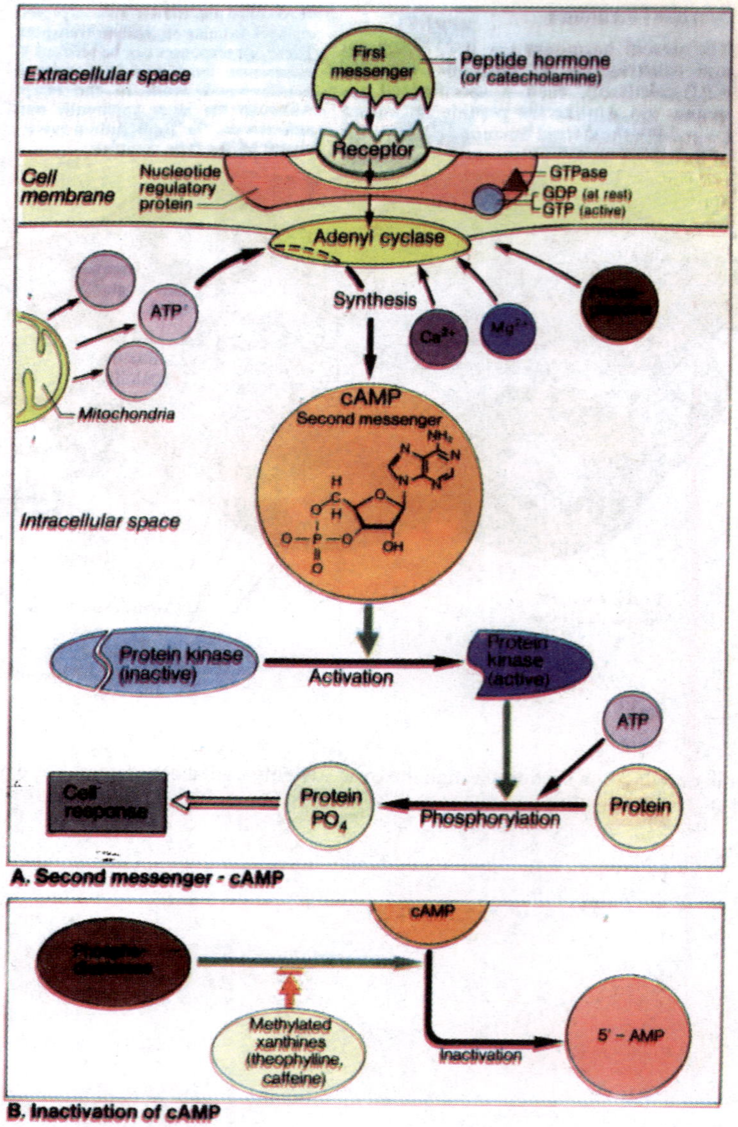

Cyclic AMP as Second Messenger.

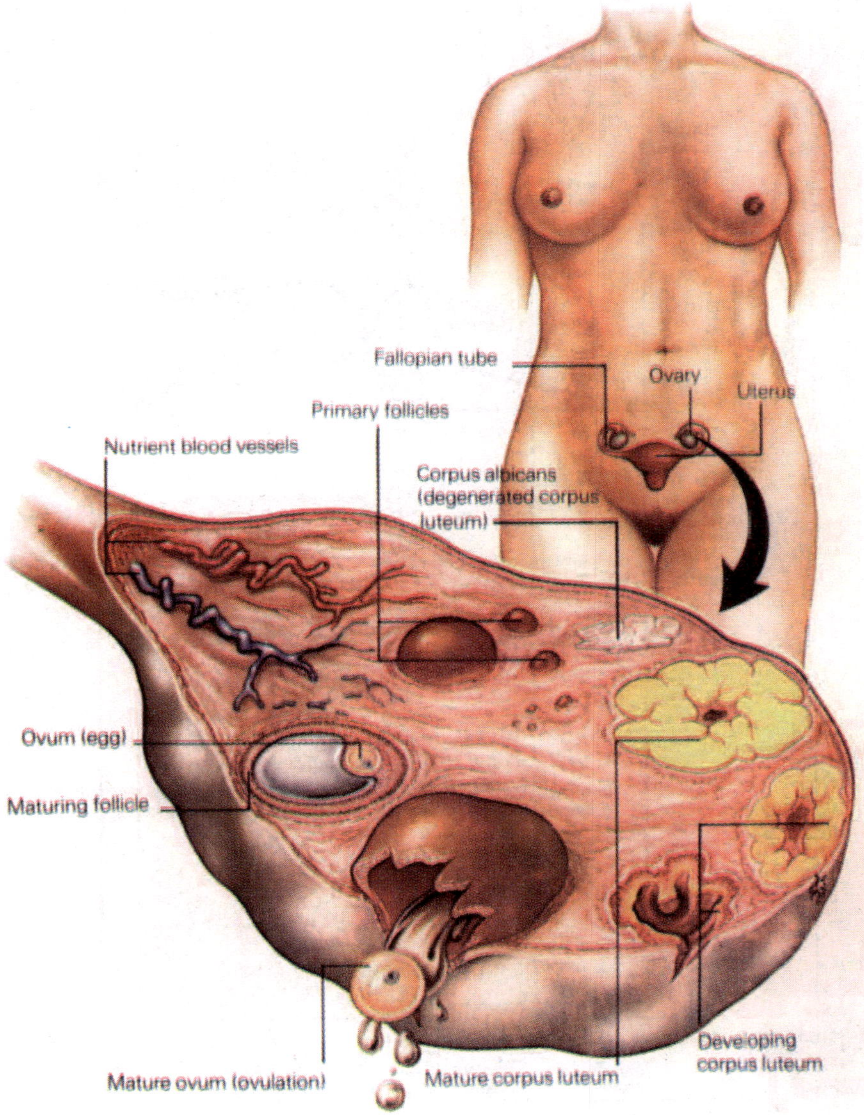

Site, structure and function of the ovaries.

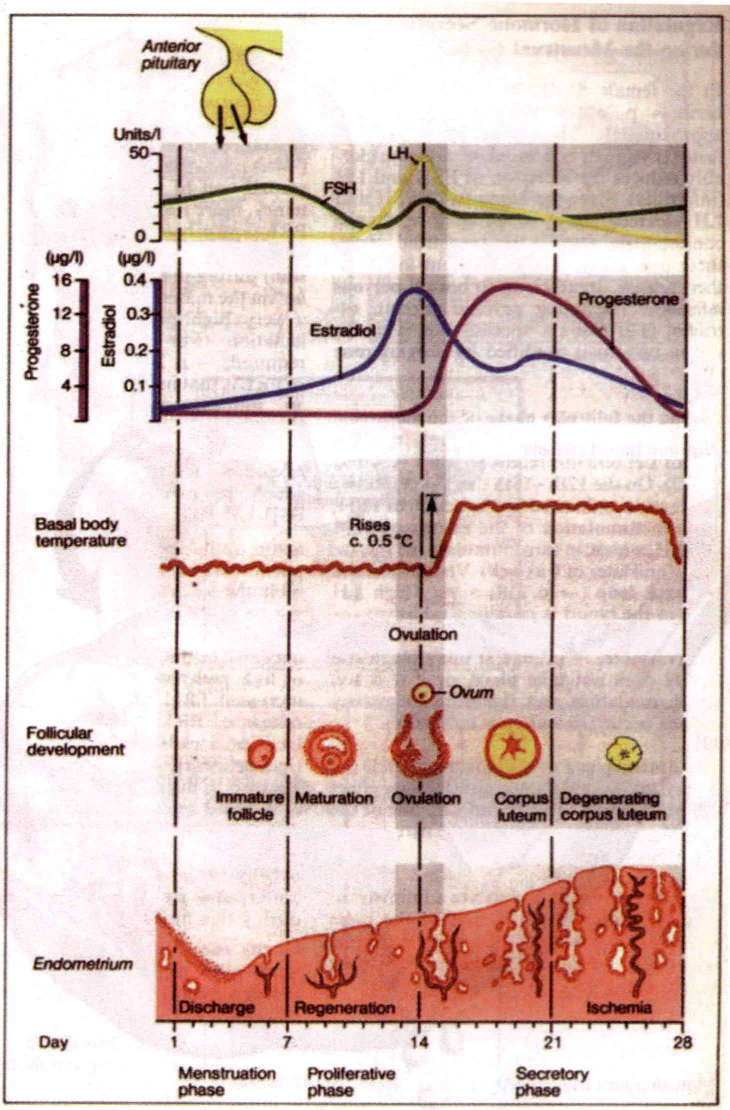

Human menstrual cycle.

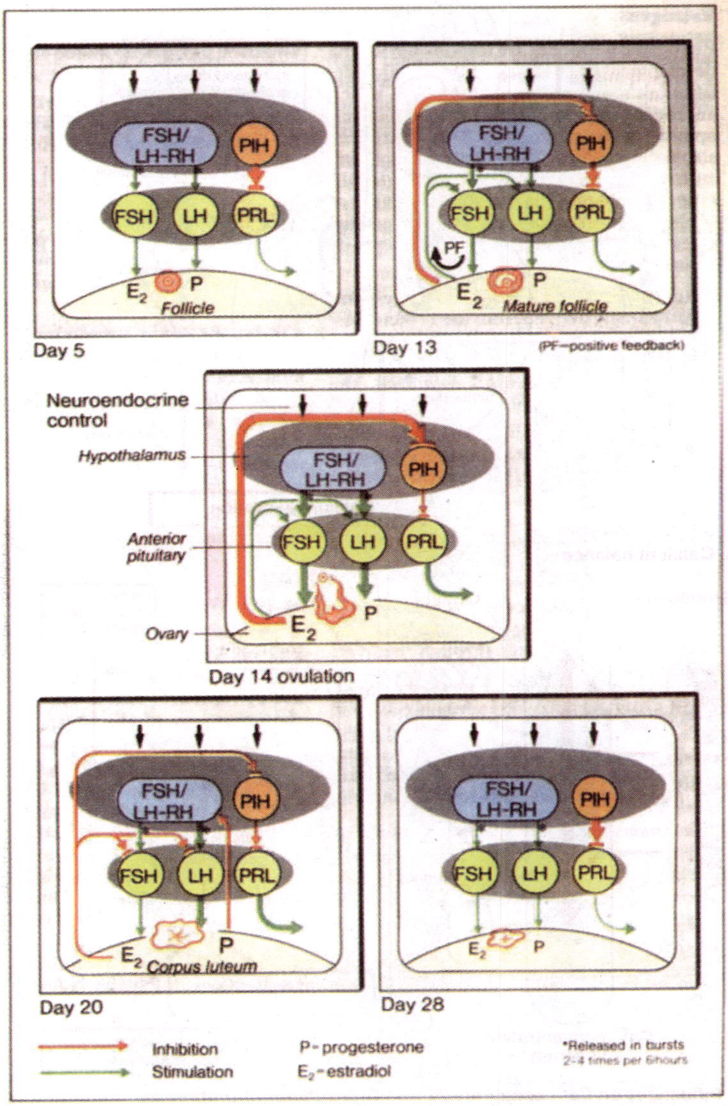

Hormonal interactions during the menstrual cycle.

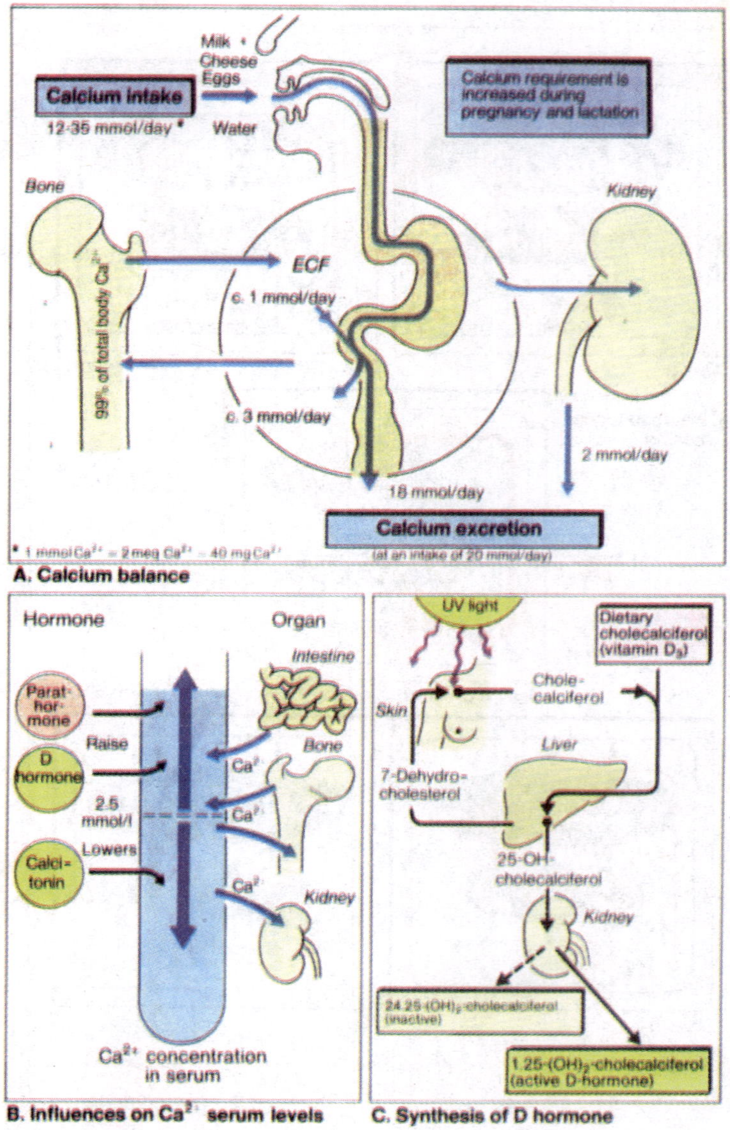

Photographs of Calcium Homeostasis.